The Care Home Handbook

The Care Home Handbook

Edited by

Professor Graham Mulley
DM, FRCP
Emeritus Professor of Elderly Medicine
University of Leeds
Leeds, UK

Professor Clive Bowman
BSc, MbChB, FRCP, FFPH
Honorary Visiting Professor
School of Healthcare Studies
City University
London, UK

Dr Michal Boyd
RN, NP, ND, FCNA(NZ), FAANP
Nurse Practitioner and Senior Lecturer
School of Nursing and Freemasons' Department of Geriatric Medicine
The University of Auckland
Auckland, New Zealand

Dr Sarah Stowe
BSc (Hons), MBChB, MRCP
Locum Consultant Physician
Airedale NHS Foundation Trust
Keighley, UK

WILEY Blackwell

This edition first published 2015
© 2015 by John Wiley & Sons, Ltd

Registered Office
John Wiley & Sons, Ltd, The Atrium, Southern Gate, Chichester, West Sussex, PO19 8SQ, UK

Editorial Offices
9600 Garsington Road, Oxford, OX4 2DQ, UK
The Atrium, Southern Gate, Chichester, West Sussex, PO19 8SQ, UK
111 River Street, Hoboken, NJ 07030-5774, USA

For details of our global editorial offices, for customer services and for information about how to apply for permission to reuse the copyright material in this book please see our website at www.wiley.com/wiley-blackwell

Library of Congress Cataloging-in-Publication Data
The care home handbook / edited by Graham Mulley, Clive Bowman, Michal Boyd, Sarah Stowe.
    p. ; cm.
  Care home handbook
  Includes bibliographical references and index.
  ISBN 978-1-118-31462-3 (pbk.)
I. Mulley, Graham P., editor of compilation.   II. Bowman, Clive, editor of compilation.   III. Boyd, Michal, editor of compilation.   IV. Stowe, Sarah, active 2014, editor of compilation.   V. Title: Care home handbook.
[DNLM: 1. Geriatric Nursing–methods–Handbooks.   2. Geriatric Nursing–standards–Handbooks.   3. Health Services for the Aged–ethics–Handbooks.   4. Health Services for the Aged–standards–Handbooks.   5. Homes for the Aged–standards–Handbooks.   6. Nursing Homes–standards–Handbooks. WY 49]
  RC954
  618.97′0231–dc23

                                                                                          2013043840

A catalogue record for this book is available from the British Library.

Wiley also publishes its books in a variety of electronic formats. Some content that appears in print may not be available in electronic books.

Cover image: © iStock.com/swilmor
Cover design by hisandhersdesign

Set in 9/11 pt Palatino LT Std by SPi Publisher Services, Pondicherry, India
Printed and bound in Malaysia by Vivar Printing Sdn Bhd

1 2015

Contents

Forewords

I was asked to write the foreword for *The Care Home Handbook* when I was Chief Executive Officer of Australia's Aged Care Standards and Accreditation Agency Ltd. This was the organisation in Australia charged with responsibility for promoting quality in residential aged care through the Australian government's accreditation scheme and industry education. In my role I had the opportunity to observe residential and nursing care and the methods of evaluation of those services in Australia and other countries.

My contact was Dr Clive Bowman, who was then the international medical director with Bupa. Clive, whom I have known for many years and whose passion for aged care is well known, assured me the Handbook would be comprehensive and user friendly.

He was correct. This Handbook is an easy to read guide that in becoming easy to read has not sacrificed the key messages. It can be taken as the 'how to' guide to residential and nursing aged care from beginning to end. It is comprehensive and focuses on applied practice. The inclusion of referenced material enables further exploration by the reader who wishes to pursue a particular interest. To my knowledge, no other such comprehensive book is available.

Ageing is a global phenomenon. In the next generation, more than 25% of people around the globe will be over 65 years of age and with that will be an increased demand for services for elderly people.

While the rates of ageing vary from country to country, the demand will be significant enough to render any debate about the actual numbers as moot.

As the world's population ages there will be increasing demand for services for older people. The increasing percentage of the population aged over 85 years and the migration of children away from their parents as they seek jobs and a better life will create an increased demand for residential care where older people live with other older people in institutions variously known as care homes, nursing homes and hostels.

Residents of these institutions will have increasing complex care needs which cannot be provided in their home. Arguably, some nursing homes will take on the characteristics of a sub acute hospital for a cohort of residents with high care needs and the nursing home (their home) is their preferred place to die.

It is these institutions that provide one of the ways for the younger generations to pay their debt to their forefathers and mothers by ensuring they have the best life possible and that rather than consider the nursing home as 'God's waiting room', it is a place where older citizens can live life to the fullest and in a way they choose.

The general public knows very little about aged care. Staff rarely know much before they commence their first role in aged care. The ratio of tertiary qualified staff to personal care workers in care homes is quite low compared to a hospital. Equally, opportunities for professional interaction and professional development are a challenge for care home staff.

The aged care workforce is predominately personal care workers whose level of training is quite variable. These are the staff with the most frequent interaction with residents and who support residents with the activities of daily living – eating, dressing, going to the toilet, etc.

There are few courses in nursing or management that adequately prepare nurses and managers to contend with the diversity of activity that is required in a nursing home on a daily basis. This will range from the entry paperwork through to complaints by relatives, high level clinical services and end of life care.

The team approach has always been the basis of nursing. However, 'nursing' homes are about much more than clinical services.

The Care Home Handbook is not a nursing text. It is a book that reflects the multi-disciplinary team based approach that is necessary to achieve positive outcomes for residents from a whole of life perspective. It reports contemporary best practice in what is a very diverse endeavour.

So what can the reader learn from this Handbook? It goes a long way in filling the gap between formal training and the realities of the workplace. At the very least, it brings any formal training into the care home context.

The breadth of the book reflects the best practice approach to the management of care homes. Residents are seen as people, individuals who have not lost their human rights on entry to their new home; who must be provided with the support to age with dignity and in the way of their choosing; and where quality of life is measured from the residents' perspective – not an externally imposed measure where management purport to know what is best for the resident.

Quality of care and services is seen as an input directed to ensuring the resident is able to enjoy the best possible quality of life, not as an end in itself.

The early chapters reflect the very important aspects of working in a care home with residents each of whom is unique. Sections on values, standards, ethics and probity reflect the underlying considerations when a resident considers their life in the home.

The latter sections contextualize the many clinical activities which are daily activities in a care home.

Good clinical care is of limited utility unless provided in a caring environment where the human rights and dignity are at the forefront of the providers' and their staff's minds.

While the content is directed towards those people working in care homes, much is relevant to people providing services to older people in the older person's own home.

It is written with UK care homes as the reference point. Many of the references are to UK legislation. A focal point is necessary to give some of the advice a context. However, based on my experiences of looking at elderly care systems in many countries, I am convinced that this focus does not detract from the book and that the advice can be readily adopted.

It also provides guidance in the established aged care systems and a benchmark for those countries where residential care is not well established.

I congratulate the editors on being able to harness the energies of such a group of expert contributors and in doing so, create a text that will be more than a significant contribution to the quality of life for older citizens.

Mark Brandon
Chief Executive Officer, Aged Care Standards and Accreditation Agency (2002–2013)
Chair Organizing Committee and Convener, International Society for Quality in Healthcare, Quality in Social Care for Older Persons special interest group
Former Board Member, Australian Centre for Evidence Based Aged Care
Sydney, Australia

People's expectations of care homes are changing. Current generations of older adults have become accustomed to more independence. Many of them and their families also want more choice about the kinds of services they receive and how these are delivered. People want a more personalised approach to their care.

There is evidence emerging that many older adults who come into residential or nursing care do so at later stages in life when their needs are greater and they have become frailer. Consequently many people have multiple and complex needs that present a different set of challenges for individualised care.

There is much more scrutiny of care and greater opportunities for family and staff to report poor, unsafe and inappropriate care. This, of course, is a good thing and reinforces the desire to improve care assessment and delivery in care homes.

The Care Home Handbook provides an up to date approach to personalisation in care. It helpfully starts with the journey that a prospective resident makes into a care home and covers the emotional challenges of such an experience. Unusually for this kind of handbook, it also addresses the question of discharge which is not ordinarily covered but may well be the outcome from a care home stay.

The sections covered in the handbook are comprehensive and nothing about care home life is left untouched. Additionally, there is an external focus on engagement with working with other professionals in the health and care systems.

Each section is helpful, brief and accessible and reports the topics through the personalisation lens. This book should be used in the way the authors intended. It is not a handbook that must be read from cover to cover but rather to be used as a navigational aid when needed and relevant to the issues.

The contributing authors reflect a wide array of talents and experience linked to the care of elderly and frail people. They have, by providing brief oversight of the salient themes, assured the most up to date approaches to meeting the needs of care home residents. The opportunity to have one's practices shaped, helped and reinforced by the contributing authors is a privilege for all and one that will benefit care home residents and their families.

Alan Rosenbach
Special Policy Lead
Care Quality Commission
London, UK

Preface

The purpose of this handbook is to improve the care, well-being and safety of people who are resident in care homes.

Care homes provide a vital role in the support of the health and care for older people internationally. The role of the care home continues to evolve greatly from a 'housing' solution to a place where often very frail people with complex health needs live permanently or for short periods.

The practice of care in care homes largely relies on established manuals and practices from hospital and community care. Typically, these are polarised either to a very clinically-driven hospital model or one dominated by social care values. We have not been able to identify a practical, succinct handbook specifically tailored for care homes. For example, standard texts often do not address several of the Geriatric 'Giants' – such as dementia, delirium, falls, stroke or impaired mobility. Many other important elderly care topics (such as fits, visual impairment, restraint, dignity and privacy) are not given the attention that they merit.

There are other considerations: regulators, accreditation organisations and others seek demonstrations of competency and safe practice. While there are some proprietary policies and procedures, they are densely worded and voluminous and not practicable for front line clinical staff. As a result, many homes are littered with a variety of cards and notices on how best to do things.

So, in this handbook, we have attempted to distil good practice into concise chapters that champion resident-centred nursing care. The handbook is not a conventional text book, nor a substitute for formal education and training, but it is a support to good safe practice. Similarly, the chapters are not exhaustive (nor exhausting) but the contributory authors have risen to the challenge of providing short accounts that blend evidence with experience so that a reader should able to remind themselves about good practice.

In reading chapters in the editing process, we all gained new insights and believe that while most of what is presented should be familiar, there will be some new 'nuggets' of information to be gained.

The handbook's approach emphasises the importance of a holistic approach, embracing social, ethical, legal, psychological as well as clinical aspects of care. It is principally aimed at staff nurses, more senior nurses and care home managers. Nursing aides and senior carers may also profit from reading it.

We have tried to ensure that the handbook is free from jargon and hope that it will remind, inform, prompt and refresh, as well as offer guidance on when to ask for help and describe what information might be needed by professional colleagues. As editors, we believe that reducing variations in practice and emphasising the best in contemporary geriatric nursing will facilitate better communications between all health professionals involved in care homes and reduce failures.

The contributors are acknowledged experts (both academics and clinical staff, with input from many care home nurses) as well as rising stars in elderly medicine from the UK, mainland Europe, the USA, Canada, Australia and New Zealand. Nurses are co-authors, co-editors or advisors for almost every topic.

Compiling this first edition started with a modest list of topics that grew. We have aimed to produce a comprehensive guide, but as editors we anticipate there may be some omissions. We very much hope that readers will provide feedback and suggestions. Please email your comments to nursingeducation@wiley.com

**Graham Mulley, Clive Bowman,
Michal Boyd and Sarah Stowe**

List of Contributors

Dr Ahmed H. Abdelhafiz, Consultant Geriatrician and Senior Clinical Lecturer, Rotherham General Hospital, Rotherham, UK

Dr Katie Athorn, Consultant Geriatrician, Hull and East Yorkshire Hospitals NHS Trust, Hull, UK

Dr Pauline Bailey, Senior Clinical Lecturer (Elderly Medicine), Newcastle University Medicine Malaysia, Johor, Malaysia

Tanya Bish, Quality and Professional Development Nurse Leader, Aged Residential Care, Waitemata District Health Board, Takapuna, North Shore, New Zealand

Professor Clive Bowman (Co-editor), Honorary Visiting Professor, School of Healthcare Studies, City University, London, UK

Dr Michal Boyd (Co-editor), Nurse Practitioner and Senior Lecturer, School of Nursing and Freemasons' Department of Geriatric Medicine, The University of Auckland, Auckland, New Zealand

Dr Mark Bradley, Elderly Medicine, Leeds Teaching Hospitals NHS Trust, Leeds, UK

Pauline Breslin, Registered General Nurse and Registered Manager, Sunnyside Nursing Home, Castleford, UK

Helen Brooks, Brain Attack Nurse Specialist, Leeds Teaching Hospitals NHS Trust, Leeds, UK

Beverley Brown, Senior Sister, Elderly Acute Medical Unit, Leeds Teaching Hospitals NHS Trust, Leeds, UK

Louise Brown, Specialist Speech and Language Therapist, Harrogate and District Foundation Trust, Scarborough Hospital, Scarborough, UK

Mary Burke, Director of Care, Killure Bridge Nursing Home, Waterford, Ireland

Professor Alistair Burns, National Clinical Director for Dementia, NHS England; Professor of Old Age Psychiatry, University of Manchester; Vice Dean, Faculty of Medical and Human Sciences, University of Manchester; Clinical Director, Manchester Academic Health Science Centre (MAHSC); Consultant Old Age Psychiatrist, Manchester Mental Health and Social Care Trust, Manchester, UK

Eileen Burns, Consultant Geriatrician, Leeds Teaching Hospitals NHS Trust, Leeds, UK

Rosie Callaghan, Tissue Viability Nurse, Stourport Health Centre, Stourport on Severn, UK

Elaine Carr, Sister, Elderly Acute Medical Unit, Leeds Teaching Hospitals NHS Trust, Leeds, UK

Dr Gurjit Chhokar, Geriatric Speciality Registrar, Yorkshire and Humber Deanery, Harrogate, UK

Dr Josie Clare, Consultant Acute Physician / Geriatrician, Cork University Hospital, Ireland

Carole Clifford, Physiotherapist, Leeds Community NHS Trust, Leeds, UK

Dr David Cohen, Consultant Stroke Physician, Northwick Park Hospital, Harrow, UK

Dr Ronan Collins, Director of Stroke Service / Associate Professor in Stroke Medicine, Consultant Physician in Older Adult and Stroke Medicine, Adelaide and Meath Hospital, Dublin, Ireland

Dr Simon Conroy, Geriatrician, University Hospitals of Leicester NHS Trust, Leicester, UK

Dr Laura Cook, Registrar in Geriatric Medicine, Leeds Teaching Hospitals NHS Trust, Leeds, UK

Dr Oliver J. Corrado, Consultant Physician in Geriatric Medicine, Leeds Teaching Hospitals NHS Trust, Leeds, UK

David Cowley, Detective Inspector, West Yorkshire Police, Leeds District Safeguarding Unit, Leeds, UK

Dr Alison Cracknell, Consultant in Medicine for Older People, Leeds Teaching Hospitals NHS Trust, Leeds, UK

Fiona Cristol, Director, Northwood Nursing and Care Services Ltd, Northwood, UK

Professor Peter Crome, Honorary Professor, Department of Primary Care and Population Health, University College London, London, UK

Professor Steven Curran, Consultant and Professor in Old Age Psychiatry, South West Yorkshire Partnership NHS Foundation Trust, Wakefield; Centre for Health and Social Care Research, University of Huddersfield, Huddersfield, UK

Dr Paul Diggory, Consultant Geriatrician, Croydon University Hospital, Croydon, UK

Dr Rose Ann DiMaria-Ghalili, Associate Professor of Nursing, Drexel University, Philadelphia, PA, USA

Lynda Dorsey, Staff Nurse, Leeds Teaching Hospitals NHS Trust, Leeds, UK

Aidan Dunphy, Older Persons Research Nurse, University Hospitals of Leicester NHS Trust, Leicester, UK

Ceri Edwards, Senior Clinical Nurse, Older People's Hospital Mental Health Team, Leeds and York Partnership NHS Foundation Trust, York, UK

Carol Fletcher, Senior Sister, St James's Hospital and Leeds General Infirmary, Leeds, UK

Anne Forbes, Growing Old Gracefully Project, RC Diocese of Leeds, Leeds, UK

Amanda Foster, Heart Failure Specialist Nurse, Calderdale and Huddersfield NHS Trust, Huddersfield, UK

Dr Gillian Fox, Consultant in Elderly Medicine, St James's University Hospital, Leeds, UK.

Cath Gilpin, Community Matron, Pudsey Health Centre, Leeds, UK

John Gladman, Professor of Medicine of Older People, University of Nottingham, Nottingham, UK

Dr Karen Goodman, Consultant Physician in Elderly Medicine, York Teaching Hospital NHS Foundation Trust, York, UK

Dr Adam Gordon, Consultant and Honorary Associate Professor in Medicine of Older People, Nottingham University Hospitals NHS Trust, Nottingham, UK

Helga Goutcher, Senior Operations Manager, St Philip's Care, Scotland, UK

Suzanne Green, Clinical Nurse Specialist in Stroke, Tallaght Hospital, Dublin, Ireland

Dr Natalia Gunaratna, Registrar in Geriatric Medicine, Leeds Teaching Hospitals NHS Trust, Leeds, UK

Verity Hallam, Registered Manager/Director, The Byars Nursing Home, Nottingham, UK

Dr Daniel Harman, Consultant Community Geriatrician, Hull and East Yorkshire Hospitals NHS Trust, Hull, UK

Dr Rachel Hepherd, Specialty Registrar in Elderly Medicine, Hull and East Yorkshire Hospitals NHS Trust, Hull, UK

Dr John D. Holmes, Senior Lecturer in Liaison Psychiatry of Old Age, University of Leeds, Leeds, UK

Sandra Horton, Provectus (UK) Limited, Mansfield Woodhouse, Nottingham, UK

Dr Anne Houghton, GP and Associate Clinical Director, Leeds South and East Clinical Commissioning Group, Leeds, UK

Dr Rhiannon Humphreys, Specialist Registrar in Geriatrics, Hull Royal Infirmary, Hull, UK

Dr Amy Illsley, Geriatric Medicine Registrar, Yorkshire and the Humber Deanery, Bradford, UK

Sadia Ismail, Consultant Geriatrician, Leeds Teaching Hospitals NHS Trust, Leeds, UK

Sandra Jackson, Clinical Director, Provectus (UK) Limited, Mansfield Woodhouse, Nottinghamshire, UK

Miranda Jacobs, Geriatric Physiotherapist, Radboud University, Nijmegen Medical Centre, The Netherlands

Professor David Jolley, Personal Social Services Research Unit, The University of Manchester, Manchester, UK

Dr Angela Juby, Associate Professor, Department of Medicine, Division of Geriatrics, University of Alberta, Edmonton, Alberta, Canada

Caroline Kane, Clinical Nurse Specialist for Neurological Disability and Rehabilitation, Peamount Healthcare, Ireland

Dr Soma Kar, Specialist Trainee Registrar, Care of Elderly Medicine, Hull and East Yorkshire Hospitals NHS Trust, Hull, UK

Dr Sandra Kavanagh, General Practitioner, South Terrace Continuing Care Centre, Edmonton, Alberta, Canada

Jean Lawrence, Retired Infection Prevention and Control Nurse, (IPS) Yorkshire, UK

Dr Dagmar Long, Consultant Community Geriatrician, Leeds Community Healthcare NHS Trust, Leeds, UK

Dr Shona McIntosh, Retired Geriatrician, Leeds, UK

Professor Finbarr Martin, Consultant Geriatrician, Guy's and St Thomas' NHS Foundation Trust, London, UK

Dr Marissa Minns, spr Geriatric Medicine, Leeds Teaching Hospitals NHS Trust, Leeds, UK

Jackie Morris, British Geriatrics Society Dignity Champion, Consultant Physician, Honorary Research Associate, Faculty of Biomedical Sciences, University College London Medical School, London, UK

Sarah Morris, Critical Care Outreach Sister, Leeds Teaching Hospitals NHS Trust, Leeds, UK

Professor Graham Mulley (Co-editor), Emeritus Professor of Elderly Medicine, University of Leeds, Leeds, UK

Dr Martin Mulroy, Consultant Geriatrician, Our Lady of Lourdes Hospital, Drogheda, Co. Louth, Ireland

Dr Sangeeta Naraen, ST7 Geriatric Medicine, St James's Hospital, Leeds, UK

Pauline Newsome, Clinical Educator, Leeds Teaching Hospitals NHS Trust, Leeds, UK

Dr Sean Ninan, Specialty Registrar, Geriatric Medicine, Yorkshire and the Humber Deanery, UK

Professor Desmond O'Neill, Consultant Physician in Geriatric and Stroke Medicine, Trinity College Dublin, Dublin, Ireland

Sean Page, Consultant Nurse for Dementia and Senior Lecturer, Betsi Cadwaladr University Health Board and University of Bangor, Glan Clywd General Hospital, Rhyl, UK

Dr Steven Parke, Specialist Registrar in Geriatric Medicine, Leeds Teaching Hospitals NHS Trust, Leeds, UK

Sandra Parry, General Manager, West Ridings Residential and Nursing Home, Wakefield, UK

Dr Mahwesh Rafique, Foundation Trainee, Pinderfield Hospital, Wakefield, UK

Dr Lauren Ralston, Care of the Elderly Consultant, Bradford Teaching Hospital Foundation Trust, Bradford, UK

Audrey Redshaw, Trust Lead – Manual Handling, Royal Bournemouth and Christchurch NHS Foundation Trust, Bournemouth, UK

Dr Ed Richfield, Elderly Medicine, Leeds NHS Trust; Research Fellowship, Hull; York Medical School, UK

Dr Stephanie Robinson, Specialist Registrar in Geriatric Medicine, Department of Age Related Healthcare, Adelaide and Meath Hospital, Tallaght, Dublin, Ireland

Melanie Rogers, Advanced Nurse Practitioner and Senior Lecturer, University of Huddersfield, Huddersfield, UK

Peter Rogers, Consultant Nurse (Clinical Governance and Research), Bupa Care Services, Leeds, UK

Claire Rushton, Lecturer in Nursing and NIHR Fellow, Keele University, Keele, UK

Debra Sagar, Ward Sister, St James's University Hospital, Leeds, UK

Katherine Sage, Dentist in General Practice, Rudheath Dental Health Centre, Northwich, Cheshire, UK

Dr Baldeep Sagu, GP trainee, Riverside GP Vocational Training Scheme, London, UK

Dr Zuzanna Sawicka, Specialty Registrar in Elderly Medicine, St James's University Hospital, Leeds, UK

Steven Searby, Health Improvement Specialist, South West Yorkshire Partnership NHS Foundation Trust, Halifax, UK

Dr Ben Shaw, Higher Specialist Trainee, Old Age Psychiatry, Royal Bolton Hospital, Bolton, UK

Mary E. Shaw, Chair of the RCN Ophthalmic Nursing Forum, University of Manchester, Manchester, UK

Professor Alan Sinclair, Professor of Medicine and Dean, Bedfordshire and Hertfordshire Postgraduate Medical School, University of Bedfordshire, Luton, UK; Director, IDOP, Putteridge Bury, Luton, UK

Claire Sissons, Registered General Nurse and Clinical Lead, Highfield Nursing Home, Tadcaster, UK

Dr Helen Slater, Care of the Elderly, Leeds Teaching Hospitals NHS Trust, Leeds, UK

Julie Spencer, Community Matron, Armley Moor Health Centre, Leeds, UK

Andrew Stanners, Consultant Physician, Mid Yorkshire Hospitals NHS Trust, Wakefield, UK

Dr Sarah Stowe (Co-editor), Locum Consultant Physician, Airedale NHS Foundation Trust, Keighley, UK

Deborah Sturdy, Director of Care, Red and Yellow Care, London, UK

Dr Evelyn Tan, Geriatrics, Leeds Teaching Hospitals NHS Trust, Leeds, UK

Dr Catherine Tandy, Consultant Physician, Department of Elderly Medicine, St James's University Hospital, Leeds, UK

Louise Taylor, Home Manager, Park Lodge Care Home, Roundhay, Leeds, UK

Dr Tharani Thirugnanachandran, Consultant Stroke Physician, Leeds Teaching Hospitals NHS Trust, Leeds, UK

Rachel Thompson, Dementia Project Lead, Royal College of Nursing, Nursing Department, London, UK

Dr Marianne van Iersel, Geriatrician, Radboud University, Nijmegen Medical Centre, The Netherlands

Dr Michael Vassallo, Consultant Physician, Royal Bournemouth Hospital, Bournemouth, UK

Stephanie Verity, Speech and Language Therapist, Friarage Hospital, Northallerton, UK

Dr Adrian Wagg, Professor of Healthy Ageing, University of Alberta, Edmonton, Alberta, Canada

Heather Waterman, Professor of Nursing and Ophthalmology, University of Manchester, Manchester, UK

Professor John Wattis, Visiting Professor of Old Age Psychiatry, Centre for Health and Social Care Research, University of Huddersfield, Huddersfield, UK

Maureen A. Whittaker, Staff Nurse, Hull and East Yorkshire Hospitals NHS Trust, Hull, UK

Lisa Wickens, District Nurse, Intermediate Care Team, Hull and East Yorkshire Hospitals NHS Trust, Hull, UK

Dr Michi Yukawa, Associate Professor of Medicine, Medical Director of Community Living Center, University of California San Francisco and San Francisco VA Medical Center, San Francisco, CA, USA

Dr Tajammal Zahoor, Specialist Registrar Stroke and Geriatric Medicine, Edinburgh Royal Infirmary, Edinburgh, UK

Ewa Zalewska, Staff Nurse, Intermediate Care/Rapid Response/IV Therapy, Mid Yorkshire Hospitals NHS Trust, Wakefield, UK

Review Panel

Tanya Bish, Quality and Professional Development Nurse Leader, Aged Residential Care, Waitemata District Health Board, Takapuna, New Zealand

Sharon Blackburn, RGN RMN, Policy and Communications Director, National Care Forum, UK

Helen Bowen, Nurse Practitioner (Older Adults), Waitemata District Health Board, Takapuna, New Zealand

Pauline M. Breslin, Registered General Nurse and Registered Manager, Sunnyside Nursing Home, Castleford, UK

Cherie Cook, Gerontology Nurse Specialist, Aged Residential Care, Waitemata District Health Board, Takapuna, New Zealand

Helga Goutcher, Senior Operations Manager, St Philip's Care, Scotland, UK

Dr Hazel Heath, Independent Nurse Consultant and Chair of RCN Older People's Forum, London, UK

Nicola Hills, RN, Quality Manager, Bupa Care Services, Leeds, UK

Sandra Parry, General Manager, Bupa Care Services, Leeds, UK

Sue Roberts, Consultant Nurse, Clinical Leadership Unit, Bupa Care Services, Leeds, UK

Peter Rogers, Consultant Nurse (Clinical Governance and Research), Bupa Care Services, Leeds, UK

Isabella Wright, Director of Nursing/Gerontology Nurse Practitioner, The Selwyn Foundation, New Zealand

List of Abbreviations

6 Ps	Pain, Paraesthesia, Pallor, Pulselessness, Paralysis, Perishing Cold
ABC	Airway, Breathing, Circulation
ABCDE	Airway, Breathing, Circulation, Disability, Exposure
ACP	Advance Care Plan
AF	Atrial Fibrillation
AIDS	Acquired Immunodeficiency Syndrome
BMI	Body Mass Index
BPM	Beats Per Minute
BTE	Behind The Ear Hearing Aids
CAM	Confusion Assessment Method
CCF	Congestive Cardiac Failure, also known as Congestive Heart Failure
CD	Controlled Drug
CDI	*Clostridium difficile* (*C. difficile*) Infection
CHF	Chronic Heart Failure
CHLS	Care Homes Liaison Service
CJD	Creutzfeldt Jacob Disease
CLI	Critical Limb Ischaemia
COPD	Chronic Obstructive Pulmonary Disease
COSHH	Control of Substances Hazardous to Health
CPR	Cardiopulmonary Resuscitation
CQC	Care Quality Commission
CRI	Cardiac Resynchronisation Therapy
DKA	Diabetic Ketoacidosis
DNAR	Do Not Attempt Resuscitation
DVT	Deep Vein Thrombosis
ECG	Electrocardiogram
FRAT	Falls Risk Assessment Tool
GCS	Glasgow Coma Scale
GDS	Geriatric Depression Scale
GSF	Gold Standards Framework
HETF	Home Enteral Tube Feeding
HIV	Human Immunodeficiency Virus
ICD	Internal Cardiac Defibrillators
IM	Intra-muscular
IMCA	Independent Mental Capacity Advocate
ITE	In The Ear Hearing Aids
IV	Intra-venous
LCP	Liverpool Care Pathway
MAR	Medicines Administration Record
MDI	Metered Dose Inhaler
MEWS	Modified Early Warning Score
MRSA	Meticillin-Resistant *Staphylococcus aureus*
NG	Nasogastric
NICE	National Institute for Health and Clinical Excellence
NMC	National Midwifery Council
NPSA	National Patient Safety Agency
NSAID	Non-Steroidal Anti-Inflammatory Agents
OT	Occupational Therapists
PD	Parkinson's Disease
PDNS	Parkinson's Disease Specialist Nurses
PEG	Percutaneous Endoscopic Gastrostomy tubes
PFT	Pulmonary Function Tests
PPE	Personal Protective Equipment
SC	Sub-cutaneous
SLT	Speech and Language Therapist
SMART	Specific, Measureable, Agreed, Realistic, Time limited
SSRI	Selective Serotonin Reuptake Inhibitors
STI	Sexually Transmitted Infections
TB	Tuberculosis, or *tubercle bacillus*
UI	Urinary Incontinence
UTI	Urinary Tract Infection
WHO	World Health Organization

Section A

The Resident's Journey

Chapter 1

Admissions and Discharges

1.1 Admissions and discharges: principles, processes and planning

Peter Rogers

Bupa Care Services, Leeds, UK

Key points

- Moving into a care home can be a distressing time for both residents and their families.
- Particular sensitivity and emotional awareness are most important at this time of transition.
- One way of delivering consistent care that meets medical as well social and emotional needs is the Nursing Process.
- This is a systematic problem-solving approach to planning and delivering care.
- It involves assessment (both subjective and objective); diagnosis; identifying outcomes; planning; implementation; and evaluation.
- The Nursing Process necessitates accurate, up-to-date documentation.

People move into a care home for different reasons and periods of time, and with varying degrees of preparation. For some, it is a short-lived experience for convalescence, respite or palliative care. For many others, it is a long-term solution to their need for social and nursing care, which has been arrived at either after careful consideration of the options available, or suddenly, following a precipitous decline in independence.

The circumstance surrounding the admission will inevitably influence how the resident, their family and friends respond. For many, particularly those contemplating permanent residency, the journey into a care home can be an emotionally difficult one both for them and those close to them.

New long-term residents have much to feel sad and anxious about; leaving a familiar environment to join a new social group, giving up many of their possessions and coming to terms with the loss of independence the admission represents, all contribute to make the move into a care home a difficult transition for many people, whatever their age.

Relatives too often have mixed emotions. While the decision might be greeted with a sense of relief that the care needs of a loved one will be recognised and met by competent staff in a safe and comfortable environment, at the same time the move can give rise to feelings of failure, guilt and intense sadness.

Whatever the particular circumstance surrounding an admission, it is crucial that the care home staff have the emotional insight and understanding necessary to sensitively and appropriately support the new resident's transition into life in the home.

The Nursing Process

The Nursing Process is one approach to the management of effective individualised care. It involves:

- the assessment of each resident's needs,
- the planning of care interventions,
- the delivery of care interventions,
- the evaluation of the resident's response and hence the effectiveness of the care provided.

In its original form, this 'systematic problem solving approach' comprised four phases of activity: assessment, planning, implementation and evaluation. In more recent times, the desire to emphasise the importance of setting out a concise statement of a person's actual or potential problems (nursing diagnosis), and the need to clearly express the intended outcomes of care – activities which were once subsumed within assessment and planning – have resulted in the now widely recognised six-step nursing process (Figure 1.1.1); a process that serves as a

The Care Home Handbook, First Edition. Edited by Graham Mulley, Clive Bowman, Michal Boyd and Sarah Stowe.
© 2015 John Wiley & Sons, Ltd. Published 2015 by John Wiley & Sons, Ltd.

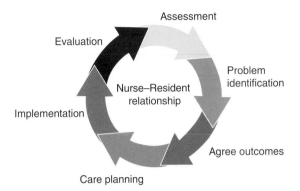

Figure 1.1.1 The six-step nursing process.

better reminder to those who use it that it is the resident or patient who is the focus of attention.

Although presented as a series of steps, the nursing process should be regarded as continuous cycle of discussion, negotiation, decision-making and review that takes place between the nurse and the resident (and at times others), in order to match care to the resident's needs and preferences.

The focus here is on the importance of assessment, the collection and interpretation of resident data as the foundation for person-centred care. However, it is important to recognise that assessment data also serve other, not necessarily complementary purposes. For example, data might be used to:

- Determine the cost of a care package and an individual's entitlement to government funded subsidies and/or financial support.
- Enable commissioners/assessors to place residents in the facilities they regard as appropriate for that person's needs.
- Provide anonymised data for public health, government and corporate planners and also academic research.

Further reading

Frauman AC, Skelly AH. 1999. Evolution of the nursing process. *Clinical Excellence for Nurse Practitioners* 3: 238–44.

Funnell R, Koutoukidis G, Lawrence K. 2009. *Tabbner's Nursing Care*, 5th edn. Elsevier, Australia, p. 72.

1.2 Assessment on admission to the care home

Peter Rogers

Bupa Care Services, Leeds, UK

Key points

- A comprehensive assessment on entry to the home will help to identify individual care needs.
- It is important to allow time for residents and their caregivers to familiarise themselves with the care home.
- A holistic assessment will include physical, psychological and social needs.
- A focused assessment can be optimised by the use of validated rating scales.
- Tips are given on the assessment of residents who are admitted for short-term care.

Whatever the particular circumstances surrounding the admission, the individual care needs of all new residents must be recognised and addressed by the nursing staff. This can only be achieved by undertaking an assessment that is sufficiently broad and appropriately detailed.

Allow time for adjustment

Whether it started before or immediately after admission, the process of familiarisation is a crucial part of the new resident's adjustment to their surroundings. This is especially true on the day of admission, when it is important not to rush into a detailed and intimate assessment of abilities and needs.

Allowing the new resident and their relatives a little time to become orientated to the new surroundings will have a positive effect on their all-important first impressions of the home and the staff. The greeting on introduction of a resident to their new home sets the tone for what is a crucial relationship; remember to smile and be friendly!

Wherever possible, new residents and their relatives should be:

- Greeted by the staff that they have already met or talked to.
- Shown around the home and introduced to a few of the staff and other residents.
- Given time to settle into their room and organise the belongings they have brought with them, and spend a little time alone with their relatives.

- Offered the chance to talk to the home manager, their named nurse or key worker about life in the home and ask to any questions they might have.
- Encouraged to take as much time as they need to reassure themselves that their loved one is settled before they leave.
- Fully informed of the visiting and telephone contact arrangements for the home.

The initial holistic assessment

The need to ensure a sufficiently broad appreciation of the new resident's needs is addressed by ensuring that the initial assessment is 'holistic' in nature, that is to say it considers the resident's physical (or biological), psychological and social needs and abilities.

The idea of a holistic approach to nursing care became established as an alternative to what is regarded by many in the profession as the paternalistic and disempowering 'medical model', which defines those who use healthcare services in terms of their problems, diagnoses and treatment needs.

The holistic approach represented below (Figure 1.2.1) recognises that a person's needs arise out of the interaction between their individual physical, psychological and social circumstances, and that by seeking to understand those interactions through the assessment process, we have a better chance of providing care that is appropriate, effective and acceptable to the recipient.

The Care Home Handbook, First Edition. Edited by Graham Mulley, Clive Bowman, Michal Boyd and Sarah Stowe.
© 2015 John Wiley & Sons, Ltd. Published 2015 by John Wiley & Sons, Ltd.

- Activities of daily living
- Pain control
- Mandatory risk assessments, e.g. pressure ulcer risk, nutritional status, fall risk
- Medical history and current health problems and medications and treatments

- Personal, social and family relationships
- Social, educational and economic history – 'Map of Life'™, 'Who am I'™
- Culture and ethnicity considerations
- Preferences about forms of address, daily routines and the provision of assistance
- Favourite activities, interests and hobbies

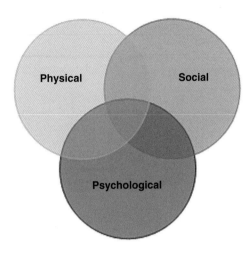

- Intellect, cognition, orientation (place and time) and memory
- Motivation, mood and emotion
- Spirituality
- Loss, change and adaptation
- Behaviours that challenge

Figure 1.2.1 Aspects of holistic assessment.

There are a number of generic assessment tools, each reflecting the emphasis of the particular nursing model or theory upon which they are based. However, whatever the nuances of the underpinning theory, adopting a holistic approach is essentially about recognising that *each individual amounts to more than just the sum of their physical parts.*

Focused assessments

Focused assessment tools are designed to provide a detailed understanding of a resident's abilities and needs in relation to a specific risk or problem. The use of these tools is largely triggered by the results of the initial holistic assessment. However, such is the impact of some healthcare deficits on older people generally that several of these specific tools now form a routine part of the initial holistic assessment.

It is now common practice to routinely screen all new residents using pressure ulcer, falls and nutritional risk assessment tools, and also to repeat these assessments periodically.

Examples of some specific assessment tools nurses might use to produce a personal care plan that fully and accurately reflects the residents needs include:

Cognitive Assessment	• Mini Mental State Examination (MMSE)
	• Abbreviated Mental Score (AMT) & AMT 4
Conscious Level	• Glasgow Coma Scale
Nutritional Status	• MUST, Malnutrition Universal Screening Tool
	• MNA, Mini Nutritional Assessment
	• NHS Oral Health Assessment tool
Mobility	• Falls Risk Assessment Tool (FRAT)
	• Dewing Tool for Wandering Assessment
Pain	• Abbey Pain Scale
	• Visual Analogue Scales
Pressure Ulcer Risk	• Waterlow Score
	• Braden Risk Assessment Scale
	• Norton Scale

Note: This is not an exhaustive list.
For details of these and other scales, see Appendix 1: Rating Scales.

Problem identification

The result of the assessment phase should be a set of clear statements setting out the actual and potential problems facing the resident at that point in time that have, wherever possible, been discussed and agreed with the resident. For example:

> Anxiety due to admission into unfamiliar surrounding indicated by verbal comments and increased heart rate.

This example illustrates the problem the resident is experiencing (anxiety), the likely cause (unfamiliar surroundings) and how it is manifested (verbal comments and increased heart rate).

When they are expressed in this way, problem statements provide the basis for a modified SMART approach to the later steps in the nursing process. They prompt the expression of anticipated outcomes (a reduction in anxiety), provide an indication as to what the planned care should address (familiarisation with the new environment, other residents and staff) and suggest criteria that can be used to evaluate the success or not of the planned interventions (changes in the resident's expressed feelings and heart rate).

This example also highlights the value of involving the resident. Nursing and care staff might make the reasonable assumption that most new residents will experience some degree of anxiety, however it is just as important to recognise the underlying cause. A resident might be more concerned about how their care will be financed or the fate of a pet than their new surroundings. In each case, the interventions detailed in the care plan will be very different.

Short-stay admissions

In addition to those taking up permanent residence in a care home, others are admitted for what is intended to be a brief interlude. Residents admitted for convalescence, intermediate or respite care may stay for a few days or several weeks, and come with needs that vary from rest, rehabilitation and a good diet to 24-hour nursing care.

While the principles of assessment remain the same for these residents, the priority assigned to different aspects of the assessment and the emergent needs may be different.

For someone admitted for one or two weeks of respite care, it may be more important to focus on ensuring that their physical needs are identified and met than devoting the time required to gain a detailed insight into their social history in the way one would with a new permanent resident. Of course, if the period of respite is the first of what might be many, then the social history and family relationships assume a greater significance and will demand more attention.

It is up to the nurse conducting the assessment to exercise discretion over what is prioritised, and to work with the resident and family to ensure the care is both appropriate to the resident's needs and aligned with their expectations of the stay and the respite or convalescence care provided.

Top Tips: Short-stay check list for care home staff

Very often the same documentation is used whatever the resident's anticipated length of stay; however some issues assume more significance in short-stay situations and are worth emphasising. These include:

- Emergency contact information for the resident's family or friends.
- Contact details of the resident's GP.
- Medication, including nutritional supplements – what is prescribed and how will it be provided?
- What medical consumables will be required, for example incontinence pads, wound dressings, stoma bags and so on, and how will these be provided?
- Resident specific information: allergies, preferences about diet, meal times, sleep patterns, washing/bathing/showers and so on.
- Have any necessary items of equipment been provided, for example specially adapted cutlery, walking frames?
- Does the resident have sufficient clothes and toiletries for the stay?
- Departure date and time, transport arrangements.

Further reading

RCN, London, 2004. *Nursing Assessment and Older People. A Royal College of Nursing toolkit.* www.rcn.org.uk/_data/assets/pdf_file/0010/78616/002310.pdf [Accessed October 2013]

1.3 Assessment of residents before admission to the care home

Peter Rogers

Bupa Care Services, Leeds, UK

Key points

- Each potential resident should have a detailed, sensitive, compassionate pre-admission assessment.
- Pre-admission assessments should ideally be done in private, and the potential resident should be asked whether or not they want someone else to be involved in the discussion.
- This assessment includes confirming biographical data, ascertaining why admission is being sought, determining the individual's specific likes and dislikes, their cultural preferences and other needs, as well as obtaining details of possible infections and their investigations.
- A list of practical tips is given to facilitate this assessment.

Location

The pre-admission assessment usually takes place wherever the potential resident is at the time of referral. Ideally, this will be somewhere that is familiar to the future resident. This helps to make the process less stressful, and also means relatives or friends can be present to contribute to the assessment.

Unfortunately this is not always possible. The assessment may take place in hospital, with the pressure to agree a discharge date and free a bed competing with the need to get a clear understand of the future resident's potentially complex and still emerging needs.

Confidentiality

While many of those contemplating a move into a care home will appreciate the contribution that their family and friends can make to their assessment, others will not. Rather than make assumptions about the older person's wishes, the nurse conducting the assessment should start the process in private and ask the resident who they want to be involved. (See Chapter 4.6.)

The purpose

Wherever it is conducted, and whatever the competing issues, the pre-admission assessment is an important stage in any planned admission to a care home, primarily because it is about deciding whether or not a particular home is the right place to meet the resident's particular needs. For all of these reasons, it is a job that requires a confident and experienced nurse who is able to focus on the future resident's actual and potential needs and how these will need to be met.

In the pre-admission assessment, you should concentrate on:

- Confirming essential biographical information.
- Understanding the key reason for admission being sought to a care home.
- Gathering information about the individual's significant needs (whether clearly identified or only suspected), including specific requirements, such as equipment.
- Gaining insight into the individual's socio-cultural expectations and preferences.
  Where the pre-admission assessment takes place in hospital, pay particular attention to:
  - The level of observation the patient is subject to, and whether this reflects their actual care

The Care Home Handbook, First Edition. Edited by Graham Mulley, Clive Bowman, Michal Boyd and Sarah Stowe.
© 2015 John Wiley & Sons, Ltd. Published 2015 by John Wiley & Sons, Ltd.

needs or is the way in which the risks associated with the hospital environment are being managed.

○ The nature of confirmed or suspected infections, and whether there are any outstanding results from specimens taken for culture and sensitivity.

The need for compassion

Although coming to the right conclusion about where a person's needs might best be met is the whole point of the pre-admission assessment, it is also important that the nurse conducting the assessment manages it sensitively. The encounter may be the first time that the prospective resident, rather than their family, has met any of the staff who might become responsible for their care.

Some pre-admission assessments will culminate in the decision that the individual would be better cared for elsewhere. Most, however, will lead to an admission. It is therefore important for the nurse conducting the assessment to appreciate that this early contact is frequently where the process of building a professional relationship based on honesty and openness with a resident and their relatives starts.

A pre-admission assessment is a useful precursor for both care home staff and future residents; however it is not always possible.

For some older people, the admission to a care home is an urgent response to a sudden change in personal circumstances or care needs. For these residents, the process of relationship-building starts when they arrive in the care home. It is at best a stressful time, but one made all the more so by the precipitating factors, whatever they are, and the speed with which the change in the resident's world is effected; something the staff managing the admission have to keep in mind.

Top Tips: Pre-admission assessment in hospital

Organising a pre-admission assessment in hospital can be difficult. Some things to consider are:

• Contact the Charge Nurse, Sister or Ward Manager to arrange an appropriate time to visit. If this person is not available, try to speak to the patient's named nurse. If unsuccessful, find out when they will be available, leave a message and call back.

• When arranging your visit, check that there are no imminent plans to move the patient to another ward, and whether any off-ward investigations are booked.

• Make a note of the name of the nurse who will be in charge on the day of your visit.

• Agree that you will call to check your visit is still OK to go ahead before setting off to the hospital. It is useful to make a note of the ward's direct line telephone number.

• If appropriate, inform the patient's relatives of the arrangements in advance.

• Finally if you are not familiar with the hospital, check out the parking provision and the location of the ward before you set off.

Further reading

Centre for Policy on Ageing. 1996. Entering care. Chapter 3 in: *A Better Home Life*. www.cpa.org.uk [Accessed October 2013]

1.4 Supporting and dealing with families

Clive Bowman

School of Healthcare Studies, City University, London, UK

Key points

- Admission of a loved one to a care home can be a time of emotional distress for the family.
- Care home staff should welcome family members, sensitively obtain important information, and answer any questions about the care home.
- The resident's cultural and religious background should be understood and respected.

For many families, strong emotions surround the admission of a loved family member to a care home. Many relatives will have previously been entirely responsible for their loved one's care, but their escalating dependency has made a care home admission a reluctant necessity.

Your prime responsibility is to your resident, but helping a family come to terms with a care home is an important part of care. Make sure they are welcome.

Some families will be so physically and mentally exhausted that they need 'time out' and it is crucial that, for these families, the care home provides them with the confidence to allow them to recharge their batteries.

Many families – and particularly partners – will want to make sure that their intimate knowledge of your new resident is fully understood. This information can be pure gold in helping you develop a good care plan. For the many residents with limited capability to express themselves, the experience of longstanding carers to help craft an initial care plan is absolutely essential. There may also be aspects of care that they have provided that it is not appropriate for care staff to provide in the same way. In such circumstances, it is good to explain why and how you will be providing the care.

Most families talk to each other and share their understanding, and therefore a family view develops and whichever family member you speak to there will be a common understanding.

However, if several family members are getting slightly different information from different staff members, and they do not have a common understanding, then uncertainty can arise. Sometimes, the concerns that can arise are best dealt with through a family conference. Often, one family member may be the point of contact and take responsibility for sharing information.

Capacity

Where a resident has mental capacity (or even diminished mental capacity) but still has the ability to make choices, then their choices and wishes should prevail and families need to understand this (see Chapter 4.6).

Where individuals lack capacity to make most choices, the input of a family member or legal advocate is most important. There are times when no such advocate is identifiable; in such cases, the person or commissioner who made the placement should be asked who has the necessary authority.

Very occasionally, family members behave very badly, and theft, acts of abuse and other crimes can be committed. There should be no hesitation in involving the police if you suspect such crimes.

Cultural and religious considerations

Living in a diverse multicultural society can bring new challenges to care home staff. As a care provider, if you are unsure what course of action is desirable in respecting a given culture (especially surrounding death and dying), ask the family. Often, they will have precise wishes and, if a religion requires particular management, liaising with the priest, minister or other chosen cleric should help ensure that cultural sensitivities are respected (see Chapter 16.8).

Further reading

Bauer M, Nay R. 2003. Family and staff relationships in long term care. A review of the literature. *Journal of Gerontological Nursing* 29: 46–57.

Gaugler JE, Ewen HH. 2005. Building relationships in residential long term care: determinants of staff attitudes toward family members. *Journal of Gerontological Nursing* 31: 19–26.

Weman K, Fagerberg I. 2006. Registered nurses working together with family members of older people. *Journal of Clinical Nursing* 15: 281–289.

1.5 Documentation and record-keeping

Zuzanna Sawicka[1] and Ewa Zalewska[2]

[1]*St James's University Hospital, Leeds, UK*
[2]*Mid Yorkshire Hospitals NHS Trust, Wakefield, UK*

Key points

- High quality record-keeping is central to providing good care.
- All documentation must be legible, accurate, intelligible and factual.
- Avoid abbreviations and jargon.
- Always include your signature, printed name and the date.
- Do not remove, delete or destroy records.

Good record-keeping is an integral part of nursing and practice. It is vital to the provision of safe and effective care.

Documentation is important, whether at an individual, team or organisational level. It can have many important purposes:

- It helps improve accountability and demonstrates decision-making processes and how judgements have been made.
- Good documentation promotes better communication and sharing of information between members of the multi-professional healthcare team, while making continuity of care easier.
- It may also help to identify risks, and enable early detection of complications.
- Documentation can be invaluable when providing evidence to address complaints or in legal processes.

The UK Data Protection Act 1998 defines a health record as:

'consisting of information about the physical or mental health or condition of an identifiable individual made by or on behalf of a health professional in connection with the care of that individual.'

The principles of good record-keeping apply to all types of records, regardless of how they are held.

These can include: handwritten clinical notes, emails, letters, laboratory results, printouts from monitoring equipment, incident reports and statements, photographs and audio-visual data (including tape-recordings of telephone conversations or text messages) (Figure 1.5.1).

As defined by the UK Nursing and Midwifery Council:

1. Handwriting should be legible and any records should be easily readable when photocopied or scanned.
2. All entries to records should be signed and the person's name and job title should be printed alongside any entry.
3. All records should be dated and timed. They should be recorded in real time and in chronological order.
4. Records should be accurate and easily understood.
5. Records should be based on facts. Avoid the use of unnecessary abbreviations, jargon, meaningless phrases or irrelevant speculation.
6. All relevant assessments and reviews should be recorded, including any arrangements and details of any future and on-going care.
7. Identify and record any risks or problems that have arisen, and show the action taken to deal with them.
8. Do not alter or destroy any records without being authorised to do so. In the unlikely event that you need to alter your own or another healthcare professional's records, you must give your name and job title, and sign and date the original documentation and the alteration clearly.

The Care Home Handbook, First Edition. Edited by Graham Mulley, Clive Bowman, Michal Boyd and Sarah Stowe.
© 2015 John Wiley & Sons, Ltd. Published 2015 by John Wiley & Sons, Ltd.

Mrs Jane Walker

Date of Birth: 27.06.1924

28.02.2012 09.15 hrs

Mrs Walker appears to have had a pleasant morning. No signs of anxiety noticed. Assisted with all hygiene needs. Pressure areas checked and intact. Nursed in bed on air pressure relieving mattress. Catheter remains in situ, urine output recorded. Diet and oral fluids taken and tolerated well.

(Signature)

DIKENS RN

28.02.2012 12.55 hrs

Mrs Walker took her tablets without difficulty. No complaints of pain voiced. Had her bowels opened – soft stool. Catheter emptied, urine clear, not concentrated. Encouraged with oral fluids.

(Signature)

DIKENS RN

Figure 1.5.1 An example of good record-keeping.

Further reading

Schnelle JF, Bates-Jensen BM, Chu L, Simmons SF. 2004. Accuracy of nursing home medical record information about care-process delivery: implications for staff management and improvement. *Journal of the American Geriatrics Society* 52: 1378–1383.

Schnelle JF, Osterweil D, Simmons SF. 2005. Improving the quality of nursing home care and medical record accuracy with direct observational technologies. *Gerontologist* 45: 576–582.

1.6 Generating a care plan

Peter Rogers

Bupa Care Services, Leeds, UK

Key points

- A care plan follows the comprehensive assessment of needs.
- The plan specifies the aims, agreed anticipated outcomes and the best-practice interventions.
- Care plans change and plans will need to be reviewed when circumstances alter.
- This documentation must be signed, with the date and time clearly stated.
- Care pathways are established agreed standards of care that are based on evidence and which can reduce clinical variability and improve outcomes.
- Meeting the needs of residents involves genuine care, concern and compassion, as well as formal care planning.

Personalised care planning is driven by the results of the nursing assessment. Each actual or potential problem should give rise to a care plan, which sets out the aims of care in the form of anticipated outcomes, agreed where possible with the resident, and the 'best practice' interventions necessary to achieve them.

Like all resident documentation, care plans must be factual and accurate, and written in a clear and legible manner, free from abbreviations and jargon. They should reflect the guidance set out by the appropriate regulatory body, for instance, by the UK, the Nursing & Midwifery Council.

- All entries must be dated, timed and signed; discontinued actions should be clearly indicated – for example by being crossed through (but still readable), signed and dated.
- Correction tape/fluid should not be used.
- A signature list, which associates staff signatures with their printed names, should be maintained for each resident's care record.

Anticipated outcomes

Each actual or potential problem should be accompanied by a concise statement of the intended outcome. Wherever possible these should reflect the SMART approach by being:

- **Specific** to the resident's problem.
- **Measureable** to enable progress toward achievement to be judged.

- **Agreed** with the resident, wherever possible.
- **Realistic**, given the resident's condition and abilities as indicated by the holistic assessment.
- **Time limited** – while rigid timeframes are rarely appropriate, it is often helpful to convey a sense of how long it should take to achieve the agreed outcome.

Planned interventions

These are the actions set out in the plan that the resident's named nurse has determined are necessary in order to achieve the anticipated outcomes agreed for each problem. The precise nature of the planned actions relies on the clinical judgements made by the nurse and reflects his/her understanding of the resident's particular needs and preferences, his/her knowledge of current best nursing practice and his/her expertise in aged care provision.

What the plan cannot convey is the way in which nurses and carers go about their work. If the resident's experience is going to be positive, they must trust their carers not only to do right things for them, but to do them in the right way, that is with an attitude which conveys genuine care and compassion for the resident. Knowledge and technical skill are vital, but professionalism in nursing requires an attitude of respect for the resident and a concern for their dignity and self-esteem (see Chapter 3.4).

The Care Home Handbook, First Edition. Edited by Graham Mulley, Clive Bowman, Michal Boyd and Sarah Stowe.
© 2015 John Wiley & Sons, Ltd. Published 2015 by John Wiley & Sons, Ltd.

Key aspects of the care planning process

- Care planning requires professional nursing expertise, particularly the capacity to recognise and manage clinical risks.
- A named nurse will produce and update each resident's plan of care.
- The individual resident, their needs and preferences are at the centre of the process and so promote choice; wherever possible, care plans should be produced with the resident and, where appropriate, shared with their family.
- Do ensure that the care of residents with complex needs is well coordinated, and that the contribution of different healthcare professionals is recorded and communicated to others.
- Planned interventions should be based on current best practice.
- Nurses writing care plans must have access to up-to-date evidence and information on which to base their plans.
- Where necessary, care plans should indicate which interventions are the responsibility of the registered nurse.
- Care plans should include appropriately frequent evaluations of the resident's response to the care provided.
- Long-term residents should have their complete care package regularly reviewed. This might take the form of a quarterly meeting, to which the resident/relatives/advocate are all invited.

Care pathways

Care pathways, sometimes called clinical or integrated care pathways, set out the anticipated care to be provided to a specific group of residents who share the same problem or diagnosis. They establish the agreed standards of care based upon the available evidence and set out an appropriate timeframe.

Often, locally defined care pathways are useful multidisciplinary tools to improve both the quality and coordination of healthcare which, along with their focus on particular conditions, perhaps explains why they have had a limited impact on the care home sector. The exceptions are those pathways that have either been developed or adopted nationally (for example the NICE Pressure Ulcer Pathway) (Appendix 1). The Liverpool Care Pathway has been withdrawn in the UK.

Further reading

Nursing and Midwifery Council, London 2010. Record keeping guidance for nurses and midwives. Available at: www.nmc-uk.org [Accessed September 2013]

Care Quality Commission 2012. Meeting the health care needs of people in care homes. Available at: http://www.cqc.org.uk/public/reports-surveys-and-reviews/reviews-and-studies/meeting-health-care-needs-people-care-homes [Accessed September 2013]

1.7 Nursing handover

Peter Rogers

Bupa Care Services, Leeds, UK

Key points

- Effective communication between nurses can improve practice and resident outcomes; poor communication at handover can cause errors in care.
- The nursing handover is a crucial part of efficient and effective clinical care.
- It involves passing on clear, relevant, accurate, resident-related information.
- Tips are offered to help improve the structure of the nursing handover.

Effective communication is fundamental to the quality of nursing care – wherever it takes place. Perhaps the most frequent routine communication interactions within a care home are the change of shift handovers between nursing and care staff. These are a crucial part of ensuring the quality of resident care: a good handover enables the incoming shift to start their work immediately, whereas an inadequate report can delay the provision of care by as much as two hours.

Nursing handover reports can take several forms: verbal, written or a combination of both. Whether they are restricted to the care staff or involve those residents who are able and willing, if they are to be effective they should:

- Use a consistent standardised approach: as well as the times and place of the handover, the World Health Organisation recommends the use of the SBAR model to structure the content (see box).
- Include all of the care staff and offer the opportunity to ask and resolve questions about residents' care needs.
- Allow sufficient time for the communication of all important resident information, and in particular any changes including:
  - Resident's condition.
  - Medications.
  - Care plans, including specific safety issues, advanced directives or DNA CRP decisions (see Chapters 4.5, 16.1 and 16.3).
- Reflect a pragmatic approach; the nurse must exercise professional judgement in deciding the extent of the exchange of information necessary to ensure the safe provision of care.

Top Tips: The 'SBAR' model for structuring handover communications

- **Situation** — Summary of resident's current status/condition, nursing and care needs, recent changes and current specific issues or concerns.
- **Background** — Pertinent to the resident's current status and care needs, significant issues in the medical and social history.
- **Assessment** — Outline of the basis on which the statement of the 'situation' has been reached.
- **Recommendation** — Statement of what actions are required, including specific aspects of care, for example commence fluid balance observations, obtain a stool specimen, liaise with the next of kin.

Note: This structured approach to providing resident information is also useful when liaising with GPs and other healthcare professionals in relation to your concerns about a resident.

The Care Home Handbook, First Edition. Edited by Graham Mulley, Clive Bowman, Michal Boyd and Sarah Stowe.
© 2015 John Wiley & Sons, Ltd. Published 2015 by John Wiley & Sons, Ltd.

As well as the need for the content of handover reports to be structured to ensure the efficient transfer of resident information, it is also important to manage the context of the handover. Currie's 'CUBAN' acronym is useful in this respect (Currie, 2002). Handover communications should be:

- **Confidential**
  Ensure handover reports cannot be overheard. If staff make notes, they should remain on their person at all times and be destroyed at the end of the shift. They must not be taken out of the home.
- **Uninterrupted**
  Handovers should take place in a quiet area where there are no distractions. If the handover includes the resident, it should take place in their own room or somewhere equally private. They should commence on time, at the beginning of the shift.
- **Brief**
  Keep the information concise and focused. Too much detail is confusing and easily forgotten.
- **Accurate**
  Check that the handover information is correct, current and that all residents have been included. Information should be clear and free from jargon and irrelevant or unethical comments.

- **Named nurse**
  In the interest of continuity of care, the nurse responsible for the resident's care should be the one who provides the handover report. Care plans should be up to date at the end of each shift.

References

Currie J. 2002. Improving the efficiency of patient handover. *Emergency Nurse* 10: 24–27.

World Health Organisation, 2007. *Patient Safety Solutions*. 1.3 Communication during patient hand-overs.

Further reading

Conwy and Denbighshire NHS Trust 2008. Nursing handover for adult patients. Guidelines: http://www.wales.nhs.uk/sitesplus/documents/861/Additional%20Info%20048.pdf [Accessed September 2013]

Hansten R. 2003. Notes from the field: streamline change-of-shift report. *Nursing Management* 34: 58–59.

Scovell S. 2010. Role of the nurse-to-nurse handover in patient care. *Nursing Standard* 24: 35–39.

1.8 Discharge arrangements

Peter Rogers

Bupa Care Services, Leeds, UK

Key points

- Residents might move out of a care home to be cared for in hospital, in another care home or in the community.
- Discharge planning should give early confirmation of the date and time of discharge, transport arrangements and (if necessary) give time for registration with the new GP.
- A comprehensive discharge letter can help optimise care in the target destination.
- Practical tips are offered on the content of the discharge summary.

Although many residents move into a care home with the intention of it being a permanent arrangement, many do subsequently move out. This might be for one of several reasons including:

- A change in health, such that the resident requires care in an acute hospital or hospice.
- A return to their own home or into the care of a relative.
- Transfer to another care home or higher level of residential care, such as specialist dementia care.

The reason for discharge and the resident's destination after leaving the home will affect what arrangements need to made and the time available to make them. A well-planned discharge is important to ensure the smooth transition of care to the next provider, and to give a positive conclusion to the current therapeutic relationship. It will require close liaison with the resident, family and possibly the destination organisation. Important things to consider include:

- Early confirmation of the date and time of discharge, communicated to the contracts office, to enable timely termination of the agreement between the resident and provider organisation.
- Transport arrangements for the resident and also their personal effects, particularly bulky items such as furniture,
- Arrangements for transferring registration between general practitioners.
- Production of a discharge summary for future care providers.

The last of these points – the preparation of a discharge summary – is particularly important, outlining as it does the assessment of the resident's on-going care needs at the point of discharge. The summary should ideally be prepared in consultation with the resident, and a copy should be provided to them or their next of kin. A copy should also be retained in the resident's care home records, as well as being shared with the GP and the destination organisation if applicable.

The Care Home Handbook, First Edition. Edited by Graham Mulley, Clive Bowman, Michal Boyd and Sarah Stowe.
© 2015 John Wiley & Sons, Ltd. Published 2015 by John Wiley & Sons, Ltd.

Top Tips: Discharge summary contents

The discharge summary is important in ensuring the continuity of a resident's care – whether in another home, hospital or in the community.

- Details of the destination address and the key contact there.
- Next of kin contact details.
- Diagnoses.
- Summary of physical and mental state.
- Summary of usual care needs, including mobility and personal care needs, feeding and continence care.
- Referrals made/required with dates and details of the relevant contacts to:
  - Social services and needs assessment services
  - Physiotherapy
  - Chiropody or podiatry
  - Continence advisor
  - Nurse specialist, for example tissue viability (wound care), district nurses
  - Community continuing care or intermediate care team.
- Medication
  - List of medication and number of days supply provided (usually seven days).
  - Ability to self-medicate (see Chapter 11.2)
  - Provision of medication administration record (MAR) (see Chapter 11.1) included in GP correspondence.
- GP home or surgery visit requested (date).
- Equipment required, for example walking frame, commodes, home adaptations.
- Continence aids provided (anticipated rate of use).
- Meals on wheels.

In addition to the discharge summary being signed by the nurse completing it, it is also good practice to ask the resident or their relative to sign a copy, after having discussed the contents, to confirm that they are in agreement with the assessment it offers.

Further reading

Medicare. 2012. Template for residents and their families: Your discharge planning checklist: for patients and their caregivers preparing to leave a hospital, nursing home or other care setting. Available at: www.medicare.gov/publications/pubs/pdf/11376.pdf [Accessed September 2013]

Murtaugh CM. 1994. Discharge planning in nursing homes. *Health Services Research* 28: 751–769.

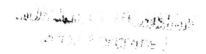

Chapter 2

Life in a Care Home

HARROW COLLEGE
Learning Centre

2.1 Healthy lifestyles

Mark Bradley

Leeds Teaching Hospitals NHS Trust, Leeds, UK

Key points

- Healthy behaviours (especially relating to food, fluids, exercise, alcohol and smoking) are important for residents – whatever their age.
- All new residents should have a nutritional screen on entry to the care home.
- Try to keep fatty and sugary snacks to a minimum.
- Balance the wish of residents to smoke or drink with the possible harm that these can cause.
- Smoking can cause fires, which may be fatal.

If we could give every individual the right amount of nourishment and exercise, not too little and not too much, we would have found the safest way to health.
                                        Hippocrates

It is important to offer residents help and advice on healthy eating, moderating alcohol, stopping smoking and staying as active as possible. In Britain, Age UK and NHS choices have useful resources – see below.

Eating well

It is never too late to start eating healthily and a healthy diet doesn't have to be boring.

Carry out routine nutritional screening (see Chapters 2.4 and 5.1) on all residents and formulate an appropriate care plan for anyone identified as a nutritional risk.

A balanced daily menu provides:

- one portion of starch food at each meal (bread, rice, pasta, potato or chapati),
- two portions of vegetables,
- two portions of fruit per day (glass of fruit juice = one portion),
- two portions of dairy foods (yoghurt, milk, custard, cheese),
- two portions of protein (meat, fish, eggs, beans).

Try and use locally sourced ingredients and make food look appetising. Limit high saturated fat or sugary foods, such as butter, ghee, biscuits, sweets, sausages, pies and pate.

Staying hydrated

Not drinking enough can lead to dehydration (see Chapter 5.3), constipation, headaches and tiredness. Try to remember the following.

- Residents should drink six to eight cups (2.5 pints, 1200 ml) of water, juice, squash, tea or coffee per day (alcohol isn't included and not too much caffeine).
- Fruit such as oranges, melons, peaches, pears all count towards their daily fluid intake, as do soups and jellies.
- Hot weather, temperatures and exudates from wounds increase fluid requirements.
- *Be aware that older people may not feel thirsty due to altered thirst recognition and may try and avoid drinks because of continence worries.*

Alcohol and smoking

Access to alcohol and cigarettes in care homes is a complex issue. This is because there is a need to balance a healthy lifestyle with an individual's right to

---

The Care Home Handbook, First Edition. Edited by Graham Mulley, Clive Bowman, Michal Boyd and Sarah Stowe.
© 2015 John Wiley & Sons, Ltd. Published 2015 by John Wiley & Sons, Ltd.

autonomy and choice, along with a desire to provide a 'homely' atmosphere. Remember that smoking and excessive drinking are associated with adverse health outcomes.

Apart from the 2007 Smoke Free legislation in the UK, there are no clear guidelines and policies are usually left to individual homes.

The UK Department of Health recommends the following for alcohol consumption.

- *Men* should drink no more than 21 units of alcohol per week (and no more than four units in any one day).
- *Women* should drink no more than 14 units of alcohol per week (and no more than three units in any one day).

What is a unit of alcohol?

- Half a pint of beer, lager or cider.
- A small pub measure (25 ml) of spirits.
- A standard pub measure (50 ml) of sherry or port.

There are one and a half units of alcohol in a small glass (125 ml) of wine.

Alcohol misuse does occur in care homes. Alcohol can interact with medicines, which can put people at risk. However it's important to try and provide a sensible and pragmatic approach to these matters.

You should give consideration to the following.

- An individual assessment and care plan for residents, especially those with alcohol problems or cognitive impairment.
- Decide if alcohol can be allowed in bedrooms or if it needs to kept separately/securely.
- Offer small amounts of alcohol with main meals.
- Offer occasional trips to pubs or clubs or hold pub/happy hour evenings.
- Provide alcoholic drinks for special occasions and parties.
- In order to accept Local Authority funded residents in England, you might be required to have a clear alcohol or smoking policy, so check with them.

Moving into a care home might be seen by some residents as an opportunity to stop smoking or reduce alcohol consumption. In such a situation it would be sensible to seek advice from the resident's GP – particularly in terms of nicotine replacement aids and therapy and problems arising from alcohol withdrawal.

In the UK, there is Smoke Free (2007) legislation; other counties have similar laws and the following advice may apply.

Are residential care homes and hospices covered by the legislation?

Yes. It covers the public areas of residential care homes and hospices. This means that sitting rooms, dining areas, reception areas, corridors and all other communal areas that are enclosed places and structures that are 'substantially enclosed' are legally required to be smoke free. In addition, work vehicles used by more than one person will also have to be smoke free.

Can residents smoke in their bedrooms?

Yes, but only if it's the management's policy. Care homes are allowed to let residents smoke in bedrooms or a special smoking room, but there are some restrictions and certain conditions have to be met.

Advice from the Fire Service

A fire can happen when you least expect it and *more people die in fires caused by smoking than any other single cause*. By taking a few simple precautions you can protect yourself, your staff, residents and business.

- Don't allow residents to smoke if they are drowsy, on prescription drugs or have been drinking.
- Don't allow residents to smoke in bed.
- Provide proper ashtrays for those who smoke.
- Make sure each cigarette is stubbed out properly.
- At the end of the day, wet ash and cigarette butts and dispose of them in a safe container.

Useful web sites

Age UK http://www.ageuk.org.uk/ [Accessed September 2013]

National Care Standards www.nationalcarestandards.org/74.html [Accessed September 2013]

NHS Choices www.nhs.uk/livewell/Pages/Livewellhub.aspx [Accessed September 2013]

2.2 Religion and spirituality

John Wattis[1], Steven Curran[1] and Melanie Rogers[2]

[1]Centre for Health and Social Care Research, University of Huddersfield, Huddersfield, UK
[2]University of Huddersfield, Huddersfield, UK

Key points

- Good nursing involves spiritual care of residents – understanding each individual's life experiences, helping them on their spiritual journey, treating them with respect.
- Spirituality includes a sense of mystery and wonder, a sense of purpose in life.
- Religion is one reflection of spirituality. It usually involves beliefs and practices which give meaning to life and belief in a higher power.
- Staff should take care of their own spiritual needs in order to provide compassionate care to others.

What is the difference between religion and spirituality? Definitions of spirituality often emphasise a sense of connectedness, meaning and purpose in life. A useful definition comes from life coach Duncan Coppock:

> Spirituality is about having a sense and appreciation of the underlying mystery of life and a quality of connection to a deeper source of strength and wisdom than comes from just thinking and logic alone. It is also about how you treat others and about how you are being in the moment.
>
> Coppock (2005)

- We get our sense of meaning in life from a variety of sources, but the most important are relationships, our work and ultimately our attitude to life, especially when we are suffering (Frankl, 2004).
- Religion is one of the ways in which people express spirituality. Religions are organised approaches to human spirituality that usually involve a set of beliefs and practices that help people give meaning to their lives and usually make reference to a higher power or truth.

Spirituality in practice

- Spirituality is distinct from religious practice, and spiritual care should be delivered to all residents, regardless of their religious beliefs or lack of them. It begins with respect for the other person.
- In dementia care this is seen in the approach pioneered by Tom Kitwood and his colleagues and described in *Dementia Reconsidered: The Person Comes First* (Kitwood, 1997).
- Spiritual care plans are not only concerned with the resident's religious beliefs. Nursing care that is delivered person-to-person is itself a spiritual exchange. Spiritual care is concerned as much with *how* care is delivered as *what* care is given. Staff who are talking to each other about the weekend, over the head of an old person they are helping, are NOT delivering spiritual care.
- Those who do their best, in any activity, to engage with and respect the individual they are caring for ARE delivering spiritual care.

Organisations encourage high quality care when they emphasise the personal aspect of caring. They make spiritual care harder when they 'industrialise' care tasks, putting the emphasis on the task rather than the personal interaction that goes with it.

Staff should take care of their own spiritual needs if they are to deliver good quality spiritual care. People need to be respected, supported and to feel connected if they are in turn to give a feeling of being respected, supported and connected to those they care for.

The Care Home Handbook, First Edition. Edited by Graham Mulley, Clive Bowman, Michal Boyd and Sarah Stowe.
© 2015 John Wiley & Sons, Ltd. Published 2015 by John Wiley & Sons, Ltd.

Activity

Take five minutes to think of the care that you give to a particular resident. How far is the care an opportunity to interact respectfully with another human being and how far is it just a 'job to be done'? How can you personalise the care giving in a way that will increase its value to yourself and the recipient of care? Make a habit of thinking about this for all the individuals under your care.

Religious care in practice

Nobody can be an expert in all religions. The starting point in offering religious care is to recognise the person's religion (if any) and what it means to them. Some religions will prescribe a particular diet or particular ways of dealing with death and dying (Chapter 16.8). They may also prescribe particular prayers or other religious observances at particular times or on particular days. Ask the person, their family and (when appropriate) members of their faith community about what is appropriate.

The Christian Council on Ageing (http://www.ccoa.org.uk) also publishes an excellent range of booklets that includes one on different faith practices: 'Religious Practice and People with Dementia' edited by Brian Allen. This resource is designed to assist those caring for people with dementia in understanding what might be of importance for members of five major world faiths: Christianity, Hinduism, Islam, Judaism and Sikhism. It contains a short summary of each religion, details of important customs and festivals and some prayers and readings that could be used with older people.

When to refer to the chaplain

Sometimes spiritual or religious questions may be beyond the staff of a residential or nursing home. Often members of the person's own faith group can help, but if they can't or if they cannot be contacted, then access to a chaplain can be of help.

Chaplains, these days, are usually trained not only in their own religious tradition but also to help people of other religions and none. They may also have access to colleagues from specific faith traditions if that is what is required.

Respect the person

Good spiritual care will always respect the other person and their religion (or lack of religion). It is not about trying to 'convert' someone to another point of view. It is about seeking to understand and respect their life experience and offering support to them in their own spiritual journey.

References

Christian Council on Ageing: resources http://www.ccoa.org.uk/index.php?option=com_ezcatalog&task=viewcategory&id=1&Itemid=42 [Accessed September 2013].

Coppock D. 2005. *The SELF Factor: The Power of Being You: A Coaching Approach*. Findhorn, Scotland, Findhorn Press (see www.self-factor.com for more information).

Frankl V. 2004. *Man's Search for Meaning: the Classic Tribute to Hope from the Holocaust*. London, Rider (Random House Group).

Kitwood T. 1997. *Dementia Reconsidered: The Person Comes First (Rethinking Ageing)*. Buckingham, Open University Press.

2.3 Mealtimes

Mark Bradley

Leeds Teaching Hospitals NHS Trust, Leeds, UK

Key points

- Each care plan should include information on food preferences.
- Listen to what residents tell you about their experiences of mealtimes and provide each individual with a service that meets their needs and wishes.
- Try to provide a quiet environment and keep distractions at mealtimes to a minimum.
- Ensure that residents have access to fruit and drinks.
- Special skill is required when feeding those who need personal assistance.

> *Ask not what you can do for your country. Ask what's for lunch!*
>
> Orson Welles

- Mealtimes are an important part of the day, both nutritionally and socially. Residents often regard them as the highlight and may rate the overall quality of a home based on their experience at mealtimes.
- It is essential to identify residents with special dietary needs and those needing extra help and assistance at mealtimes.
- Ask residents and relatives for their ideas about improving mealtimes – and put their suggestions into practice.
- If a large number of residents need assistance with feeding, it's crucial to ensure that enough staff are available. It may be necessary to run several sittings so that residents get the support they need.

Planning

- Document residents' food preferences as part of their care plan.
- Respect the need for calm and quiet at mealtimes and minimise distractions such as TV/radio.
- Try to arrange mealtimes around the needs of residents.

- Implement 'protected mealtimes' to stop non-essential activities and reschedule appointments with dentists, opticians, and so on to ensure that residents don't miss mealtimes.
- Meals should be served in courses rather than using service trays.
- Think about residents' comfort at mealtimes, for example needing to empty bowels or bladder, their seating position, oral health and dentures.

Offer residents a choice

You should give your residents a choice of:

- where to sit at a communal table,
- where to eat (bedroom, lounge, dining room),
- using a napkin or apron rather than a bib,
- using a proper cup or bowl rather than feeder cups or straws.

Also, give your residents an opportunity to:

- ask about preferred portion sizes,
- serve themselves,
- have meals with family members or relatives.

Residents with severe arthritis or those who have had a stroke may need special cutlery, particularly with a large handle – it's important to know who needs what.

The Care Home Handbook, First Edition. Edited by Graham Mulley, Clive Bowman, Michal Boyd and Sarah Stowe.
© 2015 John Wiley & Sons, Ltd. Published 2015 by John Wiley & Sons, Ltd.

Menus

- Produce menus that can be easily read and understood, for example menus with photos of food, or large print menus, and in different languages if necessary.
- Allow as much choice and variation as possible. Think about seasonal menus or rolling menus that change over a four-week cycle.
- Provide healthy snacks and drinks to have between main meals. Think about having a morning/afternoon 'tea trolley' with fresh fruit as well as drinks and biscuits.
- Provide easy access to water or juice in residents' bedrooms.
- Provide healthy finger foods for residents who may be agitated or restless at mealtimes.

If a resident needs help and assistance

Feeding a resident is a very intimate act. As a carer you can best understand this if you ask a colleague to feed you. This sounds silly, but it will teach you more than words can say.

The following tips can also help:

- Make sure that the resident is awake, alert and knows what is going to happen.
- Ensure a comfortable sitting posture, which is as upright as possible.
- Protect clothes from splatters and drips.
- Make sure that dentures, glasses and hearing aids are used (and working).
- Allow the resident to see and smell the food.
- Try to establish if the resident wants separate mouthfuls of each food or a combination, for example meat and carrots together.
- Observe if the resident is ready for the next mouthful, doesn't like the food or wants a drink, and so on.
- Allow time between mouthfuls.

Further reading

The Caroline Walker Trust. 2004. Report of an Expert Working Group. *Eating Well for Older People*. 2nd edn. Practical and nutritional guidelines for food in residential and nursing homes and for community meals. The Caroline Walker Trust. http://www.cwt.org.uk/, ..html [Accessed 30 September 2013]

2.4 Specialised diets

Michi Yukawa[1] and Rose Ann DiMaria-Ghalili[2]

[1]University of California San Francisco, and San Francisco VA Medical Center, San Francisco, CA, USA
[2]Drexel University, Philadelphia, PA, USA

Key points

- Most residents do not require specialised diets.
- Special care is needed with those who have swallowing difficulties: involve the speech and language therapist and dietitian if you have any concerns; be aware of the range of pureed and thickened liquids.
- Avoid restrictive diabetic diets in residents with diabetes mellitus.
- Avoid low fat and low cholesterol diets.
- In general, avoid low protein diets in residents with renal failure.
- Avoid weight loss medications in residents who are obese.

Most old people entering care homes do not have specialised dietary requirements. What they do need is carers to ensure that they are capable of feeding themselves and swallowing the diet that has sustained them through a long life. For the few with a long life expectancy, it is reasonable to consider a specialised diet to improve their underlying medical conditions. However, for most residents, liberalising their diet may prevent malnutrition and unintentional weight loss without compromising their underlying medical conditions. Residents of nursing homes are at increased risk of malnutrition and weight loss and thus placing them on specialised diet may exacerbate this problem.

Diabetes mellitus

The American Dietetic Association recommends that *older adults living in nursing homes should not be on a diabetic diet* (see Chapter 8.4).

- Nursing home residents should be served a regular diet with consistent amounts of carbohydrate, and should have their glycaemic control medication adjusted accordingly.
- Mean HgbA1C does not increase when diabetic residents are switched from a diabetic diet to a regular diet.

- There is no evidence to support the use of restrictive diabetic diets (such as, no concentrated sweets or no sugar added foods) for care home residents.
- Hypoglycaemic episodes are more common in nursing home residents than hyperglycemia. Hypoglycemia is more dangerous and can lead to falls (see Chapter 6.6) and cardiovascular events.

Dysphagia diets

Diets are individualised for older adults with dysphagia (swallowing difficulties) after consultation with a speech therapist and dietitian. Special diets include pureed and soft diets. In the USA, fluids that can be served in different consistencies are described as thin, nectar-like, honey-like and spoon-thick.

In the UK, a different scheme is used:

There are five categories of fluid consistency (see Table 2.4.1).

SALT teams will assess and monitor residents (see Chapter 8.2) with eating/drinking difficulties and will advise on:

- How to prevent aspiration.
- The appropriate consistency of fluids.

The Care Home Handbook, First Edition. Edited by Graham Mulley, Clive Bowman, Michal Boyd and Sarah Stowe.
© 2015 John Wiley & Sons, Ltd. Published 2015 by John Wiley & Sons, Ltd.

Table 2.4.1 Five categories of fluid consistency. Adapted from Nutrition & Diet Resources UK: Fluid Thickening Guide ref: 9091, 2005 (reviewed in 2010).

Texture	Description of fluid texture
Thin fluid	Water, tea, coffee without milk, spirits, wine
Naturally thick fluid	Product leaves a coating on an empty glass, full cream milk, cream liqueurs
Thickened fluid	Fluid to which a commercial thickener has been added to thicken consistency
Stage 1 =	• can be drunk through a straw or cup • leaves a thin coat on the back of a spoon
Stage 2 =	• cannot be drunk through a straw • can be drunk from a cup • leaves a thick coat on the back of a spoon
Stage 3 =	• cannot be drunk through a straw • cannot be drunk from a cup • needs to be taken with a spoon

- Stage 1 is also described as a syrup consistency.
- Stage 2 is also referred to as custard consistency.
- Stage 3 is also referred to as pudding consistency.

- Residents may reject pureed, soft, or artificially thickened foods due to their lack of palatability. Instead, offer foods which are naturally of a pureed consistency, such as mashed potatoes, squash or puddings.
- Residents with swallowing difficulties require one-on-one feeding to prevent aspiration.
- Carefully monitor weight, as older adults with swallowing difficulties may reduce food intake and lose weight.
- Dysphagia diets are visually unappealing and lack taste. Serve food in a visually pleasing manner: use coloured plates and serve colourful food on a plate (e.g. broccoli and carrots). During food preparation, food moulds can be used to form foods that resemble the appearance of the food being pureed.
- If the resident's life expectancy is less than five years and their quality of life is affected by soft foods, then they can continue to take regular textured food.
- There is no intervention that can consistently prevent aspiration.

Pureed diet

- Pureed diets require very little chewing and do not require formation of a bolus.
- Foods must be lump-free. Avoid fruited yoghurt, un-blended cottage cheese, peanut butter, soups and hot cereal. Fruits and vegetables: pureed with no pulp, seeds or chunks.
- Mashed potatoes: serve with gravy, sauce, butter, or margarine to moisten.
- Soups: pureed smooth.
- Eggs: souffles are allowed. Avoid scrambled, fried or hard-boiled eggs.

Soft diet

- Soft diets (mechanical soft or advanced soft) are appropriate for older adults with some chewing ability.
- Mechanical soft diets are cohesive, moist, semi-solid foods:
  - Fruits: easily mashed with fork, canned or cooked, soft ripe bananas.
  - Vegetables: well-cooked, soft, easily mashed with fork, cut into pieces smaller than 0.5 in.
  - Avoid dry food and any item difficult to chew: most bread, crackers, canned pineapple, whole grain cereal, nuts, seeds, coconut.
  - Meat: ground and cubed smaller than metric – 0.25 inch is equivalent to 6.35 mm; serve with gravy or sauce.
  - Examples: cooked breakfast cereal, soft pancakes with syrup, tuna and egg salad.
- Advanced soft diets require more chewing:
  - Easy-to-cut tender meats; fruits and vegetables without seeds. Food should be well-moistened and in bite-size pieces.
  - Avoid items difficult to chew: hard crunchy fruits and raw vegetables, sticky foods, very dry foods, corn, nuts, seeds, popcorn.

Liquids

See Table 2.4.1.

- The consistency of liquids should be individualised for older adults with swallowing problems.

Liquids are categorised as thin, nectar-like, honey-like and spoon thick.

- Thin: clear liquids, milk, commercial nutritional supplements, water, tea, coffee, soda, beer, wine, broth and clear juice. Ice cream, frozen yoghurt, and plain gelatine fall into this category.
- Nectar-like liquids are of medium thickness and include: nectars, vegetable juices, hand-made milkshakes with commercial thickener. Thin liquids can be thickened to a nectar-like consistency with commercial thickeners.
- Honey-like liquids resemble the consistency of honey at room temperature. Use commercial thickeners or commercial pre-thickened honey-like thickened products.
- Spoon-thick liquids are highly viscous and are too thick to drink with a straw. Commercial thickeners are used to prepare liquids of this consistency.
- Commercial thickeners are starch-based or gum-based.
  - Follow manufacturer directions to prepare liquids with starch-based or gum-based thickeners to obtain the appropriate consistency.
  - Fluids prepared with starch-based thickeners expand and become thicker after initial preparation. Liquids thickened with starch-based thickeners will become too thick after refrigeration.
  - Fluids prepared with gum-based thickeners are more difficult to prepare and must be shaken or blended with fluid to thicken the liquid. When mixed properly, the viscosity of liquids prepared with gum-based thickeners are stable over time.

Renal failure diet (low protein)

For a few older residents with chronic renal failure who are not on dialysis, a protein diet (0.8–1.0 g of protein/kg body weight per day) is recommended to delay the progression of renal disease.

- However, if the resident is losing weight and malnourished, then no protein restriction should be instituted.
- Also, for residents older than 80 years old, the benefit of protein restriction is outweighed by the risk of malnutrition.
- Extra protein is necessary when residents start dialysis, and thus a liberalised diet is recommended for those on dialysis.

Hyperlipidaemia and cardiac diets

The American Dietetic Association recommends that while nutritional care for older adults with cardiac disease should focus on maintaining blood pressure and blood lipid levels, eating pleasure and quality of life are more important considerations.

- Specialised diets, such as low fat and low cholesterol diets, are restrictive and can be counterproductive in long-term care, where many older adults have weight loss and are malnourished or at risk of malnutrition.
- The use of low fat and low cholesterol diets should generally be avoided in care home residents.
- Lipid lowering medications may be a more appropriate measure to lower lipids, enabling the older adult to enjoy personal food choices. However, for most residents statins are unnecessary and usually should be discontinued whenever possible.

High calorie for people losing weight

Unintentional weight loss is often a problem in older residents and often accompanies illnesses such as cancer, heart failure and dementia. Generally in such conditions, especially when they are advanced, increasing nutritional intake is ineffective. On occasions when it is indicated, high calorie and/or high protein intake can be achieved in several ways.

- Regularly served meals can be enhanced to increase the energy density of the food, for example by adding butter to mashed potatoes, the use of full fat milk and cheese in meal preparation.
- High energy, dense, between meal snacks (e.g. puddings) are of benefit.
- Oral liquid supplements can also be used to increase energy intake.
- If oral liquid supplements are not used appropriately, older adults may 'fill up' on the supplement and eat less at mealtimes, thereby negating the purpose of the supplements.
- The ideal oral liquid supplement is one that is concentrated to deliver most energy in the smallest volume of liquid.
- Oral liquid supplements should be given between meals. As with feeding, older adults will need encouragement to consume between meal snacks and oral liquid supplements.

Obesity in nursing home residents

The effects of obesity among nursing home residents have not been well studied. The following recommendations are based on the few studies of obese nursing home patients:

- Very obese residents with a body mass index (BMI) >35 kg/m² have increased risk of mortality.
- Elderly subjects with a BMI >28 but <35 kg/m² are not at increased risk of hospitalisation or increased mortality.
- Weight loss programmes for nursing home residents are controversial because of concerns about malnutrition and decrease in bone density.
- Nursing home patients with low body weight (BMI <19 kg/m²) have increased mortality rate than residents with normal weight.
- There are insufficient safety data on the use of weight loss medications, such as amphetamines, silbutramine or orlistat, for older adults with severe obesity. Therefore these medications should not be prescribed for nursing home residents with BMI >35 kg/m².

Further reading

Bradway C, DiResta J, Fleshner I, Polomano RC. 2008. Obesity in nursing homes: A critical review. *Journal of the American Geriatrics Society* 56: 1528–1535.

Darmon P, Kaiser MJ, Bauer JM, et al. 2010. Restrictive diets in the elderly: never say never again? *Clinical Nutrition* 29: 170–174.

Grabowski DC, Campbell CM, Ellis JE. 2005. Obesity and mortality in elderly nursing home residents. *Journals of Gerontology Series A* 60A: 1184–1189.

Sjoblom P, Tengblad A, Lofgrenet U-B, et al. 2008. Can diabetes medication be reduced in elderly patients? An observational study of diabetes drug withdrawal in nursing home patients with tight glycaemic control. *Diabetes Research and Clinical Practice* 82: 197–220.

Sloane PD, Ivey J, Helton M, et al. 2008. Nutritional issues in long-term care. *Journal of the American Medical Directors Association* 9: 476–485.

2.5 Activities for care home residents

Gillian Fox[1] and Carol Fletcher[2]

[1]*St James's University Hospital, Leeds, UK*
[2]*St James's Hospital and Leeds General Infirmary, Leeds, UK*

Key points

- Activities should be relevant to each resident.
- Residents should have influence and choice over their activities.
- Care should be person-centred.
- Consideration should be given to appropriate activities for people with cognitive impairment.
- Staff training in how to care for people with cognitive impairment must be a priority for every elderly care home.

- It is important, and indeed it is a legal obligation, for residents of care homes to be provided with appropriate activities.
- Many care home residents spend most of their time 'resting' – sitting and doing nothing.
- Recreation, social and community activities and personal development are essential to quality of life for people of all ages. They are of benefit to health and well-being in older people, even with advanced frailty.
- Many residents – especially those with advanced frailty or those with significant cognitive impairment – may only have limited energy or concentration, which may make adventurous activities difficult.
- Participation in activities can be just as important for an onlooker as an active participant.

Many homes engage an activity coordinator (see box) to facilitate this aspect of care, but nurses have a role to play too, in particular for one- to-one and ad hoc activities.

It is extremely important to focus on person-centred care, and on preserving the residents' individuality. It is key to be aware of the high prevalence of dementia among residents of care homes, and the changing activity needs of the person with dementia as their disease progresses. *Consideration should be given to providing staff training in working with people with dementia.*

Provision of activities should be considered in terms of the things that a person does through the day – socialising, reading, eating and drinking, worshipping – and not just in terms of formal organised activities.

Residents should have a voice in selecting the activities offered, and be able to opt out of activities that they do not enjoy.

Many homes engage an *activity coordinator*, and there are providers who come into care homes to provide activities (organised group activities).

Examples include:

- bingo
- dancing
- sing-alongs
- chair exercises and other exercises, such as Tai Chi
- quizzes
- games such as carpet bowls.

Some activities may have a functional purpose but also enjoyable and preserve the person's sense of identity, for example hairdressing or beauty therapy.

In some homes, residents are able to help with some housework or gardening, allowing them to feel they are contributing and are still valuable members of the community. Involvement in the local community may also be promoted by such events as summer/winter fairs and visits from local schoolchildren.

The Care Home Handbook, First Edition. Edited by Graham Mulley, Clive Bowman, Michal Boyd and Sarah Stowe.
© 2015 John Wiley & Sons, Ltd. Published 2015 by John Wiley & Sons, Ltd.

Person-centred care involves spending time with residents and finding out about their life and their aspirations for the future. For people with cognitive impairment, this can be more difficult. Here are some possible strategies.

1. Talk to the person: even if they have advanced dementia, their memory of events may be preserved. They may enjoy talking about past events, in addition to providing the staff with more insight into their current situation.
2. Involve the person's family: they will be able to give background information and knowledge of different aspects of a person's life, which may provide a stimulus for other conversations. They know the person best (some will have been carers for many years), and may tell you about the resident's likes and dislikes, habits, behaviours and so on.
3. Ask family and friends to bring in personal objects and photographs.
4. A memory box or scrapbook can be created with different objects and photos.
5. Group sessions for discussion, or celebration, of common memories can be enjoyable.

Some residents may wish to develop new skills, such as IT skills. They may also be able to put pre-existing skills into action, such as wood working and needlecraft, perhaps with the help of local volunteers.

It is important to value each person's social networks, and know something about their previous activities. Residents should be encouraged to receive visits from friends and family, and a quiet space should be provided for this. Residents should be encouraged to maintain interests and hobbies, and be allowed to continue with religious worship in their own chosen way.

Useful web sites

My Home life: http://myhomelifemovement.org/resources/ [Accessed September 2013]
NAPA (National Association for providers of activity for older people): www.napa-activities.co.uk [Accessed September 2013]

2.6 Intimacy, sexuality and sexual health

Karen Goodman[1] and Steven Searby[2]

[1]*York Teaching Hospital NHS Foundation Trust, York, UK*
[2]*South West Yorkshire Partnership NHS Foundation Trust, Halifax, UK*

Key points

- Care homes should ensure that the care they provide includes appreciation of residents' sexual diversity.
- Each individual's sexual needs should be sensitively discussed on admission.
- Opportunities should be provided for residents to be intimate with those with whom they have a sexual relationship.
- Safe sex should be promoted.
- If sexual behaviour becomes a problem, the incident must be carefully recorded. If there is a problem then action is needed: the flow chart provided may be helpful.
- Staff should be trained to understand sexuality in old age.

Care homes are communities where people live, work or visit. Residents should be able to enjoy their privacy, choices and fulfilment in all aspects of their lives – but the realities of facilitating this are not always straightforward. Being homosexual or bisexual creates additional anxiety compared to heterosexual individuals, and over 50% of homosexual or bisexual residents are not comfortable being identified in a care home.

Being able to show affection is a concern of individuals of any sexuality, but this is more prevalent among those who are homosexual or bisexual. This concern and anxiety in some cases extends to something as simple as holding hands with a partner.

- Care homes should aim to promote a fulfilling life in all aspects.
- Sex is one of the four primary drives, along with thirst, hunger and avoidance of pain.
- Sexuality is an integral part of the whole person.
- The over-riding principles are of individual autonomy, choice and consent (see Chapters 4.1 and 4.6).
- The more liberal attitudes of a modern society may be alien to many homosexual or bisexual elders, and while for many it may be welcome, that should not be presumed.

We will address key areas, acknowledging that the needs of carers, relatives and other residents need consideration too.

Three stages of importance in an individual's residency

1. Pre-admission:
    a. Care homes, when stating that they provide individualised care, must be quite clear that this must genuinely encompass sexual diversity.
    b. When an individual visits and commits to becoming a resident, there should be a meeting that includes consideration of the sexual/intimacy needs of that person. This discussion may involve their spouse/partner/relative.
    c. Any long-term conditions and the course of their illness which might have an impact on the above should also be considered.
2. Residency:
    a. Maintenance of relationships – this may be between couples who enter into long-term care together or are separated by need. It is important that there are facilities, such as double-rooms and other private areas, that allow for the continuation of a loving relationship.

The Care Home Handbook, First Edition. Edited by Graham Mulley, Clive Bowman, Michal Boyd and Sarah Stowe.
© 2015 John Wiley & Sons, Ltd. Published 2015 by John Wiley & Sons, Ltd.

b. Beginning/end of relationships – ageing does not preclude this; an individual's confidentiality and choice should be respected.

c. Offending public behaviour – if it involves others, this should be risk assessed in the context of capacity, appropriateness and consent. While this must be sensitively managed, it is not acceptable for other residents or staff to be subject to what in other circumstances would be considered lewd behaviour.

3. End of life:

Special consideration may be afforded to either member of a relationship as a 'final gesture' to individuals coming to the end of life, for example arranging for the partner to spend the evening/night together (Chapter 16.4).

Important considerations

- Care home staff should be aware of cultural and religious differences (see Chapter 16.8) – not only among residents and families, but also care givers. Some care home nursing staff may be ill-equipped/ embarrassed to deal with issues of sexuality because of their personal, religious beliefs – particularly on homosexuality, and relationships between people of different backgrounds.

   Therefore support mechanisms from colleagues, the care home manager and external support agencies may help to explore feelings/difficulties and develop coping strategies and skills to deal with such situations.

   First and foremost, comprehensive education and training for staff around sexuality in older people should be in place.

- A safe and secure environment should be promoted in terms of safe sex. Sexually transmitted infections, including HIV, are increasing in older age groups.

- Older lesbians, gay men and bisexuals may face (in common with older heterosexuals) health concerns, loss of a partner, friends, family members and ageism. However older lesbians, gay men and bisexuals may experience other issues/injustices through lack of legal recognition of their relationships, as well as the double discrimination of ageism and homophobia. Many gay older people kept their sexuality secret as homosexuality was frowned upon in their day, and they may harbour guilt as a result.

- The effect of medications, long-term conditions and clinical devices.
   ○ Dopamine agonists in Parkinson's disease can cause hypersexuality, including use of internet pornography. Up to 16% of people on thiazide diuretics may experience erectile dysfunction.
   ○ 'How is Billy going to manage with this in?' asked a female resident who had been catheterised for her incontinence – the implications of attachments should be discussed with individuals and explained fully.
      Specialist continence advice may be necessary.
   ○ Heart, lung and locomotor disease may place restrictions on sexual activity.
- Specialist input can be invaluable:
   ○ A geriatrician can provide a general health and medication review.
   ○ A member of the Community Mental Health Team can provide support/advice for dealing with sexual issues in people with dementia.
   ○ A social worker may become involved if there is a concern over safety of the individual or other residents.
   ○ Psychosexual counselling may be considered in some situations, for example where a resident with capacity wants to bring into the home a sex worker, or a resident who is disabled physically asks a staff member to assist him/her with masturbation
- Sexually transmitted infections (previously known as venereal diseases):
   ○ While sexually transmitted infections are often seen as a young person's problem, they can occur in any age group. Any sexual activity runs the risk of passing an infection, which in some cases may not show immediate symptoms. An example of this is Chlamydia, which is asymptomatic in most cases, or HIV, which can remain asymptomatic for several years.
   ○ If symptoms are present then these may include:
      I. pain when passing urine,
      II. unusual discharge or smell,
      III. pain in the pelvic area.
   ○ If residents have concerns regarding their risk of STIs, it is important to enable them to have access to literature/information which supports informed decisions regarding screening for STIs, and to have access to services which residents may need, such as genitourinary medicine.

When sexuality is seen as a problem

Record accurately what is happening:

- When and where did the problem occur?
- What form did the behaviour take – what did the person say or do?
- What else was happening?
- Was there anything specific that seemed to prompt this behaviour?
- Were there other people involved?
- What were the responses?

Consider whether there is actually a problem that needs to be addressed.

Figure 2.6.1 shows a flow chart to aid action planning.

Case examples

1. *A resident with capacity starts a relationship with another resident who also has capacity and is married with a wife at home*:

    These are two consenting adults who have capacity to make decisions about their relationship. The key issue here is one of confidentiality.

    Nurses should maintain the residents' confidentiality but may wish to discuss the implications

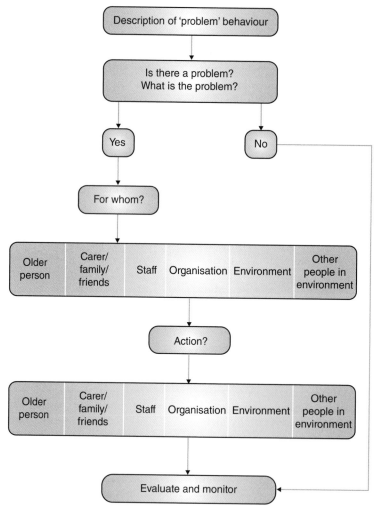

Figure 2.6.1 Flow chart to aid action planning. Reproduced from Archibald (1994), with kind permission from the RCN Publishing Company.

of their relationship to the two individuals concerned.

If confronted by the wife, the nurses should suggest that she discusses it with her husband.

The above discussions should be documented.

2. *A resident is caught masturbating openly in the communal area*:

Ensure that the resident is covered up and persuaded to return to his/her private room where he/she would be able to continue the activity.

Address any upset caused to other residents, visitors, care staff by the incident .

3. *Two men living in the home tell senior staff that they have fallen in love and want to be together. Both have mental capacity but some physicial incapacity. One of the men has adult children who contribute to the cost of his care but strongly object to their father's new relationship*:

Both men have capacity and a right to live the way they choose. Confidentiality should be maintained.

Any discrimination on behalf of the staff, other residents or visitors should be ideally prevented but, if it occurs, should be handled appropriately.

Discuss the wishes of the residents with them, make the best possible practical arrangements.

Be sensitive and supportive to the family and encourage the family to speak with their father.

There are various relevant important legal and professional frameworks for practice:

- Human and sexual rights – The Human Rights Act 1988
- Anti-discrimination legislation – The Equality Act 2006
- Sexual Offences Act (2003).

The above may be found at – www.legislation.gov.uk.

- Mental capacity – The Mental Capacity Act 2005 and Mental Capacity Code of Practice – http://www.dca.gov.uk/legal-policy/mental-capacity/mca-cp.pdfhttp://www.opsi.gov.uk/acts/acts2005/ukpga_20050009_en_1
- Nursing and Midwifery Council guidance for the care of older people – www.nmc-uk.org
- Safeguarding vulnerable adults 'No Secrets' – https://www.gov.uk/government/publications/no-secrets-guidance-on-protecting-vulnerable-adults-in-care
- Local policies/guidance within the care home.

Reference

Archibald C. 1994. Sex: is it a problem? *Journal of Dementia Care* 2(4): 16–18.

Further reading

Age UK. 'Opening Doors: Working with older lesbians and gay men' – service development resource pack.www.ageuk.org.uk [Accessed September 2013]

International Longevity Centre. 'The Last Taboo – a guide to dementia, sexuality, intimacy and sexual behaviour in care homes'. www.ilcuk.org.uk [Accessed September 2013]

Useful web sites

Royal College of Nursing – www.rcn.org.uk [Accessed September 2013]

Stonewall – www.stonewall.org.uk [Accessed 30 September 2013]

2.7 Pets

Graham Mulley

University of Leeds, Leeds, UK

Key points

- Pets can contribute to residents' well-being, yet many care homes do not allow incoming residents to bring their pets in with them.
- Those care homes that accept pets should have a written policy on practical aspects of pet care.
- Pets can benefit residents' physical and psychological health – but there are potential health hazards, particularly infections, allergies, bites and scratches.

About pets in care homes

- Approximately one quarter of people above retirement age have a pet.
- Separation from a pet can be a source of great distress and, if possible, residents should be able to take their pets into the care home. Taking a pet into a care home can ease the transition to the new residence. It is part of the philosophy of giving residents choice, independence and engagement in decision-making.
- Some countries (e.g. France, Switzerland, the USA and Norway) have laws which oblige care home providers to accept companion animals belonging to elderly residents. In others, it is left to the individual home. Some accept no pets; others accept specific animals. Some refuse permanent pets but will allow pets to be brought in by visitors.

Which pet?

Residents might enjoy the companionship of a dog, cat, bird or rabbit, and might get pleasure from an aquarium or a chicken run.

Some homes have resident pets that everyone can enjoy; others insist that the pet stays in the resident's room, to avoid possible distress to staff and other residents.

The creation of a wildlife garden can enable residents to see birds and other wildlife without having to care for an animal directly.

Benefits of pets

Though there are few hard data, anecdotal evidence shows that pets can lift depression, combat loneliness, enhance socialisation and social skills, improve physical activity, lower blood pressure and enrich residents mental well-being. In addition, in those with dementia, pets can reduce aggression, diminish agitation and reduce apathy.

Dangers of pets

The majority of adverse health problems caused by pets are minor and easily dealt with. The possibility of spreading infection (such as MRSA) has been studied – most pets that test positive for infections are unlikely to cause life-threatening disease to humans. Allergies (such as asthma and rhinitis) have not been examined in older residents.

Policy on pets

Each home that accepts pets should have a written policy. Inspecting agencies will wish to see this, as will potential residents and their families. Things to be considered are as follows:

- What arrangements are there for visits by the vet?
- Who is going to pay for the pet food, veterinary bills and pet insurance?
- Who is going to exercise the pet?

The Care Home Handbook, First Edition. Edited by Graham Mulley, Clive Bowman, Michal Boyd and Sarah Stowe.
© 2015 John Wiley & Sons, Ltd. Published 2015 by John Wiley & Sons, Ltd.

- Where will the pet sleep?
- Who is going to clean up after the pet?
- What happens if the resident dies before the pet?
- What if the pet proves to be disruptive?
- Does the owner have a certificate of immunisation?

Pet review

It is wise to ask a vet to visit every three months or so. He or she will check for worms and fleas, give vaccinations and do health checks as well as giving advice to staff.

Role of charities

Dog handlers can bring tame dogs into homes for residents to pat. Some charities provide information on which homes accept pets. Others take pets into care and keep in touch with the owners, perhaps bringing the pet in for them to see.

Further reading

Coughlan K, Olsen KE, Boxrud D, Bender JB. 2012. Methicillin-resistant *Staphylococcus aureus* in resident animals of a long-term facility. *Zoonoses Public Health* 57: 220–226.

Perkins J, Bartlett H, Travers C, Rand J. 2008. Dog-assisted therapy for older people with dementia: a review. *Australasian Journal of Ageing* 27(4): 177–182.

Useful web sites

The Cinnamon Trust is a UK national charity that cares for pets whose owners have died, or where the home does not take pets. The charity has a register of homes which accept pets. www.cinnamon.org.uk

The Society for Companion Animal studies gives help and guidance to care home providers. www.scas.org.uk

Homes for Wildlife information – how to make a wildlife haven. www.rspb.org.uk/hfw

2.8 Managing trips out of the care home

Gillian Fox[1] and Carol Fletcher[2]

[1]St James's University Hospital, Leeds, UK
[2]St James's Hospital and Leeds General Infirmary, Leeds, UK

Key points

- Trips out of the home are important for the well-being of selected residents.
- Careful planning is necessary – transport, mobility equipment, toilet arrangements, medications, oxygen, incontinence aids and glucometers should all be considered.
- Be prepared for emergencies – take a mobile phone and written details of residents' medical conditions and medications.

Many residents rate trips out as a very important aspect of their well-being, yet outings are not always organised for them.

As with all activities in the care home, outings need to be planned in a person- centred way. The residents should give their views on the choice of trips out of the home.

Some residents will be mentally and physically able to leave the care home and this should be encouraged.

Many residents will require assistance because of mental or physical disability, or both. These residents need assistance to take part in meaningful outings.

Examples of outings

- Organised visits to the seaside, markets, or local places of interest.
- Visits to places of historical interest.
- Visits to places for entertainment – the theatre, a pantomime.
- Visits to places of worship (some will have a group of volunteers who may be able to transport members of the congregation to the place of worship).
- Trips to hospital, dentist, optician, hairdressers (though many homes offer some of these services within the care home).
- Visits to relatives.
- Shopping trips.

Organising an outing

Transport

Appropriate transport needs to be arranged for residents, taking into account mobility needs and aids such as frames and wheelchairs (see Chapter 6.4). If an external provider is used, they must have the appropriate public liability insurance.

Choice of destination

Ensure that the venue can accommodate the party, and that it is accessible to people in wheelchairs and those using walking aids

Care needs during the outing

- Supplies of medication, especially PRN medications (such as GTN spray and inhalers), which may be needed for some residents.
- Portable oxygen may be needed (see Chapter 11.9).
- If residents are unable to self-administer their medications, then the medications should be given by a qualified nurse.
- A risk assessment may need to be carried out for medication.
- Diabetes care must be carefully planned, including insulin administration, blood glucose checking and provision of emergency treatment items such as hypostop (see Chapter 8.4).

The Care Home Handbook, First Edition. Edited by Graham Mulley, Clive Bowman, Michal Boyd and Sarah Stowe.
© 2015 John Wiley & Sons, Ltd. Published 2015 by John Wiley & Sons, Ltd.

- Continence problems should be planned for, with supplies of pads and spare clothing.
- Appropriate poor weather clothing should be considered.
- Plans need to be made for obtaining food and drink during the outing. These should take into account special diets (pureed, soft, etc.) and food allergies or intolerances (see Chapter 2.4).

Communication and information

Staff should have a mobile phone for communicating with the home and for use in an emergency. Staff should take written details of the residents' medical conditions, allergies and medication, in case of an emergency.

Staffing

The health and safety and requirements for adequate supervision and support are crucial; and where staff are leaving a home, there must be careful consideration that there is adequate cover for the residents remaining.

Risk assessment

A risk assessment will need to be undertaken before some outings. The care home should have a policy about when and how to do this.

Consent

Residents' ability to consent to go on an outing should be considered, and if they are unable to make their own choices it is good practice to take family views into consideration.

Emergencies

Staff must know what to do in case of an emergency (for example if a resident were to feel unwell) in order to arrange to get them back to the home or to call the emergency services.

Further reading

Popham C, Orrel M. 2012. What matters for people with dementia in care homes? *Aging Mental Health* 2(16): 181–188.

2.9 Malodour (or unpleasant smells)

Anne Houghton[1] and Pauline Breslin[2]

[1]*Leeds South and East Clinical Commissioning Group, Leeds, UK*
[2]*Sunnyside Nursing Home, Castleford, UK*

Key points

- Unpleasant smells can be caused by a resident's poor hygiene or illness, or the physical environment of the home.
- An unpleasant aroma gives a negative impression of a care home and can distress residents, staff and visitors.
- The cause of malodour should always be investigated.
- Measures that may help in improving the smell of a home include good ventilation, non-carpeted flooring and the use of fragrant aromas.

Visiting a resident who is clearly well cared for, clean and groomed, and smelling of soap, talc or perfume is reassuring and promotes positive messages of care and treatment with dignity. Conversely, walking into a care home with unpleasant smells, such as urine or strong food, does not promote confidence in care.

There are very few scientific articles on this key subject, and although care homes have statutory obligations relating to cleanliness and infection control, malodour warrants more than just an audit.

Residents benefit from feeling cared for and clean. In contrast, they may be distressed if they are aware of unpleasant smells from ostomies, infections, incontinence or the home setting itself.

Unpleasant smells or malodours in a care home can arise from an individual resident or the environment.

Tips on how to reduce smells

- *Good ventilation* ensures that the air does not become stale.
- Frequent cleaning of carpets, particularly after spillages, reduces stale smells and odour caused by bacterial overgrowth and moulds. Use *non-slip flooring* rather than carpets.
- Careful attention to cleaning and the use of air fresheners and flowers can reduce smells.

- *Air filtering/air conditioning* is not often present as it is costly to install and run.

Tips on using fragrant aromas

Encouraging fragrant smells, as well as preventing malodour in the care home, is important for residents, their visitors and the staff.

- Fragrant smells (e.g. fresh flowers, home-baked scones and newly brewed coffee) enhance taste and enjoyment of food and lift a person's mood and encourage their appetite.

Unpleasant smells can alert us to danger (e.g. leaking gas, smoke, and spoiled and unsafe foods) and are equally important for maintaining the safety of residents.

Managing malodour in individuals

Asking the question 'why does the home or individual smell?' may be key to finding diseases or problems that can be managed or improved. Unpleasant smells from residents may be both a sign and a symptom of disease – or could simply be a reflection of poor personal hygiene.

Senses of smell and taste are interlinked and diminish with increasing age. This can have an impact on the health and well-being of an older person. An impaired sense of smell can lead to reduced awareness of personal hygiene, resulting in malodour (bad breath, stale perspiration, inadequate cleansing of urine and faecal incontinence etc.) which is evident to carers and distressing to all.

Malodour can assist in making a diagnosis of disease. For example, the 'fishy' smell that may accompany a urinary infection, the smell of ketones on the breath of a person with diabetes or malnourishment (often described as the smell of pear drops) should prompt careful assessment of the individual's physical health.

Bad breath should lead to a detailed examination of a resident's mouth for signs of infection or the need for dental treatment.

Further reading

Anon. 1998. One nurse is sick of care homes that smell of incontinence. *Nursing Times* 94: 59.

Lapham DM. 1967. Odor control in long-term care facilities. *Nursing Homes* 10: 20–23.

2.10 Noise

Mark Bradley

Leeds Teaching Hospitals NHS Trust, Leeds, UK

Key points

- Noise can distress residents and should be kept to a minimum.
- Noise at night can be particularly troublesome.
- Listening to resident's concerns about noise is good practice.

The effects of exposure to noise, and how and what we perceive as noise, is very personal. It is often forgotten and overlooked by staff, but is very important to residents. Noise can cause annoyance and fatigue, interfere with communication and affect sleep. Some common sources of noise in a care home are:

- other residents
- staff members
- visitors and guests
- alarms, telephones, buzzers and call systems
- televisions and radios
- tradesmen, workmen and delivery drivers
- environment, for example floorboards, plumbing, kitchens, trolleys, lifts and doors.

Attempt to minimise noise wherever possible

Try and remember that your work environment is the residents' home environment.

- Where possible remind other residents and visitors not to make too much noise.
- Talk to workmen and delivery staff about noise levels and the timing of their work and visits.
- Warn residents about fire alarm testing and think about the locations of doorbells and buzzers and how loud they really need to be.
- Look at installing quiet door closures and quiet fill valves for water cisterns.
- Think about using silent call systems or using pagers.

Remember to talk to residents and relatives about excessive noise and consider collecting their views as part of a feedback/customer care initiative. Encourage staff and residents to report noise concerns and then act on them.

Noise at night

A study by the Joseph Rowntree Foundation (2008) identified noise at night as a particularly troublesome issue: 'The levels of noise and light during the night were too high to support good sleep for residents. Staff talked too loudly close to bedrooms and homes had noisy floorboards, plumbing and buzzer alarm systems.'

People who don't sleep well may not feel well the day after, and repeated sleep disturbance can have an adverse effect on cardiovascular health as well as exacerbating fatigue, memory difficulties and concentration.

At night try to do the following:

- Talk quietly in corridors and near people's rooms.
- Open and shut doors quietly.
- Avoid unnecessary trips up and down corridors, especially with a noisy trolley.
- Stop your keys from jangling.
- Minimise routine, indiscriminate over-checking of residents at night.

Reference

Joseph Rowntree Foundation 2008. *Supporting older people in care homes at night* [Online]. Available: www.jrf.org.uk [Accessed September 2013]

Values, Standards, Ethics and Probity

Chapter 3

Respect and Dignity

3.1 Nursing professional accountability

Deborah Sturdy[1] and Finbarr Martin[2]

[1]*Red and Yellow Care, London, UK*
[2]*Guy's and St Thomas' NHS Foundation Trust, London, UK*

Key points

- Nurses should provide a high level of care: the individual resident is your primary concern.
- You are responsible for your actions and omissions.
- It is important to keep up to date and be aware of the legal aspects of your work and changes in policy.

'People in your care must be able to trust you with their health and wellbeing' (NMC, 2008).

The responsibilities and expectations of the nursing role, and the experience needed to ensure high standards of care along with supervision of often large numbers of carers, mean that nurses have a greater degree of autonomy and, therefore, responsibility than many other healthcare professionals.

Nurses often work in care homes or individual units as the sole professional, with limited access to off-site support and help. Their responsibilities can be undervalued and overlooked.

Accountability for nursing practice is the cornerstone of the nursing profession. In all countries, registered nurses are governed by legislation that sets out areas of accountability of practice. These include accountability to patients, regulatory bodies, civil law and criminal law. Nurses are also accountable to their employer through their contract of employment.

In the UK, when legal processes review the standards upheld by an individual health professionals, the 'Bolam test' is applied. This emerged from a legal case in 1957 which states that: 'You need not possess the highest expert skill at the risk of being found negligent, it is sufficient if you exercise the ordinary skill of an ordinary competent professional exercising your particular specialty' (adapted from Bolam v Friern Barnet Hospital Management Committee 1957).

Although this legislation is specific to the UK, the underlying principles apply to all nurses working internationally. The application of what is 'reasonable' in terms of standards of performance in legal cases means that the onus is on the health professional to ensure their competence, skills and knowledge are up to date in the area of practice in which they work.

- Nurses are personally accountable for actions and omissions in their practice.
- Nurses must always be able to justify their clinical decisions.
- Nurses must always act lawfully, both in professional practice and their personal life.

The professional accountability conferred on nurses at registration provides the robust professional framework in which they are expected to practice. This sets a regulatory framework, ensures systems which monitor and manage fitness to practice, and protect the public's and the profession's interests.

Internationally, Nursing and Midwifery Councils and Boards set out the expectations for nurses on the register about their conduct and practice.

These Council and Boards act as guardians for public safety. The Codes of Conduct clearly frame the parameters of practice and public trust.

To justify the public's trust in nurses you must:

- Make sure that care of people is your first concern, treating them as individuals and respecting their dignity.
- Work with others to protect and promote the health and well-being of those in your care, their families and carers, and the wider community.
- Provide a high standard of practice and care at all times.
- Be open and honest, act with integrity and uphold the reputation of your profession.
- Be personally accountable for actions and omissions in your practice and always be able to justify decisions.
- Always act lawfully, whether those laws relate to your professional practice or personal life.

The Care Home Handbook, First Edition. Edited by Graham Mulley, Clive Bowman, Michal Boyd and Sarah Stowe.
© 2015 John Wiley & Sons, Ltd. Published 2015 by John Wiley & Sons, Ltd.

Failure to comply with this Code may bring your fitness to practice into question and endanger your registration.

Nurses in care homes are responsible for considerable amounts of supervision of care staff. This role and the responsibilities placed on nurses are significant. The delegation of duties carries great responsibility, with an expectation to make judgements about the ability of the person who is being delegated to, ensuring that the task meets required standards and supervising and supporting the person who is carrying out the tasks.

The complexity of the care home environment and typical staffing patterns means that this is a substantial part of nurses' role and working day. The need for assurance that the team members supporting residents' care are able to do their duties with diligence is an essential aspect of managing the team.

Understanding and applying principles of best practice are key to assuring your residents and yourself that care is being delivered appropriately.

Ensuring your own competence comprises several areas, which focus on the need for a clear understanding of your role in protecting the public and being a member of a privileged profession:

- Up-to-date knowledge through professional updates and current evidence-based practice.
- Awareness of policy development.
- Changing legal frameworks within which you have to work, for example:
  - Mental Capacity Acts (see Chapter 4.6).
  - Legislation regarding decisions by healthcare proxies.
  - Restraint legislation guidance and procedures (see Chapter 4.2).

Reference

NMC, 2008.Code of Conduct. Available at: http://www.nmc-uk.org/Documents/Standards/nmcTheCodeStandardsofConductPerformanceAndEthicsForNursesAndMidwives_TextVersion.pdf [Accessed September 2013]

Useful web sites

Accountability Scotland: http://www.advancedpractice.scot.nhs.uk/legal-and-ethics-guidance/accountability/accountability-to-the-profession.aspx [Accessed September 2013]

NMC, 2009. Care and respect every time; what to expect from nurses. Available at: http://www.nmc-uk.org/patients-public/Older-people-and-their-carers/Care-and-respect-every-time/ [Accessed September 2013]

NMC, 2010. Raising and escalating concerns; guidance for nurses and midwives. Available at: http://www.nmc-uk.org/Get-involved/Consultations/Past-consultations/By-year/Guidance-for-raising-and-escalating-concerns/ [Accessed September 2013]

RCN, 2004. Interpreting accountability. Available at: http://www.rcn.org.uk/__data/assets/pdf_file/0008/78605/002249.pdf [Accessed September 2013]

RCN, Delegation Healthcare Assistants http://www.rcn.org.uk/development/health_care_support_workers/accountability_and_delegation_film [Accessed September 2013]

http://www.rcn.org.uk/_data/assets/pdf_file/0010/387541/Accountability_HCA_leaflet_A5.pdf [Accessed September 2013]

http://www.rcn.org.uk/_data/assets/pdf_file/0004/361912/Fold_Out_Booklet_Web.pdf [Accessed September 2013]

http://www.rcn.org.uk/_data/assets/pdf_file/0010/400033/RCN_delegation_information_sheet.pdf [Accessed September 2013]

3.2 Unprofessional behaviour

Helga Goutcher[1] and Peter Rogers[2]

[1]St Philip's Care, Scotland, UK
[2]Bupa Care Homes, Leeds, UK

Key points

- Professionalism in nursing includes:
  - treating every individual with respect and kindness, acting as advocates for residents and not discriminating against anyone under your care
  - respecting confidentiality
  - not bullying
  - respecting professional boundaries.
- Tips are given on whistle-blowing and whether to accept gifts.

Definition

A profession is:

- a disciplined group of individuals,
- who adhere to high ethical standards, and
- uphold themselves to, and are accepted by the public as possessing special knowledge and skills in a widely recognised, organised body of learning derived from education and training at a high level,
- and who are prepared to exercise this knowledge and these skills in the interest of others.

The responsibility for the welfare, health and safety of the individual and community shall take precedence over other considerations.

In the UK, nurses are regulated by the National Midwifery Council (NMC) whose roles are:

- To safeguard the health and well-being of the public.
- To set standards of education, training, conduct and performance so that nurses and midwives can deliver high quality healthcare consistently throughout their careers.
- To ensure that nurses and midwives keep their skills and knowledge up to date and uphold professional standards.
- Have clear and transparent processes to investigate nurses and midwives who fall short of standards.

All Registered Nurses are required to comply with the NMC code. Therefore:

1. You must treat people as individuals and respect their dignity.
2. You must not discriminate in any way against those in your care.
3. You must treat people kindly and considerately.
4. You must act as an advocate for those in your care, helping them to access relevant health and social care, information and support.

Confidentiality

When sharing information, a registered nurse in a care home should always consider and be mindful of breaches in a resident's right to confidentiality.

- Do not disclose information to anyone who is not entitled to it.
- Follow the guidelines or policy on confidentiality as set out by your employer.
- Be aware of and follow the professional guidelines on confidentiality.

Bullying and harassment

It is not acceptable to bully or harass residents (this would trigger a safeguarding referral – see Chapter 4.3), relatives or other members of staff in a care home.

Examples of bullying behaviour include:

- derogatory remarks,
- rude or aggressive comments or online comments,
- insensitive jokes and pranks,
- insulting or aggressive behaviour,
- inappropriate public criticism.

Bullying includes comments on social networking sites.

NMC nurses must uphold the reputation of the profession at all times (NMC, 2008). This means that conduct online and conduct in the real world should be judged in the same way, and should be at a similar high standard. Nurses and midwives will put their registration at risk, if they:

- share confidential information online,
- post inappropriate comments about colleagues or patients,
- use social networking sites to bully or intimidate colleagues,
- pursue personal relationships with patients or service users,
- distribute sexually explicit material,
- use social networking sites in any way which is unlawful.

For example, manipulated photos that are intended to mock individuals would be considered offensive if printed and pinned on workplace notice boards, and are no less offensive when shared online, even when privately shared between friends.

Whistle-blowing

If you have concerns about anything happening where you work and the concern is serious because it might affect patients or people receiving care, colleagues or your whole organisation, it can be difficult to know what to do.

You may feel that raising the matter would be disloyal to colleagues, to managers or to your organisation. However, everyone working in health and social care has a duty to follow their Professional Code of Conduct, and put residents and other people they care for first and protect their safety.

It is always advisable and encouraged to try to resolve any concerns within your organisation first. But if unable to do this, or feel your concerns are not being heard, then speak to someone who is independent of your organisation.

Most organisations will have a policy to raise concerns/whistle-blowing policy.

However, if you need to raise a concern, guidance was issued by the CQC (England) in 2011 as follows:

- If you see something being done wrong, can you tackle it yourself, there and then? A firm, polite challenge is sometimes all that is needed.
- Talk to your line manager if possible, or someone senior in the organisation, about the problem.
- If you do not feel able to raise your concern with your line manager or other management, consult your own organisation's whistle-blowing policy, if there is one, and follow that.
- If you have tried all these, or you do not feel able to raise your concern internally, you can raise your concern in confidence with your regulator.

Failure to keep appropriate professional boundaries

It can be challenging in a care home to ensure that a professional level of involvement is maintained at all times. Keep your personal and professional life separate as far as possible.

It is key that you:

- Maintain clear professional boundaries in the relationships you have with others, especially with vulnerable adults.
- Refuse any gifts, favours or hospitality that might be interpreted as an attempt to gain preferential treatment.
- Do not ask for or accept loans from anyone for whom you provide care or anyone close to them.
- Maintain clear sexual boundaries with the people for whom you provide care, their families and carers at all times.
- Be aware of and follow the professional guidelines on maintaining clear sexual boundaries (available from the advice section on www.nmc-uk.org).

Do not use social networks to build or pursue relationships with anyone under your care, even if they are no longer under your supervision. If you receive a friendship request from a current or former patient, Facebook allows you to ignore this request without the person being informed, avoiding the possibility of giving unnecessary offence.

Receiving gifts

It is not unusual in care homes for residents and relatives to want to give you gifts. However, before accepting them, ensure you have familiarised yourself with your organisational policy on receiving gifts. You must refuse any gifts, favours or hospitality that might be interpreted as an attempt to gain preferential treatment. Nurses can receive gifts or favours from people they care for but must be confident that the giving of these gifts could not be interpreted as being in return for preferential treatment.

Finally

If you have concerns about another nurse's actions, do not be afraid to discuss it with them (in an appropriate manner).

* Tell them why it bothers you, and give them a rationale for why it isn't appropriate.
* Teach them how it affects patient care.
* Ask them to think about their comments or actions and offer suggestions on what an appropriate action would be.

If the problem is not resolved, do not be afraid to go to your manager or team leader to discuss it (they may not know it is a problem), but let the person you are having concerns about know that you are going to discuss the problem with a supervisor first, otherwise you will create unnecessary resentment. They may still be angry at you for reporting them, but they will respect you for letting them know in advance that they are being reported.

Further reading

Cleary M. 2009. Dealing with bullying in the workplace: towards zero tolerance. *Journal of Psychosocial Nursing in Mental Health Services* 47: 34–41.

Useful web sites

http://www.nmc-uk.org/Nurses-and-midwives/The-code/ [Accessed September 2013]
http://www.nmc-uk.org/Nurses-and-midwives/safeguarding/ [Accessed September 2013]
http://www.nmc-uk.org/Nurses-and-midwives/Raising-and-escalating-concerns/ [Accessed September 2013]

3.3 Aggression

Catherine Tandy

St James's University Hospital, Leeds, UK

Key points

- The small proportion of residents who are aggressive often have delirium or dementia or both.
- Violent behaviour can be prevented by an appreciation of the causes of aggressive behaviour, such as invasion of personal space.
- A resident who is violent should be assessed in detail, using the guidelines available.
- Non-drug approaches can be helpful in the management of violence.
- If there are no other options and/or a risk to safety, restraint with the minimum amount of force can be used BUT be clear what you are doing and why so that others can understand your actions. The resident's dignity and safety are paramount.
- Staff training can reduce the number and severity of aggressive episodes.
- Detail every aggressive act in writing as soon as possible after the event.

The problem

- Acts of physical or verbal aggression by residents towards staff or other residents generally occur in people with dementia, delirium or both (see Chapters 10.1 and 10.2).
- Acts of violence usually reflect the confusion and frustration of the resident and their inability to express themselves verbally or in other more acceptable ways.
- Examples of physical aggression in care homes include pushing, shoving, spitting, scratching, biting, grabbing, kicking, throwing things and hitting someone with an object.
- Aggression can cause physical harm and emotional distress to staff and residents. It must be taken very seriously – even though incidents rarely cause serious injury to staff.
- Violence is more common during the day and may be provoked by unwanted touching, wandering into another person's room or competition for a chair or TV programme. Triggers are listed in Box 3.3.1.

Management of violence

- You can prevent violence by understanding the individual's needs, habits and preferences. It is also important that staff are trained in the art of managing behaviour that is challenging. Even with excellent staff, not all violence can be prevented.
- The key question that should be asked is: 'what has led this person to act in a violent way?' This will ensure that future risk is reduced.
- The National Institute for Health and Clinical Excellence (NICE) recommends that patients with dementia who develop challenging behaviour should be specifically assessed to establish factors that may generate, aggravate or improve behaviour. Assessment should include the following:

1. the person's physical health,
2. depression,
3. undetected pain or discomfort,
4. side-effects of medication,
5. individual biography, including religious beliefs, spiritual and cultural identity,

The Care Home Handbook, First Edition. Edited by Graham Mulley, Clive Bowman, Michal Boyd and Sarah Stowe.
© 2015 John Wiley & Sons, Ltd. Published 2015 by John Wiley & Sons, Ltd.

6. psycho-social factors,
7. physical environmental factors,
8. a behavioural and functional analysis.

Prevention of violence

Carers should identify factors that may cause aggression (see Box 3.3.1) and try to influence them. For example you might:

- Provide person-centred care and build a positive relationship with the resident.
- Champion residents' decision-making, dignity and rights (see Chapters 4.1 and 4.6).

Box 3.3.1 Factors that may trigger violence

Specific activities:
Personal care – transfers, turning, bathing, dressing, feeding, toileting
Giving medicines
Activities in which the resident anticipates pain

Environmental factors:
Lack of privacy
Lack of activities – boredom

Misunderstandings:
When a resident is denied something
Not explaining care before providing it
A resident interpreting care as dangerous or threatening

Resident factors:
Dementia or delirium
Delusions and hallucinations
Psychosocial stress, such as bereavement
Pre-morbid personality
Frustration at dependency
A perception of loss of dignity
Anxiety, fear

Carer factors:
Interpersonal style of caregivers – attitude
The relationship between residents and carers
Poor communication between staff and resident
Tiredness
Pressurised
Unfamiliarity with the care home

Organisational factors:
Short staffing – only attending after active demands/having to rush care/excessive workload

---

- Use non-pharmacological interventions. There is evidence for the clinical effectiveness of aromatherapy, multi-sensory stimulation, therapeutic use of music and/or dancing, pet therapy (see Chapter 2.7) and massage in patients with dementia who have behavioural problems.
- Ensure good communication about activities that may cause violence in order to reduce misunderstanding.
- Ensure a proactive preventative approach to preventing delirium (see Chapter 10.2).

Education and training for staff

- It is proven that education and training programmes can enable staff to deal with difficult situations in ways that don't require restraint. Training can reduce the number of violent events, their seriousness, their psychological effects and give staff confidence in their management and care of residents.
- Training should concentrate on when to anticipate violence, negotiation and how to deal with difficult situations.
- To ensure best practice, there also needs to be adequate ongoing support to care staff. Counselling, support groups and debriefing to reduce stress may be helpful.

Assessment and care planning

- Individual care plans should aim to minimise violence. The individual should be fully involved in all decisions about their care and if they lack capacity (Chapter 4.6), their next of kin, friend or advocate should be included in decision-making to ensure choices are closely aligned to known preferences and habits.
- Care plans should have time limits and be reviewed regularly.
- Incidents should be reported (see Box 3.3.2) to monitor the situation and used to identify patterns or solutions through reflective learning. Tools such as the UK Royal College of Nursing work-related violence tool can be used to provide practical support in completing assessments, help you to gain more knowledge of the risks involved and subsequently have more control over reducing violence.

Box 3.3.2 Reporting aggressive behaviour

It is good practice to complete a written report as soon as possible after the incident. This might include:

- employee's name and occupation,
- location of episode,
- date, day, time,
- details of assailant,
- what the employee was doing at the time,
- circumstances of the assault,
- outcome – injuries, time off work, and damage to property,
- information on any remedial action.

From Health and Safety Executive, 1997.

Restraint of residents

- Restraint can take many forms – physical, environmental or pharmacological (see Chapter 4.2). The UK Mental Capacity Act 2005 defines restraint as 'the use or threat of force to help do an act which the person resists, or the restriction of the person's liberty of movement, whether or not they resist'.
- When considering restraint of a resident, you should respect basic human rights of dignity and freedom and these must take priority (see Chapter 3.4).
- If there are no other options and/or a risk to safety restraint with the minimum amount of force can be used BUT be clear what you are doing and why so that others can understand your actions. The resident's dignity and safety are paramount.
- In the case of those who lack capacity, for restraint to be legally acceptable it must be clear that it is carried out in the person's best interests to prevent harm. Any form of restraint should be the least restrictive action possible. If a member of staff uses excessive restraint, they could be liable to civil and criminal penalties.

Reference

Health and Safety Executive. 1997. *Violence and Aggression to Staff in Health Services: Guidance on Assessment and Management*. London, HSE Books.

Further reading

Almvik, R, Rasmussen, K, Woods, P. 2006. Challenging behaviour in the elderly – monitoring violent incidents *International Journal of Geriatric Psychiatry* 21: 368–374.

Commission for Social Care Inspection. 2007 *Rights, risks and restraints. An exploration into the use of restraint in the care of older people*. [Online]. Available: http://www.cambridgeshire.gov.uk/NR/rdonlyres/46979CAB-51B2-4305-B64B-E520165D56D7/0/Restraint.pdf [Accessed September 2013]

Department for Constitutional Affairs, 2007. *Mental Capacity Act. Code of Practice*. London, Stationery Office.

Evans D, Wood J, Lambert L. 2002. A review of physical restraint minimization in the acute and residential care settings. *Journal of Advanced Nursing* 40: 616–625.

National Institute of Clinical Evidence (NICE). 2006. *Clinical guideline 42 Dementia* [Online], Available: http://guidance.nice.org.uk/CG42 [Accessed September 2013]

Royal College of Nursing, 2008 *Work related violence*. [Online] Available: http://www.rcn.org.uk/_data/assets/pdf_file/0010/192493/003271.pdf [Accessed 30 September 2013]

Testad I, Aaland AM, Aarsland D. 2005. The effect of staff training on the use of restraint in dementia: a single-blind randomised controlled trial. *International Journal of Geriatric Psychology* 20: 587–590.

3.4 Dignity in the care home

Andrew Stanners[1] and Sandra Parry[2]

[1]*Mid Yorkshire Hospitals NHS Trust, Wakefield, UK*
[2]*West Ridings Residential and Nursing Home, Wakefield, UK*

Key points

- Dignity is fundamentally important to all people.
- Dignity is *unique* in every person.
- Residents in care homes are at risk of losing their dignity.
- Care home staff have a duty to know their residents and what makes their residents lives unique.
- Care home staff have a duty to promote dignity in their residents by helping them to live according to their chosen values.

All of us know that dignity is something to value, but it can be difficult to describe exactly what dignity is and what we should do in recognition of its importance. We also know that dignity is especially important in care settings, including care homes, but this, too, raises difficult questions about how care home staff should promote a client's dignity. This contribution first describes dignity as something that is *unique in every individual* and second, because care home residents are at particular risk of losing their dignity, it will emphasise the special responsibility of care home staff to recognise, promote and protect this fundamental value.

If asked to think of someone who is dignified we might think of an important person, such as the Queen, who conducts herself in a dignified way. We find it easy to identify *her* dignity because it is conferred by her exceptional life.

It can be harder to define dignity in other people, yet we *all* have our own unique lives, our own individual characters, history and interests, which confer dignity on each of us. All of us (providing we don't harm others) have a right to have our dignity respected. (Box 3.4.1)

Respecting dignity in the care home presents a rewarding challenge to care home staff. (Boxes 3.4.2, 3.4.3 and 3.4.4) People who live in care homes may have illnesses, such as dementia, that can alter the way they live their life, including how they make choices and communicate with others. When a person moves into a care home they may leave parts of their former

Box 3.4.1 Make Time to Reflect

Consider ten ways in which you would want your dignity respected if you were in a care home.

Box 3.4.2 Encourage *and recruit* for positive staff values

Empathy, kindness, compassion, understanding, openness, collaborativeness, thoroughness (with audit and assessment), preparedness to show leadership and challenge poor staff practice, willingness to seek and act on feedback (advocates can help with this).

Box 3.4.3 Dignity Dilemmas

- A person with dementia who no longer wants to be clean-shaven.
- A life-long vegetarian whose dementia results in a taste for meat.
- Problems arising when a person's personal values conflict with those of staff, for example walking and falling or eating and choking.

Solutions to dilemmas like these will be more acceptable and sustainable if you work in partnership with relatives and carers (and chef) to respect the client's choices.

Box 3.4.4 A good chef

- Can come up with imaginative solutions for residents with unusual tastes, for example the client who wants to eat Christmas pudding every day!
- Can involve residents in the production of meals, such as the former baker who is helped by the chef to bake and who as a result can come off sedation.
- Can accommodate the vegetarian who develops a taste for meat.
- Can help provide food for a client's regular visitors.

Box 3.4.5 Recognising dignity

- Get to know your residents as well as possible.
- Start the assessment process prior to the client entering the care home. (Identify family, friends, places, belongings, memory boxes, captioned photos, occupation etc.)
- Show respect in your client's home: knock on the door before entering and don't use mobile phones in care areas.
- Recognise the dignity of your client's visitors, who may spend a lot of time in the care home.

Box 3.4.6 Respecting individual choices

- Watching 'a TV soap' once a day.
- Writing to the local MP.
- Keeping chickens.
- Making new friends.

Box 3.4.7 Use the Six Senses Framework (Nolan, 2006)

Care home residents should have:

- a sense of security;
- a sense of continuity;
- a sense of belonging;
- a sense of purpose;
- a sense of fulfillment; and
- a sense of significance.

life behind. Therefore, to be able to respect their client's dignity, care home staff must make special efforts to know their residents and the important features that shape their residents lives – the things that make their residents unique (Boxes 3.4.5, 3.4.6 and 3.4.7).

Reference

Nolan, MR. 2006. The Senses Framework: improving care for older people through a relationship-centred approach. Available at: http://shura.shu.ac.uk/280/1/PDF_Senses_Framework_Report.pdf [Accessed 30 September 2013]

Further reading

Alzheimer's Society. 2012. What standards of care can people expect from a care home? http://www.alzheimers.org.uk/site/scripts/documents_info.php?documentID=153 [Accessed September 2013]

The Dignity in Care Network: http://www.dignityincare.org.uk/ [Accessed September 2013]

Local Government Association, NHS Confederation and Age UK, 2012. Delivering Dignity: Securing dignity in care for older people in hospitals and care homes. A Draft Report for Consultation http://www.nhsconfed.org/Documents/dignity.pdf [Accessed September 2013]'

My Home Life. www.myhomelife.org.uk [Accessed September 2013]

Chapter 4

Rights and Legal Considerations

4.1 Human rights

Jackie Morris

University College London Medical School, London, UK

Key points

- A better comprehension of the need for human rights in the care home ensures the delivery of more compassionate and humane care.
- Human rights-based care promotes a better understanding of the needs and rights of the individual receiving care and the person delivering care.
- Important features of human rights of residents are: fairness; respect; equality; dignity and autonomy.
- It is important to ensure that the resident has private space to talk to family, friends and the GP.

Human rights principles call for the full recognition of the human rights of older people to enjoy a healthy and fulfilling life by acknowledging their experience and wisdom – as well as their right to control their own lives – and more generally to participate actively in society.

Failure to deliver human rights-based care has led to scandals and well-publicised media campaigns to protect vulnerable adults. Human rights-based care ensures the delivery of true person-centred care, thus enabling resident's wishes and needs to be heard, identified and acknowledged.

Many residents have diagnosed or undiagnosed dementia; staff will therefore need to work with and listen to their next of kin and/or person with lasting power of attorney to fully respect their rights.

In the UK, the Human Rights Act was introduced in 1998 to give further legal effect to the fundamental human rights contained in the European Convention on Human Rights. Similar legislation is in place in other countries. The British government legislation introduced in 2009 ensured that care home residents in privately run care homes whose fees are funded by the state, or where the contract is arranged by the state, now have the protection of the Human Rights Act.

Knowledge and understanding about capacity and the Mental Capacity Act should complement the meaning of human rights to an older person living in a care home (see Chapter 4.6).

In the UK, responsibility for the implementation and monitoring of standards rests with the local authority funding body as well as the NHS. The Care Quality Commission inspects adherence to human rights. Other regulatory bodies perform this role in other countries *and it is important to be familiar with local legislation and regulations.*

The acknowledgment that human rights were not understood led to the introduction of the human rights-based approach to care and treatments.

In the UK Human Rights Act, the key human rights affecting older people are Articles 2, 3, 6 and 8.

FREDA stands for fairness, respect, equality, dignity and autonomy.

Article 2 – the right to life

Identifying treatable and reversible medical problems early and making sure that care home residents have easy access to food and nutrition are all part of providing care which meets the recommendations of Article 2.

Ill health causing changes in a resident's behaviour should not be attributed solely to dementia. Physical and other treatable causes must be ruled out.

True teamwork enhances the delivery of healthcare.

The use of charts to measure pain, fluid balance, food charts, weights, bladder and bowel care can help

---

staff identify early signs of ill health enabling better communication with the visiting doctor (Appendix 1).

Through the delivery of the highest possible standards of mental health and physical care, quality of life will be respected as well as enhanced.

Article 3 – the right to freedom from degrading and humiliating treatment

Seeing the world from the individual's point of view and ensuring that care is delivered in a respectful, compassionate and humane way allows the individual receiving care to feel in control. Dawn Brooker recommends (Brooker, 2006) that residents are included in conversations and helped to relate to others.

The following are examples of simple and basic things that really matter:

Always:

Say hello when walking by.
Maintain eye contact.
Make sure that hearing aids are working.
Identify hearing or visual loss.
Make sure that spectacles are clean.
Make sure that the resident's mouth and teeth are comfortable and clean.
Explain, include and involve the resident when assisting them to do the simplest activity.
Ensure that their fingernails are clean before eating.
Encourage individuals to feed themselves rather than be fed.
Make sure food and drink is easily accessible.
Make sure there is a bowel and bladder care plan rather than just saying 'please change pads regularly'.
If requested, make sure that personal care is delivered by somebody of his or her sex.
Listen to the individual and their family.
Allow them to choose their own clothes.
Ensure that all staff understand and know each individual's life history.
Ensure that movement and handling are delivered in a dignified manner, hoists used only where really necessary and ensure that the individual's modesty is protected when they are hoisted.

Making sure that all residents are treated with respect is not always easy.

A care home assistant said to a confused and unhappy resident 'how am I supposed to treat you with respect if you do not treat me with respect?' This demonstrated a lack of understanding by the resident as well as inadequate education of the care assistant.

Everybody is entitled to a fair and public hearing within a reasonable timeframe. This is particularly relevant to older people admitted to a care home who are living with dementia.

Many residents are not adequately involved and informed about their admission to a care home and on admission can feel very frightened and angry, feeling that they have been imprisoned against their will. Listening to them – as well as involving them and their families, on arrival in the home, to develop their individual care plan – will help overcome their feelings of uncertainty and give them back a sense of some control (Chapters 1.1, 1.2 and 1.3).

The importance of ensuring that residents have an equitable and fair access to healthcare interventions – such as podiatry, physiotherapy, and occupational therapy as well pain relief and medication review – cannot be over-emphasised.

Article 8 – the right to a private and family life

It is daunting to arrive in a care home and have to lead your life always surrounded by strangers.

The care home must ensure that there are facilities which allow for families and friends to see care home residents in private.

In addition, enabling a care home resident to see their GP in confidence and in private, when necessary, is fundamental.

Another marker of privacy and human rights is the use of the toilet. The British Geriatrics Society (2006) has made the use of the toilet in their 'Behind Closed Doors' campaign a marker of human rights. The British Geriatrics Society's campaign to improve continence care in care homes reminds staff *that incontinence is a sign that something is wrong* (see Chapter 5.4).

Care staff should be encouraged to ask nurses or the visiting GP to help find a treatable or remediable cause for incontinence.

It is possible that people who are restless, agitated and appear uncomfortable may need to go to the toilet; but they may not be able to tell staff. Even when people are immobile, it is better for them to be assisted to use the toilet and to be able to use it in private.

Underpinning Human Rights is the need to understand the importance of the individual's *autonomy*. The UK Mental Capacity Act (2005) states, that:

> *Every adult has the right to make his or her own decisions and it must be assumed they can unless it is proved otherwise. Also, a person must be given all reasonable help before anyone treats them as though they are unable to make their own decisions.*

Just because someone makes what might be seen as a poor decision, it should not be assumed that they are unable to make any decisions.

Any decision made for a person who is unable to so for themselves must be done in their best interests.

Any decisions made for someone else should not restrict their basic rights and freedoms.

Care home staff must have an understanding about the use of lasting power of attorney, court of protection and Independent Medical Capacity Advocates in enhancing an individual's autonomy and protecting them from neglect and or abuse.

References

British Geriatrics Society. 2006. Behind closed doors: dignity and toileting http://www.bgs.org.uk/campaigns/dignity.htm [Accessed September 2013]

Brooker D. 2006. *Person-Centred Dementia Care: Making Services Better*. London, Jessica Kingsley Publishers.

The Mental Capacity Act, 2005.

4.2 Restraint in the care home

Andrew Stanners[1] with Sandra Parry[2]

[1]Mid Yorkshire Hospitals NHS Trust, Wakefield, UK
[2]West Ridings Residential and Nursing Home, Wakefield, UK

Key points

- Restraint is anything that restricts a person's freedom.
- Restraint is undignified, can be dangerous, and should only be used as a 'last resort'.
- The need for restraint can be reduced by anticipating problems, knowing your residents, and respecting their dignity.
- Work in partnership: if you think you may need to restrain a client you should share the decision-making process.

To restrain someone is to prevent them from doing something – to restrict their freedom in any way (Box 4.2.1). At best, restraint causes loss of dignity and at worst it can cause serious injury or death. Restraint in the care home should therefore be an *absolute last resort* and everything possible should be done to avoid it.

Avoiding restraint in the care home depends on striking the right balance between a client's freedom and the risks of harm (to anyone). Particular circumstances in care homes, including illnesses

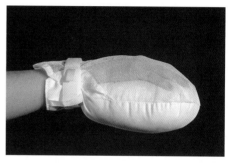

Figure 4.2.1 Mittens. Source: Medical Photography Department, Pinderfields Hospital, Wakefield.

Box 4.2.1 Restraint is *anything* that restricts freedom

- Physical restraint:
  - Mittens (Figure 4.2.1).
  - Bed-rails (Figure 4.2.2).
  - Locking doors.
  - Removing buzzers.
  - Removing aids to communication and mobility (including footwear).
  - Restricting mobility with obstacles such as furniture.
- Chemical restraint:
  - Any sedating medicine. (These can cause serious side-effects, such as falling, and their use should be audited and minimised.)
- Telling someone not to do something is restraint.
- All restraint should be a last resort and proportionate: use the least possible restraint for the shortest time.
- Always do a risk assessment.

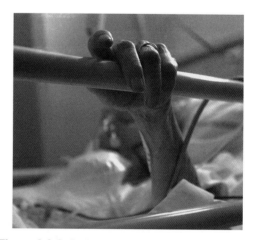

Figure 4.2.2 Bed-rails. Source: Colourbox.com (http://www.colourbox.com/image/image-1008426). Reproduced with permission.

suffered by some residents and pressures on resources, can give rise to potentially harmful situations. If staff don't anticipate these and act correctly, restraint may become necessary.

Anticipating (Box 4.2.2) and preventing (Box 4.2.3) potentially harmful situations whilst respecting client freedom requires great skill.

First, care home staff should know their residents and respect their dignity: residents should be allowed as much freedom as possible (Box 4.2.4). This may involve balancing some risks – such as falling – against others, but will build trusting relationships and lessen the potential need for restraint. Devices, such as falls monitors, can help reduce risk in some circumstances.

Second, staff should recognise triggers to potentially harmful behaviour and respond to them.

Third, staff should work in partnership with other people, such as family members, carers and outside experts, to prevent a need to restrain.

Last, staff should show leadership to other staff through good practice and sharing expertise. They should also follow correct procedures – such as audits –

Box 4.2.2 Anticipate situations that may escalate and necessitate restraint

- Look for reasons behind potentially harmful behaviour: consider hunger or behaviours associated with your client's former life, including their occupation.
- Urinary and respiratory infections demand a rapid response because they can trigger agitated behaviour.
- Audit your use of chemical restraint and ask for reviews of treatment.
- Falling should prompt a review of treatment.

Box 4.2.3 Prevent the need for restraint

- Plan ahead for problems – write a 'challenging behaviour' or 'escalation care plan'.
- Work in partnership:
  ○ discuss measures with families
  ○ consult the care homes liaison team (or equivalent) based in your local Mental Health Trust.
  ○ ask for a pharmacist, GP, geriatrician or psychiatrist to review your client's medication and care.
- Avoiding the need for restraint can start in the pre-assessment process: anticipate and avoid potential conflicts between residents.

Box 4.2.4 Respect your residents dignity

- Treat your residents as individuals and build trusting relationships.
- Allow freedom to move about.
- The 'party line' should be no restraint.
- Have a secure front door but keep everything else open – even the garden.
- Sensitively use devices such as sensors, CCTV, alarms on doors and crash mats.

Box 4.2.5 Show good leadership

- Use the 'Early Warning' audit tool to identify when restraint has been used.
- Keep good records of accidents and incidents.
- Hold a Clinical Review Meeting every week to look at falls, medication, and challenging behaviour.
- Use previous care home scandals – such as Winterbourne View – in staff training discussions.
- Good leadership can help prevent staff practices from deteriorating.
- 'Blow the whistle' if you see abuse or if you experience problems that prevent you from working properly.

Box 4.2.6 An example of justified restraint

A tissue viability nurse and general practitioner were both involved in a decision to use mittens for a woman whose scratching was preventing the healing of sores.

---

and be prepared to challenge inappropriate staff practice (Box 4.2.5).

Further reading

Care Quality Commission. 2010. *Essential Standards of Quality and Safety*, March 2010, part 2 outcome 7, p.94 – 99. http://www.cqc.org.uk/sites/default/files/media/documents/gac_-_dec_2011_update.pdf [Accessed September 2013]

Care Quality Commission. 2011. Review of Compliance for Winterbourne View, 2011, http://www.cqc.org.uk/sites/default/files/media/documents/1-116865865_castlebeck_care_teesdale_ltd_1-138702193_winterbourne_view_roc_20110517_201107183026.pdf [Accessed September 2013]

RCN Publication. 2008. *Let's Talk About Restraint*. http://www.rcn.org.uk/__data/assets/pdf_file/0007/157723/003208.pdf [Accessed September 2013]

4.3 Abuse

Deborah Sturdy[1] and Finbarr Martin[2]

[1]Red and Yellow Care, London, UK
[2]Guy's and St Thomas' NHS Foundation Trust, London, UK

Key points

- Abuse is absolutely unacceptable.
- Abuse of vulnerable adults is a complex and challenging area of practice.
- The need for expert advice and stringent protocols is essential for the management of both the victim and the suspected perpetrator of the alleged incident.

A widely accepted definition of abuse is 'the violation of an individual's human rights and civil rights by any other person or persons'. Abuse can take place anywhere and is an abuse of the authority, trust and power of the perpetrator.

Abuse can be:

- sexual
- financial and material
- psychological
- neglect or omission
- institutional
- physical.

The recognition of abuse and the need for the widest awareness by all staff will help in both its detection and prevention.

When to suspect abuse

Some key pointers that should make you concerned about the possibility of abuse include:

- Frequent minor injuries, such as bruises, abrasions, welts or other unexplained marks.
- Unexplained bruising, particularly in well-protected areas.
- Burns in unusual places.
- Families where there is a history of mental ill health or alcohol dependency.
- High dependency, social isolation or stress of caring.
- Excessive repeat prescriptions, indicating over use of medication.
- Poor living conditions and low income.
- The informal carer appearing to resent the person, being angry or frustrated and having a sense of loss of their own ambitions.
- The informal carer is defensive and wants to accompany the person at all times.

Some facts about abuse from the UK are listed below (however, these would be similar internationally) (http://www.hscic.gov.uk/).

- 41% of cases of abuse were in the person's own home.
- 34% of abuse was in a care home.
- 25% was by a family member.
- 25% was by a member of social care staff.
- 13% of the alleged abusers were other vulnerable adults.
- 12% were recorded as either a friend or neighbour, volunteer, other professional or a stranger.
- 3% of abusers were health care workers.

What to do

Being aware of the possibility of abuse and recognising it is key to a stopping it and protecting the victim of abuse. The response and the action taken will ensure both the victim and accused will be supported to ensure a fair and proper process of investigation. Seek advice from the safeguarding adult lead within your locality, know their number and use their expertise (see Chapter 17.8).

Key actions

As a registered nurse:

- You have a responsibility to act appropriately in safeguarding vulnerable adults.
- You should be aware of your local adult protection policies and procedures and clear about your own role within these.
- You should know who is the lead person in your service for adult protection and how to contact him or her.

In your work area:

- Ensure that leaflets are readily available on how residents, carers and families can identify and report abuse.
- Ensure that the name and contact details for your local adult protection lead person are available, along with your up-to-date local multi-agency adult protection procedures.
- Consider systematically reviewing your work practices to ensure that inadequate care is swiftly identified and effectively modified.

In your practice:

- Seek feedback on your work from colleagues and service users along with appropriate supervision and mentorship.
- Maintain your clinical and professional competence and strive to give the highest standards of care based on best evidence.
- Keep up to date by reading nursing journals and seek any training or updating you need.
- Ultimately, be vigilant about identifying any aspects of your own practice, and that of your colleagues, that could potentially violate an individual's human or civil rights.

This is a key responsibility and everyone is accountable. All staff must have this information available to them.

- The recognition and management of abuse in vulnerable adults is everyone's business.
- Be aware of and acknowledge the possibility of abuse.
- Create an open culture in which abuse is discussed and where staff members feel safe to raise concerns.

We will then succeed in providing our duty of care to those for whom we care.

Further reading

Department of Health. 2010. Clinical Governance and Adult Safeguarding: An Integrated Process. Department of Health. http://www.dh.gov.uk/publications [Accessed September 2103]

Department of Health. 2011. Change for life campaign http://www.nhs.uk/change4life/Pages/change-for-life.aspx [Accessed September 2013]

Department of Health. 2011. Statement of Government Policy on Adult Safeguarding. 16 May 2011 and a suite of new guidance including Safeguarding Adults: The Role of Health Service Practitioners (March 2011). http://www.dh.gov.uk/publications [Accessed September 2013]

Department of Health. 2011. Safeguarding Adults: The role of NHS Commissioners. Department of Health (first published March 2011). http://www.dh.gov.uk/publications [Accessed September 2013]

Heath H, Sturdy D. 2007. Vulnerable adults: the prevention, recognition and management of abuse. *Nursing Standard* June 2007.

Health Services Commissioner for England, 2011. *Care and compassion?* Parliamentary and Health Service Ombudsman, London . http://www.ombudsman.org.uk/__data/assets/pdf_file/0016/7216/Care-and-Compassion-PHSO-0114web.pdf [Accessed September 2013]

NMC. 2010. Raising and escalating concerns: Guidance for nurses and midwives. London, NMC.

NMC. 2011. Safeguarding adults: if you don't do something who will? (Update April 2011). London, NMC.

Tabernacle, B, Honey, M, Jinks, A, 2009. *Oxford Handbook of Nursing Older People*. Oxford, Oxford University Press.

Useful web sites

Northern Ireland
Review of criminal records regime announced 10 March 2011 http://www.northernireland.gov.uk/index/media-centre/news-departments/news-doj/news-doj-10032011-ford-announces-review.htm [Accessed 30 September 2013]

Scotland
Protecting Vulnerable Groups Act 2007. http://www.legislation.gov.uk/asp/2007/14/contents [Accessed September 2013]

Wales
Report on the protection of Vulnerable Adults Project Board http://wales.gov.uk/about/cabinet/cabinetstatements/2011/vulnerableadults/?lang=en [Accessed September 2013] 18 February 2011 http://wales.gov.uk/docs/cabinetstatements/2011/110218vulnerableadultsen.doc [Accessed September 2013]

Protection of vulnerable adults: The Welsh government's approach http://wales.gov.uk/topics/health/socialcare/vulnerableadults/?lang=en 24 January 2011 [Accessed September 2013]

4.4 Dealing with complaints and concerns

Clive Bowman

School of Healthcare Studies, City University, London, UK

Key points

- All complaints and concerns should be taken seriously: no one can get everything right all the time, so be receptive to complaints – not defensive.
- Exactly when a concern becomes a complaint is often difficult to determine. If in doubt, ask the potential complainant.
- When listening to a concern or complaint, make sure you have understood it by 'playing it back' to the complainant, 'Can I make sure I have properly understood you?'
- Minor concerns and complaints can and should be addressed immediately – but make sure the remedy is shared with colleagues at handover and is recorded in the case notes.
- Serious complaints must be dealt with formally using a complaints policy. Make sure the care home manager or other responsible person is alerted as soon as possible.
- Keeping good records can be very helpful in investigations! Conversely, poor records can be very unhelpful.
- Complaints are often an excellent way of getting helpful information to improve a service.

Very few people expect care to be perfect all the time, but transparency when things do go wrong is always the best policy.

All concerns and complaints must be taken seriously. If complaints are addressed correctly, they can improve both the care of the individual and the confidence of family and friends.

Most concerns are not major but are about some aspect of care or service that has not met expectations, or result from a misunderstanding. Concerns can accumulate over time and, if not dealt with properly, can seriously impair the trust of either an individual resident or, more frequently, their family and friends.

It is crucial to always remember that admission to a care home of a loved family member – for whom often great commitment and care has been provided – is accompanied by strong emotions that include grief, guilt, a sense of failure and indeed anger.

Most complaints are simple matters and are made orally by family, friends and, of course, residents, who should be carefully heard: the lost sock, the cold cup of tea, may seem trivial, but if it's on the resident's or their families' mind, it is not trivial at all.

Most concerns can and should be resolved on the spot, but do make sure that whatever was the problem (be it a food or drink preference or dislike, or a particular aspect of personal care) that your response has completely satisfied the person making the complaint.

Do communicate what has been changed to colleagues at handover by ensuring that the care plan is updated.

Make clear what you have done to ensure that whatever was wrong has been, to the best of your ability, fixed.

Often, complaints seem to have a number of dimensions. It is good practice to listen and then 'replay' the concern or complaint to make sure you have heard and understood the complainant.

This may not be easy if there are communication or capacity problems. In some cases, the advocacy service (or equivalent) or an interpreter may be needed.

Sometimes people will be distressed when making a complaint and it can be very difficult to identify the key concerns. As complaints frequently require investigation, it is crucial that what the home investigates is definitely the problem that has been presented as a concern. It is worth spending time with a complainant to patiently distil what the exact problem is that will need investigation.

The Care Home Handbook, First Edition. Edited by Graham Mulley, Clive Bowman, Michal Boyd and Sarah Stowe.
© 2015 John Wiley & Sons, Ltd. Published 2015 by John Wiley & Sons, Ltd.

More formal or serious complaints made orally must be fully documented. Be aware of the complaints policy in your home, and if there are allegations of abuse (see Chapter 4.3) of any nature, make sure that the complainant has immediate access to the most senior person in the home, who will take responsibility for managing such a matter internally and for liaising with statutory authorities.

Often, complaints will be made in writing to home managers or more senior management. In these instances, you can be sure that the care records will be carefully scrutinised and all the involved individuals will be interviewed.

Good clear case notes are invaluable.

On occasion, very serious accusations may be made about your personal actions. These may seem, and indeed may be, wholly unjustified. However, you must make sure the complainant is referred to (or complaint is given to) a senior colleague.

Good complaints policies will indicate the sort of time periods that will be necessary to make investigations and determine a correct response. Many residents, families and friends simply do not understand this. Often their complaint is the first one they will have made.

If you have a leaflet on your home's complaints procedure, make it available – and also point out that there are time periods for investigation. It is crucial that when the length of the investigation means that the schedules are going to be broken, that the complainant is given clear information that they can understand.

Getting the right balance can be difficult. Some older people do not complain. It is therefore crucial that

- You should never accept that residents are worried about complaining for fear of reprisal.
- When you simply cannot satisfy a complainant, ask yourself the simple question, 'what more can I do?' If there is no obvious way forward, say so, but make sure the complaint is referred to senior management.

In the most extreme circumstances, when unjustified complaints continually undermine care homes, you may need statutory support to limit the communications. Where a complainant is a resident, there are extreme circumstances when their continued residence in the home will need formal review.

Unacceptable behaviours

A small number of complainants hinder the consideration of their own, or another complainant's, case. This may be because of unacceptable behaviour in their dealings with staff, or because of unreasonably persistent contacts that distract staff from their work but does not add anything to the complaint under consideration.

You should not have to accept abusive, offensive, deceitful, threatening or other forms of unacceptable behaviour from complainants. If such behaviour does occur, report it to a senior manager. In most cases, when someone's behaviour is considered unreasonable, a senior manager politely but firmly talking them through this can resolve the situation.

It is also reasonable to warn the complainant that if the behaviour continues, action to restrict their contact will be taken.

If the behaviour is so extreme that it threatens the immediate safety and welfare of staff, the matter may be reported to the police or legal action may be considered. In such cases, the complainant may not receive prior warning of these intended actions. In these (thankfully rare) circumstances, the complainant's behaviour may be a reflection of a mental illness, and getting the right solution in the best interests of the resident can be enormously difficult.

Restricting access

Exceptionally, senior management may find it necessary to impose a restriction of contact, which will be carefully documented and explained to the complainant. These 'rules' need to be carefully understood by the whole team and supported.

Further reading

Allen PD, Nelson HW, Gruman C, Cherry KE. 2006. Nursing home complaints: who's complaining and what's gender got to do with it? *Journal of Gerontology and Social Work* 47: 89–106.

Stevenson DG. 2006. Nursing home consumer complaints and quality of care: a national view. *Medical Care Research and Review* 63: 347–68.

4.5 Incident reporting and root cause analysis

Sarah Stowe[1] and Alison Cracknell[2]

[1] *Airedale NHS Foundation Trust, Keighley, UK*
[2] *Leeds Teaching Hospitals NHS Trust, Leeds, UK*

Key points

- Healthcare can harm the very people it is trying to help despite the best efforts of highly trained, dedicated professionals.
- An *adverse event* is any action that causes unintended injury to a resident, such as a fall, pressure ulcer or medication error. Overall, safety should be everyone's responsibility and errors should be anticipated in order to minimise harm.
- Many errors result in very little or no harm (near misses) or even go unnoticed, but they provide an opportunity to improve practice and avoid repeated mistakes.
- A *serious incident* is one that causes (or has the potential to result in) death or severe harm to an individual or property.
- A *never event* is one that causes death or severe harm in an individual and is inexcusable because it is eminently preventable with the use of precautionary measures. For example, death or severe harm of a resident due to the maladministration of insulin by a healthcare professional.
- Older people with multiple co-morbidities taking numerous medications are particularly at risk of harm from adverse events and their carers must therefore be vigilant in minimising threats to their safety.
- Investigations which consider only the actions or omissions of a culprit or individual are incomplete and misleading. Understanding what has gone wrong and why is vital to reducing the risk of adverse incidents.

Adverse incidents are often deemed to be a consequence of *human error*, but analysis of the circumstances of an incident reveals that they are rarely straightforward, but have many contributory factors (Figure 4.5.1). For example, working conditions, communication within the team and equipment failure may all play a part in creating an error-prone environment and are termed *latent system failures*. Knowledge of latent failures allows an organisation to design safer systems that minimise errors. *Active failures* are caused by errors of judgement, lapses in concentration, failure to follow a protocol correctly or a decision to act against the best interests of the resident (violation). These are often secondary to *human factors* such as tiredness, stress, distractedness and lack of knowledge and training.

Incident reporting should be actively encouraged within a non-punitive atmosphere that promotes transparency and accountability and strives for continuous improvement. Different organisations may employ electronic or written reporting methods to facilitate local and national collection of data about safety incidents. In the UK, the National Reporting and Learning System (NRLS) analyses incidents across NHS organisations in England and Wales, setting priorities to develop and disseminate actionable learning. Data from incident reporting suggest that at least 10% of hospital in-patients suffer a harmful adverse event as a consequence of their admission, and about half of these incidents are preventable. However, there is less information about safety incidents in care home residents. Organisations and individuals who are reluctant to report their own mistakes for fear of the consequences are unlikely to engage in a safety culture. Staff who report incidents should receive timely feedback on their contribution and details of action plans generated from root cause analyses.

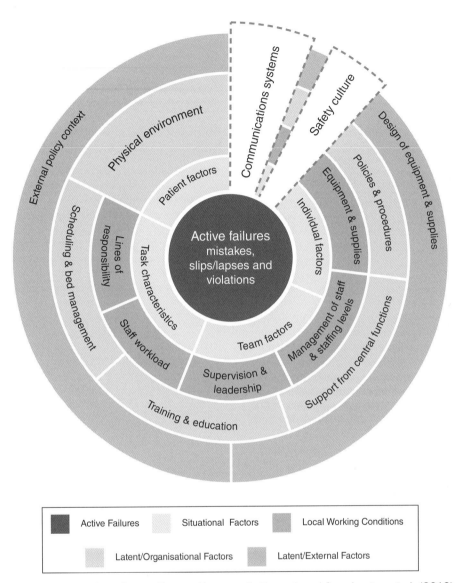

Figure 4.5.1 The Yorkshire Contributory Factors Framework. Reproduced from Lawton et al. (2012) with permission from the author and BMJ Publishing Group Ltd.

Analysis of the root cause(s) of an incident looks beyond the active failure and examines the event from a wider organisational perspective, to identify latent failures and plan who or what is required to stop errors before harm occurs. Different methods of analysis are available, and lead investigators who are responsible for local implementation of action plans following a serious incident require training in this area. See Box 4.5.1 for a worked example using a model of nine classes of contributory factors from the UK National Patient Safety Agency toolkit.

Case study of a safety incident

What happened?

- Nurse checks insulin dose for resident A and is about to administer the dose but is called away to assist with another resident who has fallen.

- Nurse returns and erroneously gives insulin for resident A to resident B.
- Resident B is at risk of hypoglycaemia. Resident A does not receive their insulin dose.
- Incident reported by nurse at the end of the shift.

Box 4.5.1 A worked example using a model of nine classes of contributory factors from the UK National Patient Safety Agency toolkit

Contributory factor	Analysis
Resident/patient factors	Resident has cognitive and multiple sensory impairments and was not able to question the nurse about receiving an unexpected injection
Individual staff factors	Nurse suffering sleep deprivation due to young baby at home. Nurse not had lunch break due to time pressures of excessive workload
Task characteristics	Administration of insulin is a high risk procedure with the potential for serious harm
Communication systems	Lack of awareness by other staff that this nurse is on drug round, so called away from this task to help elsewhere despite risk of error from distraction
Team factors: management of staff, staffing levels, safety culture	Rapid turnover of temporary agency staff has contributed to poor morale among staff Staffing levels low due to sickness, lack of senior nurses available to provide support when administering high risk drugs
Training and education	Lack of regular training on medication safety
Equipment and Supplies	Lack of signs to highlight to others that nurse performing medication round
Physical environment	Care home staff cover multiple floors
Safety culture	Implementation of safety policies not a priority, culture of 'blame' predominates

Why did it happen?

See Box 4.5.1.

Outcome of RCA

Overall analysis reveals a *system failure* rather than simply human error. In order to prevent this happening again recommendations may include:

- Introduction of a new system for highlighting a drug round in progress: signage, tabards to be worn over uniform.
- Mandatory training for all staff on medication safety with regular education updates.
- Supervised administration of certain high risk medications, such as insulin, warfarin and methotrexate.
- Recruitment of staff to cover sickness absences to alleviate stress on employees.

Reference

Lawton R, McEachan RRC, Giles SJ, Sirriyeh R, Watt IS, Wright J. 2012. Development of an evidence-based framework of factors contributing to patient safety incidents in hospital settings: a systematic review. *BMJ Quality and Safety* 21(5): 369–80.

Useful web sites

NHS patient safety resource http://www.patientsafetyfirst.nhs.uk/content.aspx?path=/ [Accessed September 2013]

NPSA Incident Decision Tree http://www.npsa.nhs.uk/idt/ [Accessed September 2013]

NPSA Root Cause Analysis Toolkit http://www.npsa.nhs.uk/rca/ [Accessed September 2013]

Never events (NRLS resource) http://www.nrls.npsa.nhs.uk/neverevents/ [Accessed September 2013]

Seven steps to patient safety (NHS resource) http://www.nrls.npsa.nhs.uk/resources/collections/seven-steps-to-patient-safety/ [Accessed September 2013]

WHO web site http://www.who.int/patientsafety/en/ [Accessed September 2013]

4.6 Capacity

Zuzanna Sawicka[1] and Ewa Zalewska[2]

[1]*St James's University Hospital, Leeds, UK*
[2]*Mid Yorkshire Hospitals NHS Trust, Wakefield, UK*

Key points

- Mental capacity is a term used to describe a person's ability to make a decision or perform an action that might have legal consequences.
- Capacity can be affected if there is a disturbance of mental function, such as dementia.
- A person is assumed to have capacity unless proved otherwise.
- People with capacity have the right to make their own decisions – even if these are unusual.
- In establishing capacity, the assessor considers whether the resident can understand the issue, retain information, has the ability to weigh it up and to communicate their decision.
- Different countries have differing laws and practices relating to capacity.

Mental capacity is a legal term for a person's ability to do something or formulate a decision which may have legal consequences (such as where they wish to live).

- Capacity is an important principle in English and Welsh law in maintaining an individual's right to independence.
- Everyone has this right and it has a bearing on the care and treatment of individuals.
- Capacity can be affected when an individual develops an impairment of, or disturbance in, the functioning of their mind or brain, such as dementia. When this impairment or disturbance is sufficient that a person is unable to make a particular decision, they are deemed to lack capacity.

The UK Mental Capacity Act

The Mental Capacity Act (MCA) 2005 applies to everyone involved in the care, treatment and support of people aged 16 and over, living in England and Wales, who are unable to make all or some decisions for themselves. (Note that the situation in Scotland is slightly different – see BMA (2009).) It is aimed at protecting and restoring power to those vulnerable people who lack capacity. The Act is underpinned by five key principles.

Principle 1: A presumption of capacity
Every adult has the right to make his or her own decisions. *Capacity is always assumed unless an individual is proved to lack the ability to self-govern their needs.*

Principle 2: Individuals must be supported to make their own decisions
Every effort should be made to support an individual in any decision-making process, for example, through using simple language or visual prompts. Even if an individual is deemed to lack capacity, it is important that the person is involved as far as possible in making their own decisions.

Principle 3: Unwise decisions
Individuals have the right to make decisions that others might regard as unwise or unconventional. Everyone has their own values, beliefs and preferences which may not be the same as those of other people. They have a right to have these respected.

Principle 4: Best interests
Decisions made on behalf of a person who lacks mental capacity must be done in their best interests.

Principle 5: Less restrictive option
Individuals who make a decision or act on behalf of a person who lacks capacity must consider whether it is possible to determine or act in a way that would interfere less with the person's rights and freedoms of action, or whether there is a need to decide or act at all.

The Care Home Handbook, First Edition. Edited by Graham Mulley, Clive Bowman, Michal Boyd and Sarah Stowe.
© 2015 John Wiley & Sons, Ltd. Published 2015 by John Wiley & Sons, Ltd.

Establishing an individual's capacity

The Mental Capacity Act states that a person is unable to make their own decisions if they cannot do one or more of the following four things:

1. *understand* information given to them,
2. *retain* that information long enough to be able to make the decision,
3. *weigh up* the information available to make the decision,
4. *communicate* their decision – this could be by talking, using sign language or even simple muscle movements.

When establishing an individual's capacity, every effort should be made to involve family, friends, carers or other professionals to help either an individual to make a decision or a decision to be made in an individual's best interests.

Any evaluation of capacity should be documented including how any conclusions have been drawn.

In the UK, a capacity decision can be made by anyone as long as they have a 'reasonable belief' that a person lacks capacity. However, in other countries (such as New Zealand), it can only be done by a qualified health professional – usually a medical practitioner.

Advocacy of an individual

Advocacy is speaking up for, or acting on behalf of, yourself or another person.

Everyone has the right to an advocate in order to help an individual make and express clearly their own views and wishes.

An advocate could be an individual's friend or a member of their family. Sometimes these advocates are previously appointed under Lasting Powers of Attorneys (known as Enduring Powers of Attorney in Australia and New Zealand). This allows individuals over the age of 18 to formally appoint one or more people to look after their health, welfare and/or financial decisions, if at some time in the future they lack capacity to make those decisions.

If an individual is without close friends, or there are conflicts between an individual's advocate and the individual, then an independent mental capacity advocate (IMCA) may be required, who will act to support an individual in making a decision or help medical/nursing professionals to make a decision in a person's best interests when they are unable to make their own decision. This is the case in the UK: it is not applicable in Australia (see http://www.racgp.org.au/afp/200610/20061004bird.pdf) or New Zealand (see http://www.ageconcern.org.nz/money/planning/enduring-power-attorney). Please check the situation in your own country.

Legal responsibilities

It is the personal responsibility of any healthcare professional proposing any form of care to determine whether an individual has the capacity to make a decision to give consent to the care to be given. If a person lacks capacity, care, such as treatment, can be given on the legal basis of necessity as it is in the best interests of an individual. In the UK, most decisions can thus be made unless they involve the following which have been deemed by the Courts as requiring High Court Rulings: cases of doubt in a person's capacity or best interests; in those with persistent vegetative states in whom hydration and nutrition is to be withdrawn.

Reference

BMA, 2009. Medical treatment for adults with incapacity. Guidance on ethical and medico-legal issues in Scotland. bma.org.uk/-/media/.../Ethics/adultswithincapacity-scotlandapril2009.pdf [Accessed September 2013]

Further reading

Hotopf M. 2005. The assessment of mental capacity. *Clinical Medicine* 5: 580–584.

Robinson L, Dickinson C, Rousseau N et al. 2012. A systematic review of the effectiveness of advance care planning interventions for people with cognitive impairment and dementia. *Age and Ageing* 41: 263–269

Walker L. 1998. Assessment of capacity to discuss advance care planning in nursing homes. *Journal of the American Geriatrics Society* 46: 1055–1056

Core Nursing and Personal Care Skills

Chapter 5

Feeding and Nutrition, Hygiene, and Promotion of Continence

5.1 Nutrition

Pauline Newsome and Oliver J. Corrado

Leeds Teaching Hospitals NHS Trust, Leeds, UK

Key points

- Malnutrition can affect anyone, but older people are among the most vulnerable.
- Nursing home residents are at particular risk of malnutrition (about 15% of care home residents are underweight) as a result of their frailty, multiple medical problems and loss of independence.
- Good nutrition is essential to maintain residents' quality of life, health and wellbeing.
- Weight loss increases the risk of a variety of problems, in particular pressure sores (sometimes called decubitus ulcers) (see Chapter 5.6) and infection.

Factors which affect nutrition in older residents

- Oral problems.
- Swallowing problems (see Chapter 5.2) (related to such illnesses as stroke, Parkinson's disease and other neurological disorders).

  These will need input from a speech and language therapist and perhaps a dietician (see Chapter 8.2).
- Poor dentition: missing teeth, caries, ill-fitting dentures, denture-induced oral trauma.

  Older people with more than 20 teeth are more likely to have a normal Body Mass Index (BMI) but few care home residents have this many teeth.
- Stomatitis and oral candidiasis (thrush).
- Reduced manual dexterity and loss of independence.

  These impair the ability to hold or manage cutlery and to feed oneself and can result from stroke, arthritis or neurological diseases (e.g. Parkinson's disease, neuropathies and cerebellar disease).
- Depression.

  This may affect an individual's interest in food.
- Malabsorption.

  As a result of previous surgery, coeliac disease and small bowel disease including fistulae, diverticulae and bacterial overgrowth.

- Dementia.

  Dementia can reduce appetite and interest in food and impair the individual's ability to feed themselves.
- Impaired sensation.

  The ageing process can impair taste, appetite and sense of smell.
- Acute and chronic disease.

  Acute illness can affect nutrition at the time and also during recovery. Residents recently discharged from hospital are at particular risk. Chronic ill health (in particular cancer) can also impair nutrition.
- Drugs and alcohol.

  Nutrition can be impaired in those who suffer from alcoholism.
- A number of medications can also reduce interest in food and appetite.
- Palliative care.

  End of life nutrition should be aimed at comfort and choice, not be concerned with weight loss.

Nutritional screening

Malnutrition is often undetected. *All care home residents should be routinely screened for malnutrition.*

There are a number of ways in which nutrition can be assessed, ranging from simple questionnaires enquiring about weight loss and food intake, to more complex assessments of nutritional intake (using food diaries) against standard dietary reference values.

The Care Home Handbook, First Edition. Edited by Graham Mulley, Clive Bowman, Michal Boyd and Sarah Stowe.
© 2015 John Wiley & Sons, Ltd. Published 2015 by John Wiley & Sons, Ltd.

These are best undertaken by a dietician.

However, the best assessment is to use a screening tool which incorporates a calculation of Body Mass Index (BMI).

BMI is calculated from the following equation:

$$BMI = \frac{weight\ in\ kilograms}{height\ in\ metres^2}$$

The BMI relies on determining the resident's weight and it is important that all homes have the appropriate equipment, including sitting scales and hoist scales, in order to weigh more dependent residents. *These scales should be checked every six months for accuracy.*

Height is measured in metres (not feet and inches). A simple method of assessing the height of those unable to stand is measurement of the digit span. Ask the resident to hold out an arm by their side at ninety degrees to the trunk. Measure the distance from the tip of the middle finger to the middle of the sternum. Multiply this by two – this will be equivalent to the resident's height.

An alternative method of estimating height is to measure ulna length in centimetres (the length of the forearm from the olecranon process at the elbow to the styloid process of the wrist). This measurement can be converted to an approximate height using a standard table (see link below).

Once the height and weight are known, the BMI can be calculated from a chart.

A good source is the following link http://www.bapen.org.uk/must-calculator.html which can be stored as a computer 'favourite'. Knowing the BMI makes it possible to determine the degree of risk a resident has for undernutrition:

High risk – score 2 – BMI < 18.5

Medium risk – score 1 – BMI 18.5 – 20

Low risk – score 0 – BMI over 20

Objective weight assessment may be supported by subjective clinical judgement, such as loose clothes or rings, or previous photographs to help assess if their weight is of concern.

Management strategies

1. Undertake a nutritional assessment to determine the risk of malnutrition, identify and act for the nutritionally 'vulnerable' person.
2. Keep food diaries.
3. Weigh residents weekly.
4. Make sure the care plan reflects a resident's needs and goals, and that all members of the team are aware of the problem. Different coloured plates or trays may raise carers' and relatives' awareness.
5. Correct remediable factors. Does the resident need to see a dentist? Many dentists will visit a home to undertake basic dental care (Chapter 17.5). A set of dentures is not permanent: with time, gums atrophy and dentures may need relining if they become loose. (To register for NHS dentist Dental Advice in the UK: Telephone 0800 298 5787.)
6. Food can be presented on smaller plates or in smaller bowls. A teaspoon may help if residents can only manage small quantities or have swallowing difficulties (see Chapter 5.2).
7. Hydration is the key to good nutrition, as anyone with dry mouth/poor oral state will struggle to eat (see Chapter 5.3). Aim for 6 to 8 glasses daily.

   It may help to offer drinks at least a half-hour before or after meals.
8. Older people may need time, help and encouragement to eat.
9. Find out what residents enjoy eating and tailor their diets accordingly. Breakfast clubs, special suppers or coffee mornings can encourage social inclusion.
10. Families can be involved in filling in diaries, providing additional 'treats' as well as assisting with feeding.
11. Connecting a person with dementia with a familiar object, stimulus or activity may have a positive effect. This may be soft music, a particular aroma or even chocolate!
12. Exercise will improve appetite and muscle strength.

Tips on food and nutritional supplements

- It is best to give smaller portions more frequently.
- Extra snacks at bedtime can be helpful because the appetite for the next meal will not be affected.
- You can add extra calories to vegetables and starches by topping them with butter, cream, olive oil, sauces or cheese.
- Sandwiches made with peanut or other nut butters, or meats augmented with slices of cheese or avocado, can improve calorie intake.
- Creamed soups are higher in calories than clear broths. Add more calories to creamed soups by add-

ing a spoonful of dry milk powder. (Maxijoule® is a dry carbohydrate that can be added to most food and is tasteless.)

- Add extra cheese to omelettes.
- Stir chopped nuts into plain yogurt and top with honey.
- Add calories with a nutritious beverage such as milk, 100% fruit juices, or vegetable juice.
- Make coffee with full fat milk.
- Calogen® (a soluble fat based additive) can be added to milk and is undetectable.
- Clotted cream (seriously fattening) and banana.
- Porridge made with full fat milk then double cream/sugar (even for diabetics).
- Ice cream made with clotted cream added to fruit smoothies/milkshakes or as a dessert.
- Shortbread biscuits, although small, are full of calories.

It is extremely gratifying when these strategies work and the resident gains weight.

Nutritional supplement drinks, such as instant breakfast mixes and canned or powdered shakes, can provide more calories and require little or no preparation. It may be easier to drink rather than to eat something. Supplements should only be used after a nutritional risk assessment has been completed and focused interventions to increase frequency of small meals and increase calorie dense foods have been attempted. A dietician can assess a resident's needs and recommend appropriate supplements.

Useful web sites

http://www.bapen.org.uk/must-calculator.html [Accessed October 2013]

www.cqc.org.uk/sites/default/files/media/documents/PCA_OUTCOME_5_new.doc [Accessed October 2013]

www.nhs.uk [Accessed October 2013]

www.scie.org.uk/publications/guides/guide15/factors/nutrition/index.asp [Accessed October 2013]

5.2 Swallowing difficulties and associated problems

Ed Richfield[1] and Louise Brown[2]

[1] Leeds NHS Trust, UK
[2] Harrogate and District Foundation Trust, Scarborough Hospital, UK

Key points

- Dysphagia (difficulty in swallowing) is very common in care home residents and has many causes.
- Dysphagia may be for solids or liquids.
- Good oral hygiene can lessen the risk of dysphagia.
- The role of the speech and language therapist in assessing and treating dysphagia, and in educating the care home team in recognising dysphagia, is very important.
- Dangers of dysphagia include aspiration (with the risk of pneumonia), subnutrition, dehydration and social isolation.
- Aspiration pneumonia is a medical emergency.

How do we swallow?

Before discussing the problems which arise when swallowing is impaired, we will consider the normal process of swallowing, something which we often take for granted until it goes wrong.

Although it may initially seem straightforward, swallowing is a complex process. Successful swallowing transfers chewed food from the front of our mouths (in the form of a soft *'bolus'*) through the pharynx, into the oesophagus, without entering the airway (trachea or naso-pharynx) along the way. This coordinated action of muscles and breathing is regulated by both conscious and subconscious areas of the brain.

Therefore, dysphagia (difficulty swallowing) may arise from diseases affecting neurological, respiratory or musculoskeletal systems, and has many possible causes.

Disruption to passage of food can also arise in the oesophagus, for example through narrowing, or neuromuscular failure. These causes of dysphagia are often considered separately.

Why is it important to recognise dysphagia?

Dysphagia is surprisingly common, it has been estimated that it affects between 50 and 75% of Nursing Home residents, and is associated with increased morbidity and mortality (RCLST, 2009; Kayser-Jones and Pengilly, 1999). Dysphagia is common in people with neurologic disease, such as stroke, Parkinson's disease or dementia.

Aspiration

Is when oro-pharyngeal contents pass in to the respiratory tract. We have all experienced this when 'something goes down the wrong way'. Aspiration can cause direct damage through corrosive effects (especially acidic stomach contents) or introduce infections, most commonly resulting in *aspiration pneumonia*. People with multiple illnesses, reduced immunity, and impaired cough reflex, including many older people in care homes, are at particular risk of developing pneumonia following aspiration (Marik and Kaplan 2003).

Malnutrition

Reduced oral intake because of dysphagia may rapidly lead to dehydration and malnutrition.

Psycho-social

Eating and drinking is a major social function and source of pleasure, we are often encouraged to 'Eat, drink and be merry'. Loss of this function can cause distress and social isolation.

The Care Home Handbook, First Edition. Edited by Graham Mulley, Clive Bowman, Michal Boyd and Sarah Stowe.
© 2015 John Wiley & Sons, Ltd. Published 2015 by John Wiley & Sons, Ltd.

How can I recognise dysphagia?

Dysphagia may be sudden or gradual in onset and may be exacerbated by inter-current illness. Awareness of the 'warning signs' will allow you to recognise dysphagia promptly. We have organised these according to urgency.

Red – Requires early referral and investigation

- Severe coughing, choking or cyanosis with food/ liquids.
- Nasal regurgitation of food/liquids.
- Wet voice or hoarseness after swallowing.
- Failure to manage secretions (i.e. gurgling and heavy drooling in absence of known cause).

Amber – Be alert, look for other evidence of dysphagia

- Food spilling from mouth.
- Taking a long time to finish meals.
- Complains of food sticking.
- Grimacing when eating.

Green – May contribute to or result from dysphagia

- Dry mouth.
- Poor oral hygiene.
- Regurgitation.
- Weight loss.

How can I assess someone's swallow?

If you are suspicious that someone may have dysphagia, it is important that they are assessed promptly and accurately. As a first step, the bedside 'sip test' is an effective way of screening, and can be conducted by non-specialists AFTER they have received appropriate training.

In the absence of appropriately trained staff, specialist assessment by a speech and language therapist (SALT) should be sought, usually via the resident's GP (Chapter 8.2).

If complications of dysphagia, such as aspiration pneumonia, are suspected urgent medical assessment is required.

Remember – The bedside screening test only assesses the ability to swallow water. If a patient already has swallowing recommendations in place (i.e. thickened fluids), testing their swallow with water may cause harm (aspiration) and should NOT be attempted. These patients require assessment by the speech and language therapist.

How can we improve swallowing?

There are many strategies to improve swallowing. Some will be implemented by the SALT, while others can be initiated by you, and should be emphasised as part of good practice. We will consider these separately.

Non-Specialist

- *Promote oral hygiene* – While improving swallow, this also promotes the resident's dignity and enhances pleasure from eating. In addition *good oral hygiene reduces the chance of developing pneumonia in the event of aspiration* (Marik and Kaplan, 2003; Eisenstadt, 2010).
- *Posture* – Emphasise safe postures when eating/ drinking.
  1. Sitting posture: sitting upright at 90 degree angle.
  2. Bed posture: backrest elevated to 90 degree angle.
  3. Chin tuck: chin tilted forward towards chest. Note – there is no agreed anatomical position for chin tuck – may require SLT advice (Okada et al. 2007).
- *Environmental modification* – reducing distraction (TV/radio) during meal times and not talking to residents while they are eating promotes good swallow.
- *Time* – Provide a 30 minute rest period before eating. It is important not to rush people when eating, especially if you are assisting them.
- *Verbal re-enforcement* – encourage residents to put into practice the techniques they have learned.
- *Diet choice* – Ensure a varied choice of diet, and encourage independence during mealtimes, for example offering finger foods and promoting independent feeding, which enhances dignity as well as improving nutrition.
- *Placement of food* – vary the placement of food according to the type of deficit; for example if left facial weakness is present, then place the food in the right side of the mouth.
- *Medications* – request the GP or nurse practitioner to review the use of sedatives or hypnotics, as they can impair the cough reflex and affect swallowing.

Table 5.2.1 Quick guide to thickening fluids.

Stage	Description
Stage 1	This consistency can be drunk through a straw or from a cup (if advised or preferred). It leaves a thin coat on the back of a spoon
Stage 2	This consistency is too thick to drink through a straw, but can be drunk from a cup. It leaves a thick coat on the back of a spoon
Stage 3	This consistency cannot be drunk through a straw or from a cup. It needs to be taken with a spoon

Reproduced with permission from Nutrition & Diet Resources UK *Fluid Thickening Guide* ref: 9091, 2005, reviewed in 2010 (www.ndr-uk.org).

Specialist

While these recommendations are usually put in place by the SALT, it is important that you understand them in order to re-enforce good practice, and assist residents where necessary. We know that it is often difficult for individuals to stick to these recommendations, *but care staff play an important role in improving concordance and reducing aspiration* (King and Ligman, 2011)

- *Thickened fluids* – see Table 5.2.1.
- *Modifying texture* – ensure that residents receive the correct diet consistency, this includes not receiving food which has been pureed unnecessarily, which may reduce the pleasure of eating (see Chapter 5.1).
- Specialist techniques are described as direct or indirect and a detailed explanation is beyond the scope of this chapter. They should always be demonstrated and explained by the SALT, with instructions provided. They are specific to individual residents and should not be applied independently. *If in doubt, seek clarification and further training*.
- *Indirect therapy* – exercise programmes without food/fluid.
- *Direct therapy* – specific postural technique or manoeuvre when swallowing food/fluid.

Box 5.2.1 has some top tips and Table 5.2.2 has some frequently asked questions. At the end of the chapter we suggest further reading if you wish to learn more.

Box 5.2.1 Top tips when modifying fluids.

Thickened fluids must be used within the recommended time (usually 30–45 minutes)

Ensure the correct ratio of thickener to fluid – different products will vary

Do not thicken boiling drinks – allow time to cool

Not all supplements thicken well – you may need to consult a dietician

If in doubt, seek advice

Table 5.2.2 Frequently asked questions.

Question	Solution
What if a resident won't take thickened fluids?	Check oral hygiene, ensure appropriate use of thickener.
What if a resident is still aspirating despite following SLT recommendations?	Requires further review. Dysphagia, despite safest feeding practice, is complex, sometimes non-oral feeding is appropriate but this requires detailed medical and ethical review.
What if family/ friends are giving normal diet to a resident who requires modified intake?	Be aware of the reasons for this: modified diet is often less enjoyable. Involve the MDT in discussions with resident and family to discuss reasons for modified diet and maximise concordance.

References

Eisenstadt SE. 2010. Dysphagia and aspiration pneumonia in older adults. *American Academy Nurse Practitioner* 22: 17–22.

Kayser-Jones J, Pengilly K. 1999. Dysphagia among nursing home residents. *Geriatric Nursing* 22: 77–85.

King JM, Ligman K. 2011. Patient noncompliance with swallowing recommendations: reports from Speech and Language Pathologists. *Contemporary Issues In Communication Science And Disorders* 38: 53–60.

Marik EP, Kaplan D. 2003. Aspiration pneumonia and dysphagia in the elderly. *Chest* 124: 328–336.

Okada S, Saitoh E, Palmer JB et al. 2007. What Is the chin-down Posture? A Questionnaire Survey of Speech Language Pathologists in Japan and the United States. *Dysphagia* 22: 204–209.

Royal College of Speech and Language Therapists (RCLST). 2009. RCSLT resource manual for commissioning and planning services for SLCN. RCLST.

Further reading

Groher ME, Crary MA. 2010. *Dysphagia. Critical Management in Adults and Children*. Mosby Elsevier.

Logemann JA. 1998. *Evaluation and Treatment of Swallowing Disorders*. Pro-Ed, Inc.

Yorkston KM, Miller RM, Strand EA. 2004. *Management of Speech and Swallowing in Degenerative Diseases*. Pro-Ed, Inc.

5.3 Hydration

Josie Clare[1] and Mary Burke[2]

[1]*Cork University Hospital, Ireland*
[2]*Killure Bridge Nursing Home, Waterford, Ireland*

Key points

- Dehydration – a lack of fluid in the body – is common in residents but can be difficult to recognise.
- Signs of dehydration include a dry mouth, sunken eyes, delirium, constipation, hypotension, lethargy, reduced function and dark urine.
- Access to palatable drinks is most important.
- Dehydration may occur because of reduced fluid intake (many old people have a reduced sensation of thirst) or increased fluid loss. The cause(s) must always be sought.
- The use of subcutaneous fluids can reduce the need for hospital admission.

Dehydration is a lack of fluid in the body.

Adequate hydration is critical to body functions. It is important for carrying oxygen and energy to the body, as well as carrying away waste products.

Dehydration is common in older adults. Older people often have a decreased thirst sensation and renal function and reduced total body water. All of these factors increase the risk of becoming dehydrated.

Fluid intake in older people

For sedentary living, a formula to determine appropriate fluid intake is as follows:

- 1.5 l for the first 20 kg of body weight.
- 15 ml additional fluid for every additional kg of weight.

Therefore a 40 kg person should have a fluid intake of 1.8 l and an 80 kg person an intake of 2.4 l.

Most older patients take up to a litre of fluid in the form of solids.

Fluid intake should increase if the older person is exposed to higher temperatures inside or outside of the care home.

Causes of dehydration in older people

Poor fluid intake, for example:

1. Acute illness such as infection (e.g. urinary tract or chest infection).
2. Impaired access to drinks, poor mobility and decreased functional ability, which can result in difficulty reaching for fluids, holding a glass or drinking.
3. Lack of thirst sensation, for example in advanced dementia.
4. A poor swallow technique. This may be a result of stroke, dementia, or general illness.
5. Fear of incontinence and therefore a reluctance to take fluids.
6. Sedation secondary to medications, such as sleeping tablets.
7. Depression.

Losing too many fluids, for example:

1. Vomiting or diarhoea.
2. Fever and perspiration.
3. Medications – especially diuretics.
4. Warm climate or increased room temperature.

Dehydration in younger adults is often recognised by decreased skin turgor and a dry mouth. Because older adults lose skin elasticity, it can be more difficult

The Care Home Handbook, First Edition. Edited by Graham Mulley, Clive Bowman, Michal Boyd and Sarah Stowe.
© 2015 John Wiley & Sons, Ltd. Published 2015 by John Wiley & Sons, Ltd.

to assess skin turgor. Mouth breathing is more common and therefore a dry mouth is not necessarily a sign of dehydration.

Common symptoms or signs suggesting dehydration

1. Delirium (increased confusion) (see Chapter 10.2).
2. Lethargy.
3. Decreased functional ability.
4. Constipation or faecal impaction.
5. Dark or concentrated urine.
6. Weight loss.
7. Low blood pressure.
8. Sunken eyeballs.
9. The individual looks dry.

Requirements to ensure adequate hydration

1. Ensure that fresh fluids are readily available, for example by having accessible water dispensers and jugs.
2. Consider adding additional fluids to meals, for example extra milk to rice pudding.
3. Regular toileting of residents who are at risk of incontinence will reduce the fear of it.
4. Ensure that oral hygiene is maintained (see Chapter 17.5).

Managing dehydration

1. Discuss medication with the resident's GP. It may be possible to reduce or stop diuretics (e.g. Furosamide or Bumetanide).
2. Commence a fluid balance chart to monitor intake.
3. Encourage oral fluids.
4. If there is concern about swallow safety, then a review by a Speech and Language therapist may be necessary (see Chapter 5.2). Thickened fluids may be advised to make swallowing easier and safer.
5. Some residents may require intermittent use of subcutaneous fluids.
6. A blood test may be necessary to confirm the extent of dehydration.

Using subcutaneous fluids (hypodermoclysis)

Administering fluids subcutaneously is an alternative option to the traditional intravenous route for giving fluids. It can benefit the older person who is unable to take a sufficient oral intake of fluid during periods of infection or other inter-current illness. It can help to avoid the need for admission to hospital.

Giving fluids subcutaenously involves the insertion of a small gauge butterfly cannulae under aseptic conditions into subcutaneous tissue.

Local protocols for the use of subcutaneous fluids should be available.

Case history

Mrs A is an 85 year old resident. She has a history of osteoarthritis and very limited mobility. Her most recent MMSE is 20/30. Over the past few days, she has been generally unwell, lethargic and less interactive. She does not recognise her family members. Her bowels have not openend for three days. Her oral intake of fluids is now less than 400 ml per day. On examination, her urine is dark and dipstick testing shows protein, leucocytes and nitrates.

Impression

A urinary tract infection may have contributed to a diminished sensation of thirst. Dehydration will have compounded her constipation. Constipation will further reduce her sensation of thirst.

Mrs A has features of delirium (see Chapter 10.2). The factors contributing to her delirium are infection, dehydration and constipation. Unfortunately, the delirium will also further reduce her sensation of thirst.

Plan

Mrs A should be gently encouraged to take oral fluids throughout the day. A fluid balance chart should be kept. It is likely that she will need subcutaneous fluids for at least a few days to ensure that she has a minimum fluid intake of 1.5 litres per day. Mrs A will benefit from a medication review. She will need an antibiotic for her urinary tract infection and laxatives for her constipation.

Outcome

Following the treatment of her urinary tract infection, constipation and dehydration, Mrs A will hopefully slowly improve over a number of days. She may not return to her normal self for a few weeks. It is important to remain alert to the likelihood that her dehydration and constipation may recur and continue to encourage oral fluids and monitor fluid balance.

Further reading

Barton A, Fuller R, Dudley N. 2004. Using subcutaneous fluids to rehydrate older people: current practices and future challenges. *Quarterly Journal of Medicine* 97: 765–768.

Chidester JC, Spangler AA. 1997. Fluid intake in the institutionalised elderly. *Journal of the American Dietary Association* 1: 23–28.

5.4 Urinary incontinence

Adrian Wagg

University of Alberta, Edmonton, Alberta, Canada

Key points

- Ask all residents if they have any problem with continence. If it is difficult to obtain an answer, then seek information from family or friends, or other care home staff.
- A comprehensive continence assessment is highly desirable to inform care plans and ensure incontinence products, such as pads, are appropriately used.
- Proactively seek to treat continence problems: evidence suggests benefit, even in the most frail elderly people.
- There is probably no reason to assume that interventions which work in community dwelling older people (pelvic floor exercises, bladder training) should not do so in frail elderly residents, but regard should be made to potential benefits, harm and feasibility.

Urinary incontinence (UI) assessment

- *Obtain a history* – obtain type and timing of signs and symptoms. These signs and symptoms are divided into three main categories: *bladder storage* problems, *voiding* and *post-micturition (post-voiding)* problems, such as urinary retention (Box 5.4.1).
- *Treat, or arrange for treatment, of underlying causes* – If the incontinence is new, consider causes which might be reversible (Box 5.4.2).
- Do *not* treat asymptomatic bacteriuria (a positive urinalysis or mid-stream specimen of urine with 10^5 bacteria); it won't help and just exposes an individual to the risk of more complex infection.
- Think about other medical problems which the resident has which might affect continence status (Box 5.4.3). Assess and refer as appropriate.
- *Make a diagnosis* – patterns of symptoms which lead to common urinary incontinence diagnoses are shown in Box 5.4.4. Some residents may not empty their bladder fully. This may be of no importance, but may lead to increased frequency, or – if the bladder is continually full – to overflow incontinence, where there is a constant, frequent dribbling loss. Remember to feel the abdomen to estimate the size of the bladder but, more importantly, *if you suspect that the resident may not be emptying their bladder, arrange for a measurement of post-void residual volume using a bladder scan.*

Sometimes very confused or immobile residents may urinate in inappropriate places, but otherwise may be continent – this is called *functional incontinence.*

Ensure the toilets are clearly labelled and familiarise residents with their location.

Think about using urinals for convenience and a secure bedside commode for night time.

Box 5.4.1 Lower urinary tract symptoms

Storage	Voiding	Post-micturition
Frequency (>8)	Hesitancy	Incomplete emptying
Nocturia (>2)	Straining	Post-micturition dribbling
Urgency	Intermittent stream	
Urgency incontinence	Poor stream	
Exertional (stress) incontinence	Terminal dribble	

The Care Home Handbook, First Edition. Edited by Graham Mulley, Clive Bowman, Michal Boyd and Sarah Stowe.
© 2015 John Wiley & Sons, Ltd. Published 2015 by John Wiley & Sons, Ltd.

Box 5.4.2 Reversible causes of urinary incontinence

- **D**elirium
- **I**nfection (acute urinary tract infection)
- **P**harmaceuticals (review medicines)
- **P**sychological (depression, withdrawal)
- **E**xcess urine output (polyuria)
- **R**educed mobility
- **S**tool impaction
  (and other environmental factors)

Box 5.4.3 Co-existing medical conditions potentially affecting continence status

- *Functional impairment*
- *Cognitive impairment*
- Recurrent urinary infection
- Constipation
- Arthritis
- Falls/hip fracture
- Contractures
- Peripheral vascular disease
- Stroke
- Parkinson's disease
- Dementia
- Diabetes mellitus
- Congestive heart failure
- Venous insufficiency
- Chronic lung disease

Box 5.4.4 Characteristics of common types of incontinence

Characteristic	Stress incontinence	Urgency incontinence
Exertional loss (coughing, straining)	Common	Untypical (but resident may have 'mixed incontinence')
Sudden uncontrollable urge	Uncommon	Common/typical
Frequency	Uncommon	Common
Nocturia	Uncommon	Common
Volume lost	Typically small	May be large

Diagnosis

There is no harm in making a symptomatic diagnosis of the cause of urinary incontinence and starting treatment based upon that while you await a more detailed assessment. Remember, *management* should take into account the *degree of bother* to the resident and/or carer, their *goals for care*, level of cooperation, and the *overall prognosis and life expectancy*.

Red flag findings

Remember the things that should immediately prompt your referral to a specialist:

- *pain on passing urine (dysuria)* (see Chapter 8.6),
- blood in the urine (haematuria),
- a visible bulge beyond the opening of the vagina (prolapse).

Treatment

The initial treatment for urinary incontinence in frail older people (DuBeau et al., 2010) is shown in Figure 5.4.1.

Initial treatment should be individualized and influenced by *goals of care, treatment preferences*, and *estimated remaining life expectancy*, as well as the most likely clinical diagnosis.

For some residents, management with pads may be the only possible solution for UI (after treatment of contributing co-morbidity and associated factors). This is especially true for residents who have no or minimal mobility (require the assistance of at least two people to transfer) or have advanced dementia (unable to state their own name).

Maintenance of mobility is extremely important and valuable in continence management for the frail elderly resident (see Chapter 6.1).

Conservative and behavioural therapy for UI includes:

- adequate hydration,
- caffeine restriction,
- weight maintenance,
- bladder training for the more fit or alert residents,
- prompted voiding (Box 5.4.5) for those who are frailer and more cognitively impaired,
- for selected, more cognitively able frail persons, pelvic muscle exercises may be considered, but they have not been well studied in this population.

For urgency incontinence, ask the physician about a trial of anti-muscarinic drugs such as darifenacin, fesoterodine, propiverine, solifenacin, tolterodine or trospium, avoiding high dose oxybutynin. These are all effective agents, but common side-effects include dry mouth, constipation, heartburn and, occasionally, blurred vision.

Similarly, α-blockers such as tamsulosin or alfuzosin may be cautiously considered in frail men with suspected outlet obstruction from prostate disease. Care needs to be taken as some people experience postural hypotension with these drugs (see Chapter 6.6). The first dose should ideally be given just before bed.

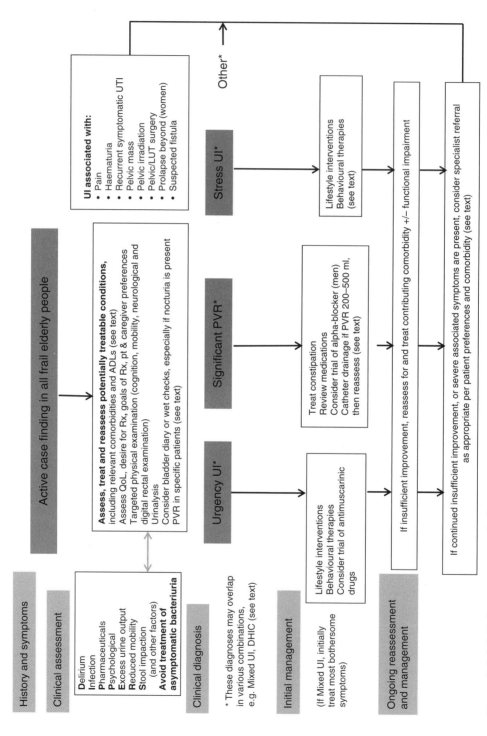

History and symptoms

Clinical assessment

Delirium
Infection
Pharmaceuticals
Psychological
Excess urine output
Reduced mobility
Stool impaction
(and other factors)
Avoid treatment of asymptomatic bacteriuria

Clinical diagnosis

* These diagnoses may overlap in various combinations, e.g. Mixed UI, DHIC (see text)

Initial management

(If Mixed UI, initially treat most bothersome symptoms)

Ongoing reassessment and management

Active case finding in all frail elderly people

Assess, treat and reassess potentially treatable conditions,
including relevant comorbidities and ADLs (see text)
Assess QoL, desire for Rx, goals of Rx, pt & caregiver preferences
Targeted physical examination (cognition, mobility, neurological and digital rectal examination
Urinalysis
Consider bladder diary or wet checks, especially if nocturia is present
PVR in specific patients (see text)

UI associated with:
• Pain
• Haematuria
• Recurrent symptomatic UTI
• Pelvic mass
• Pelvic irradiation
• Pelvic/LUT surgery
• Prolapse beyond (women)
• Suspected fistula

Urgency UI*

Significant PVR*

Stress UI*

Other*

Lifestyle interventions
Behavioural therapies
Consider trial of antimuscarinic drugs

Treat constipation
Review medications
Consider trial of alpha-blocker (men)
Catheter drainage if PVR 200–500 ml, then reassess (see text)

Lifestyle interventions
Behavioural therapies (see text)

If insufficient improvement, reassess for and treat contributing comorbidity +/- functional impairment

If continued insufficient improvement, or severe associated symptoms are present, consider specialist referral as appropriate per patient preferences and comorbidity (see text)

Figure 5.4.1 Initial management of urinary incontinence in frail older people. *Post-voiding residual urine.

Box 5.4.5 Behavioural management of UI

Prompted voiding:

involves prompts to toilet with positive reinforcement when successful, and is designed to increase resident requests for toileting and self-initiated toileting, and decrease the number of UI episodes.

Habit retraining:

requires the identification of the incontinent person's individual toileting pattern, including UI episodes, usually by means of a bladder diary. A toileting schedule is then devised to pre-empt UI episodes. There is no attempt in habit retraining to alter the voiding pattern.

Timed voiding:

involves toileting an individual at fixed intervals, such as every 3 hours. This is considered a passive toileting programme; no attempts are made at patient education or reinforcement of behaviours, or to re-establish voiding patterns. Other terms used to describe timed voiding are scheduled toileting, routine toileting, and fixed toileting.

Combined toileting and exercise therapy:

functional intervention rtaining incorporates strengthening exercises into toileting routines by nursing assistants. Another combination intervention, administered by occupational or physical therapist, involves toileting and mobility skills.

DDAVP (vasopressin) used to treat nocturia or nocturnal polyuria has high risk of causing hyponatraemia (low serum sodium levels) and should be only used in specialist hands with close monitoring.

Pads, catheters and appliances

The use of pads, catheters and appliances may be a pragmatic solution to the management of intractable incontinence when all other methods have failed, or at end of life.

Due regard should be made to the pattern of incontinence when pad choice is made, and a combination of sizes and absorbencies may be needed for discrete, acceptable use by day and night.

The resident's manual dexterity should be taken into account if self changes are required.

The use of bedside commodes and male or female urinals may make continence an achievable goal in an otherwise intractable condition.

An additive super absorbent powder such as 'Vernagel' may be very useful to avoid spillage from urinals. Your continence advisor should be able to give practical advice on the availability of appliance.

Ongoing assessment and management

Optimal UI management can usually be achieved by a combination of the above approaches. If initial management does not provide sufficient improvement, then the first step should be to reassess for and treat contributing co-morbidity and/or functional impairment.

A template referral letter to a continence advisor is in a later section (see Chapter 17.9).

References

DuBeau, CE, Kuchel GA, Johnson T, et al. 2010. Incontinence in the frail elderly: report from the 4th International Consultation on Incontinence. *Neurourology and Urodynamics* 29: 165–178.

Further reading

Newman DK. 2004. Incontinence products and devices for the elderly. *Urology Nursing* 24(4): 316–333; quiz, 334.

Ostaszkiewicz J, Johnston L, Roe B. 2005. Timed voiding for the management of urinary incontinence in adults. *Journal of Urology* 173: 1262–1263.

Palmer MH, 2005. Effectiveness of prompted voiding for incontinent nursing home residents, in *Evidence-based Practice in Nursing & Healthcare: A Guide to the Best Practice*, EF-O BM Melnyk,(Ed.), Lippincott Williams & Williams, p. 20–30.

Palmer MH, 2004. Use of health behavior change theories to guide urinary incontinence research. *Nursing Resources* 53(6 Suppl): S49–55.

Roe B, Milne J, Ostaszkiewicz J, et al. 2007. Systematic reviews of bladder training and voiding programmes in adults: a synopsis of findings on theory and methods using metastudy techniques. *Journal of Advanced Nursing* 57: 3–14.

Schnelle, JF, MacRae PG, Ouslander JG, et al. 1995. Functional Incidental Training, mobility performance, and incontinence care with nursing home residents. *Journal of the American Geriatric Society* 43: 1356–1362.

van Houten P, Achterberg W, Ribbe, M. 2007. Urinary incontinence in disabled elderly women: a randomized clinical trial on the effect of training mobility and toileting skills to achieve independent toileting. *Gerontology* 53: 205–210.

5.5 Faecal soiling, constipation and stoma care

Stephanie Robinson[1] and Rónán Collins[2]

[1] Department of Age Related Healthcare, Adelaide and Meath Hospital, Dublin, Ireland
[2] Adelaide and Meath Hospital, Dublin, Ireland

Key points

- All residents should have a bowel habit record.
- Faecal impaction is the commonest cause of faecal incontinence.
- Any change in bowel habit should prompt a comprehensive assessment.
- Management is multi-disciplinary involving nursing, clinical nutrition, medical, physiotherapy, occupational therapy and pharmacy staff.
- Medications commonly affect bowel function and should be reviewed regularly.

Constipation, diarrhoea and faecal incontinence are common in care homes and are at the core of nursing care planning.

Principles of promoting a normal bowel habit in the care home

- All health and care providers supporting people resident in care homes have an obligation to promote faecal continence.
- Residents should have a bowel chart with an individualised bowel programme.
- Exercise and physical activity are encouraged to promote physiological bowel function.
- Residents should be encouraged to toilet coinciding with maximum intestinal motility. This is usually after breakfast or mealtimes, taking advantage of the gastro-colic and gastro-duodenal reflexes.
- Residents should be accompanied to the toilet, if possible, rather than using a commode or bedpan.
- Ensure that toilet facilities are private, comfortable and can be used safely and without rush.
- A clinical nutritionist should play a role in meal planning where bowel health is problematic.
- Encourage fluid intake in all residents, except when there is a medical contraindication, such as fluid restriction in heart failure.
- Avoid constipation-causing medications (see Table 5.5.1).
- Avoid over-zealous use of laxatives.

Constipation

Constipation is very common in older adults but can generally be prevented in the care home. The term itself covers an array of symptoms including: reduced frequency of defecation, abnormally hard stool, reduced volume of stool, difficulty with passing stool and a sense that the rectum is not fully emptied. Residents and their carers often differ in their perception of the problem.

Diarrhoea

Diarrhoea is an increase in the frequency of bowel motion to more than three per day (see Chapter 13.7). It is often associated with an increase in stool fluid consistency. It should be categorised as an *acute* or a *chronic* problem according to the presence of symptoms for less than, or greater than, a period of three weeks.

Acute diarrhoea should always be presumed infectious in origin until proven otherwise.

Faecal soiling and incontinence

- Faecal incontinence is often a precipitating factor in a person's admission to care.
- It is a symptom, not a disease, and usually occurs in conjunction with urinary incontinence.

Table 5.5.1 Causes and solutions of faecal incontinence.

	Cause	Solutions
Constipation 30% of cases	• Overflow diarrhoea • Inadequate fluid/fibre • Immobility	• Treat constipation • Prevent recurrence • Involve clinical nutrition support in meal planning
Neurological disease Central or local	• Dementia • Stroke • Multiple sclerosis • Autonomic neuropathy (e.g. diabetic) • Spinal cord lesions	• Continence promotion policies • Individual programmes for patients
Gastrointestinal disease	• Diverticulitis • Diarrhoea • Infection • Inflammatory bowel disease (e.g. Crohn's, ulcerative colitis) • Rectal prolapse • Colonic or rectal tumours • Radiation enteritis • Prior surgical trauma	• Recognise symptoms early • Guided by acute clinician assessment
Environmental & lifestyle	• Immobility • Prolonged bed rest • Unsuitable toileting facilities • Alcohol intake	• Timely response to call bell • Promote comfort and privacy
Medications	See list in this section	Regular medications review

Table 5.5.2 Clinical assessment of bowels.

	To include:
History	Normal bowel habit, acute change(s), duration of new symptoms, precipitant(s), impact on quality of life.
Physical examination	General condition of the resident, including hydration status. External skin condition, external haemorrhoids, skin tags, rectal prolapse, gaping anus (may include a digital rectal examination to assess anal tone, sensation, presence of tumour or hard faeces).
Functional assessment and cognitive screen	Impaired cognition is common. Screen for superimposed delirium.
Medication review	See guidelines below.

- It is prevalent in nursing homes and is estimated to affect between 20 and 60% of residents.
- Incontinence affects quality of life and may lead to embarrassment and shame.
- Healthcare professionals can actively reduce the incidence of incontinence, and when it occurs work to alleviate its impact on patients' quality of life.

Faecal incontinence is 'the involuntary and inappropriate passage of bowel motion'. It can be divided into two subgroups; *urge incontinence* where the patient is aware of the need to pass faeces but is unable to hold it and *passive incontinence* where the person is unaware of the defecation process.

Understanding the causes of faecal incontinence is paramount to its management (Table 5.5.1).

Constipation with overflow diarrhoea is often associated with faecal staining.

Sudden changes in bowel pattern

A sudden change in bowel habit should always prompt a comprehensive clinical assessment as it usually indicates the development of bowel pathology (Table 5.5.2).

Medications and bowel pattern

Many medications interfere with normal bowel motility and should be reviewed regularly (Table 5.5.3).

Table 5.5.3 Medications interfering with bowel patterns.

Constipating drugs	Diarrhoea causing drugs
Codeine-based analgesics	Laxatives
Opiates	Antibiotics
Iron preparations	Antacids
Anti-cholinergics	Proton pump inhibitors
Diuretics	Non-steroidal anti-inflammatory drugs
Anti-depressants	Cholinergics, e.g. anti-dementia drugs
Anti-hypertensives	
Anti-spasmodics	

Stoma care in the care home

- Skin irritation and leakage are the most frequent problems encountered with stoma care.
- The fear of the latter is often a cause of great distress to patients.
- Skin damage arises from contact irritation or from trauma when removing the stoma bag.
- Regular hygiene, barrier creams and good stoma changing practices usually resolve issues.
- Avoid risk of leakage by ensuring an appropriately fitted appliance is used. Expert advice should be sought from the nearest stoma care specialist nurse.

Further reading

Fauci AS, Harrison TR. 1998. *Harrison's Principles of Internal Medicine*. McGraw-Hill, Health Professions Division.
Madoff RD, Parker SC, Varma MG, et al. 2004. Faecal incontinence in adults. *Lancet* 364(9434): 621–632.
Ouslander JG, Schnelle JF. 1995. Incontinence in the nursing home. *Annals of Internal Medicine* 122(6): 438–449.
Wagg A, Lowe D, Peel P, et al. 2008. Continence care for older people in England and Wales: data from a national audit. *Journal of Wound, Ostomy and Continence Nursing* 35: 215–220.

Useful web site

National Institute for Health and Clinical Excellence: The management of faecal incontinence in adults www.nice.org.uk/CG49 [Accessed September 2013]

5.6 Skin care

Rosie Callaghan

Stourport Health Centre, Stourport on Severn, UK

Key points

- Every resident should have a skin assessment on entry to the care home.
- Pressure ulcers affect the quality of life of many residents.
- The main aim of pressure ulcer management is prevention.

The functions of the skin

The skin is the largest organ in the body. It is made up of three layers:

- epidermis
- dermis
- subcutaneous tissue.

The functions of the skin are shown in Figure 5.6.1.

Skin changes with age

The elderly resident is more susceptible to skin damage and slower wound healing rates. Age-related skin changes include:

- *Pigmentation:* A decrease in the production of melanocytes causes this and increases the risk of skin cancer.
- *Thickness:* The dermal thickness reduces by 20% and the subcutaneous tissue has fewer fat cells.

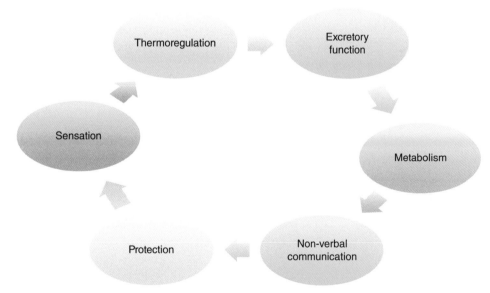

Figure 5.6.1 Functions of the skin.

The Care Home Handbook, First Edition. Edited by Graham Mulley, Clive Bowman, Michal Boyd and Sarah Stowe.
© 2015 John Wiley & Sons, Ltd. Published 2015 by John Wiley & Sons, Ltd.

- *Moisture:* There is a reduction in the number of sweat glands and the skin becomes dry, rough and flaky.
- *Turgor:* The skin tents/stands up when pinched.
- *Texture:* Increase in the number of creases and lines.

Extrinsic factors also affect the skin. These include:

- smoking
- chronic illness
- environmental pollutants
- ultra violet light
- decreased mobility
- drug-induced disorders.

All residents should have their skin assessed as part of their holistic assessment on admission. Principles of good skin care can be found in Figure 5.6.2.

This should be documented using a body map and a plan of care worked out.

We should endeavour to:

- Use warm, not hot, water.
- Use soap minimally, as soap changes the pH of the skin.
- Use soap after faecal incontinence.
- Avoid excess rubbing of fragile skin.
- Pat the skin dry.
- Keep the skin clean and dry:
  - Avoid wet wipes containing alcohol, as these dry the skin.

- Apply emollient regularly.
- Gently apply emollients; do not rub them into the skin.

Wound healing

There are three types of wound healing:

- Primary: these usually do not involve tissue loss (for example surgical wounds).
- Secondary: this involves tissue loss and heals by secondary intention (for example pressure ulcers).
- Tertiary: these can be left open for several days to allow drainage or oedema to subside and they heal by tertiary intention.

In order to achieve wound healing you need to:

- Be sure of your aim.
- Know what type of wound you are dealing with.
- Complete a comprehensive assessment.

Figure 5.6.3 illustrates what should be included in this assessment.

The wound assessment should include:

- Type of injury: acute or chronic.
- Accurate history of the wound.
- Category of wound: leg ulcer, pressure ulcer, laceration and so on.

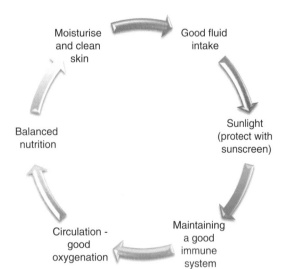

Figure 5.6.2 Principles of good skin care.

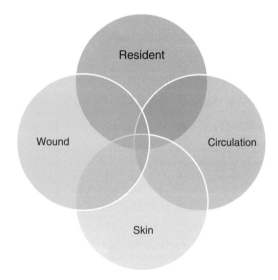

Figure 5.6.3 Assessment of wound healing.

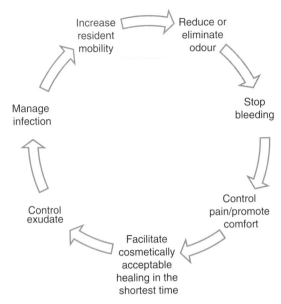

Figure 5.6.4 Know what your wound objectives are.

- Position of the wound.
- Size of the wound.
- Method of closure, drains and so on.
- Clinical appearance:
  - colour of the wound bed
  - colour and amount of exudate
  - pain assessment
  - signs of infection.

See Figure 5.6.4. Dressing selection can then be made in order to meet these objectives.

Remember:

- The wound must be kept warm, at an optimum temperature for wound healing.
- The wound must be kept moist and not dry or excessively wet with exudate.
- The wound should be left as undisturbed as possible.
- *There is not one wound dressing that satisfies all wounds and the dressing may not take a wound through all the phases of wound healing.*

Dressing selection

First establish what you need your dressing to do. Is it to:

- Remove necrosis?
- Remove slough?
- Promote granulation?
- Promote epithelialisation?
- Control exudates?
- Control the bacterial load?

The appropriate dressing can then be selected.

Pressure ulcers (previously called pressure sores/decubitus ulcers/bedsores)

- Pressure ulcers affect about 20% of care home residents.
- A resident's risk of developing a pressure ulcer should be assessed on admission to the care home, then monthly (more often if there is a deterioration in their health).
- Most pressure ulcers are avoidable and the best management is prevention.
- Most pressure ulcers occur over bony prominences, the most common of these being the sacrum and heels.
- They can also occur where medical devices, such as masks or catheters, press into the body.
- They can be painful and unpleasant and can affect the quality of life of residents.
- The total cost of treatment in the UK is estimated to be £1.4–£2.1 billion annually, comprising 4% of total NHS expenditure.

The causes of pressure ulcers are shown in Figure 5.6.5.

- *Pressure* usually occurs over a bony prominence, such as the hip, sacrum or heel. However, pressure can occur wherever the tissue becomes compressed, such as with the use of a splint.
- *Shear* is where the skeleton and underlying tissue move but the skin remains stuck to a point on the surface, as can occur when the resident slips down the bed. This dragging effect occludes the blood vessels.

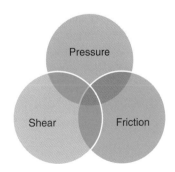

Figure 5.6.5 Causes of pressure ulcers.

- *Friction* is where two surfaces move or rub across one another, as occurs with a new pair of shoes and the development of a blister. This can cause superficial tissue damage.

These processes can occur in isolation or together.

Other intrinsic factors that also are known to contribute to the development of pressure ulcers are:

- extreme age
- limited mobility
- vascular disease
- sensory impairment
- malnutrition
- dehydration
- previous pressure damage.

Assessment and management of pressure ulcers

It is important to accurately assess the resident and the pressure ulcer. This should include assessment and documentation of:

- Category of ulcer.
- Location.
- Size, shape and any undermining/ tracking (were the ulcer travels under the skin surface, often horizontally).
- Wound bed: type of visible tissue, for example necrotic, granulation.
- Exudate level and consistency.
- Pain.
- Skin condition around the wound.
- Malodour (see Chapter 2.9).
- Signs of infection.

The European pressure ulcer advisory panel (see Useful web sites) is the most widely used system for describing the depth and extent of the ulcer:

Category 1

Non-blanchable redness of intact skin, usually over a bony prominence. There may be:

- discoloration of the skin
- warmth
- oedema
- hardness or pain compared to the adjacent tissue.

Category 2

Partial thickness (superficial) skin loss or blister.

Category 3

Full thickness tissue loss (deep).
Subcutaneous fat may be visible, but no underlying structures such as tendon or bone are visible.

Category 4

Full thickness tissue loss with bone/tendon/underlying prosthesis visible.

It is important to remember that red means danger.

If the red area goes white when finger pressure is applied, and then returns red, this is a warning to relieve the pressure or damage will occur.

If the red area stays red when finger pressure is applied, then the microcirculation has already been damaged and it is a category 1 ulcer.

All residents should be encouraged to change position regularly. There is no set regime for this, as every resident will have different needs.

Following a risk assessment, and taking into account the resident's mobility, if a pressure ulcer is present then the appropriate pressure relief mattress and chair cushion should be selected.

Useful web sites

European Pressure Ulcer Advisory Panel
http://www.epuap.org/guidelines/Final_Quick_
    Treatment.pdf [Accessed 30 September 2013
www.judy-waterlow.co.uk [Accessed September 2013]
Information, facts and advice, with details of 'Your Turn', a
    UK national movement working to reduce the number of
    pressure ulcers.
National Institute for Health and Clinical Excellence (NICE).
    The Prevention and Treatment of Pressure Ulcers.
    National clinical guidelines on the prevention and treat-
    ment of pressure ulcers 29 September 2005
www.nice.org.uk/nicemedia/pdf/CG029publicinfo.pdf
    [Accessed September 2013]

5.7 Personal grooming

Angela Juby[1] and Sandra Kavanagh[2]

[1]*Division of Geriatrics, University of Alberta, Edmonton, Alberta, Canada*
[2]*South Terrace Continuing Care Centre, Edmonton, Alberta, Canada*

Key points

- Personal grooming can make a resident look and feel better.
- Ascertain the previous grooming habits of the resident.
- Grooming is best done by a caregiver who knows the resident.
- Patience and flexibility is vital – grooming should not be rushed.

Personal grooming includes those aspects of care that ensure that residents have a neat, tidy and pleasant appearance. Examples are hair care, attention to nails and teeth, personal preferences with clothing, removal of ear wax, use of make-up, and shaving or removing facial and body hair.

Personal grooming is often done with the help of care assistants, but it is important that trained nurses are also involved as this is an opportunity to listen to individuals' concerns and look for changes in their general condition.

While residents usually enjoy being groomed, some may resist attempts to help them look attractive.

Grooming procedures

A team approach to grooming is important as it allows for care to be performed when the resident is most amenable (such as *nail cutting and shaving*).

Cleaning hearing aids regularly and checking battery function as well as inspecting the *ear canal* for wax is important for optimal hearing function.

Cleaning *spectacles* is similarly important to maximise safe function and independence. Eye glasses should be clearly labelled to prevent a mix up with other residents, as the dementia resident may not be able to verbalise their lack of visual function caused by wearing incorrect glasses – or not wearing their customary spectacles.

Hair care can include regular washing, cleaning, styling, gentle brushing or combing to remove tangles. In the early stages of dementia, hair styling can

significantly enhance the resident's mood, self-esteem and quality of life. The scalp should be examined during washing for any skin lesions or infections.

Make-up use is best based on the resident's previous normal practice. If this was something they used to do, those still able should be encouraged to still apply their own. In others, simple application of lipstick can enhance the mood, self-esteem and behaviour of residents.

Shaving should be personalized: some men prefer wet shaving, others electric razors; some wish to be shaved once a day, others twice; some may wish to have a day without being shaved. Women who have troublesome facial hair may prefer depilatory creams to being shaved: ask the resident for their preference and ensure that the procedure is done in private in a sensitive way to minimise embarrassment.

Oral/dental care

Dental care is the most important aspect of grooming, as dental health affects global health (see Chapter 17.5). For people with dementia this can be very challenging because it may cause anxiety and resistance.

Those residents with teeth

Most residents will have some of their own teeth.

Preventing gingivitis (red, swollen, bleeding gums) is important. Gingivitis is due to deposition of plaque, from food debris on the teeth that becomes infected. If left untreated the deposits of plaque harden to form tartar (hard, chalky, white substance). This is not

The Care Home Handbook, First Edition. Edited by Graham Mulley, Clive Bowman, Michal Boyd and Sarah Stowe.
© 2015 John Wiley & Sons, Ltd. Published 2015 by John Wiley & Sons, Ltd.

removable with simple brushing and will require the intervention of a dental professional. Thus, good *early preventive dental care* is important.

The approach to residents for dental care will depend on the stage of dementia, as well as the presence of any behavioral problems. More specific information is provided by Alzheimer's UK (see Useful web sites).

Residents with dentures

Oral care is also important for individuals who have *dentures*. Dentures loosen over time as the gum bones shrink (a natural part of ageing, worsened when there are no teeth present). Loose dentures may make eating more difficult than not wearing dentures at all and just using the gums to eat a soft diet. Each resident will need to be individually assessed in this regard.

When dentures are worn for eating, it is not unusual for food to become lodged underneath the denture plate. This leads to increased oral bacteria (and the health risks mentioned for those with unclean teeth) but can also cause agitation and distress as it is very uncomfortable.

Oral infections can also occur under the denture, including oral thrush (candidiasis). This can be extremely painful and uncomfortable for the resident, and could result in a blood infection if left untreated.

Dentures should be removed and cleaned after every meal or snack. They should be removed and soaked in denture cleaner overnight. Oral care still needs to be done in the mouth (once the dentures are removed) to ensure no trapped food debris remains between the gums and cheeks.

Residents with dementia should be given the opportunity to insert and remove their own dentures when they are able, as this is much easier and more comfortable for them.

Cleaning the mouth with an antiseptic oral mouthwash is useful for all residents and will reduce the level of bacterial colonisation in the mouth.

Personal grooming of residents who have behavioral problems

Personal grooming of a resident can be extremely challenging if the person is delirious of demented, or if, for other reasons (such as deafness), the individual misunderstands what the caregivers are trying to do

to them. Some residents resist attempts to groom them, and the procedure can be distressing both to the resident and staff.

Decreasing resident resistance

- The method of approach to the resident is paramount.
- The demeanour of the care provider sets the tone for whether this care will be possible.
- Taking time is important to reduce the risk of resistance.
- A calm and friendly approach helps put the resident at ease.
- Staff should adapt to the resident's schedule and not have a preset agenda of their own.

Promoting safety

Given the proximity to eyes, nose and mouth, safety of both the care provider and resident is important to prevent injury to either party.

Suggestions for improving safety when helping the resident with hygiene include:

- Encourage cooperation through providing a personal approach for each resident.
- Provide a distraction by conversation with the resident, or singing a song that is familiar to them. Give them enough time to do as much as possible for themselves, for example encouraging them wash their face; placing their clothes on their bed in a logical order.
- The presence of the family, or a familiar person, can be helpful in challenging situations.
- Prioritise the care. For example, oral care should take priority over shaving or nail care. Pneumonia is a common illness in nursing homes. Research has shown that *good oral care significantly reduces the number of cases of pneumonia in this vulnerable population*. Data also suggest that *a healthy oral state may reduce the development and severity of systemic diseases such as heart disease and diabetes*.

Useful web sites

http://www.agedcareaustralia.gov.au/internet/agedcare/publishing.nsf/Content/Tips+for+carers-2 [Accessed September 2013]

http://alzheimers.org.uk/site/scripts/documents_info.php?documentID=138 [Accessed September 2013]

5.8 Washing and dressing

Pauline Breslin[1] and Anne Houghton[2]

[1] Sunnyside Nursing Home, Castleford, UK
[2] Leeds South and East Clinical Commissioning Group, Leeds, UK

Key points

- Sensitivity in dealing with the intimate procedures of washing and dressing is paramount for a continuing good relationship with the resident.
- Always ask the resident's permission before helping them to wash or dress.
- Use this opportunity to listen to the resident's concerns and to look for signs of dehydration or disease.
- If the resident requires two people to help with bathing or dressing, do not attempt to do these tasks single-handedly.

Washing and dressing

- These everyday activities provide the healthcare professional with an opportunity to observe, assess and listen to residents.
- They are intimate acts of care which require permission, cooperation and confidence in the carer's ability, and are often an opportunity to assess the wider health needs of the resident. Use this opportunity to ensure that the axillae are moist, that there are no pressure sores (check the buttocks, sacrum and heels)(Chapter 5.6), the abdomen is soft and that there are no breast lumps.
- Talking and listening to the resident while carefully performing these basic tasks can often elicit important information as to how the resident feels.

Preparation

Before washing and dressing a resident:

- Check the care plan for recommended skin care and application of prescribed topical preparations.
- Remember that soap has a drying effect and is not always the desired toiletry - soap substitutes may be used.
- Ensure the environment is comfortable, with no draughts from open windows, and that the door is closed.
- Promote privacy and dignity. Some residents may never have been seen without their clothes on and are vulnerable. Bath towels can be used to provide as much cover and warmth as necessary.
- Consideration should be given to involving same sex carers, if they are available.

Care staff should check skin, nails, hair and ears while assisting a resident to wash.

- Look for changes in colour and texture of skin.
- Use warm water and always clean thoroughly, ensuring folds and skin creases are included.
- Never rub vigorously, as ageing skin can become dry and fragile. Rubbing can cause skin tears and bruising.
- Keep finger nails trim and clean (with permission).
- Do not cut toe nails as this is the role of the chiropodist (podiatrist). (Remember that in residents with diabetes or with poor circulation, trauma to the feet can have severe consequences.)
- Remove hearing aids if necessary to clean the ears, but remember that the resident cannot now hear you. Check the ears for accumulated wax (discuss clearing wax with the resident's GP) and reinsert the aids, ensuring that they are working properly and that the resident can now hear you.
- Check the condition of the hair and scalp and organise hair washing or visit to the hairdresser for cutting and styling.
- Check if the eyes are sticky and, if so, gently wipe them with moist cotton wool.
- Always dry the resident carefully and thoroughly with attention to skin folds.

The Care Home Handbook, First Edition. Edited by Graham Mulley, Clive Bowman, Michal Boyd and Sarah Stowe.
© 2015 John Wiley & Sons, Ltd. Published 2015 by John Wiley & Sons, Ltd.

Dental care

- Offer tooth brush and paste to the resident or gently and thoroughly brush teeth.
- Ensure dentures are removed, cleaned and fitted back into the mouth correctly.
- Check the mouth for infection or soreness. As residents age, their gums can shrink and dentures become loose and rub. Ill-fitting dentures cause pain and an inability to enjoy and eat food properly, and can make residents miserable and lead to weight loss.
- Dentures can become mislaid or mixed up. Prompt referral to the dentist may be required (see Chapter 17.5).

Independence

Residents will have varying levels of independence and some may be able to perform some washing and dressing activities unaided.

Offer support in order to promote as much independence as possible, as this contributes to a resident's self-esteem. Offer choice in selection of clothing and ensure that dressing is assisted if required.

Take care with moving arthritic and paralysed limbs, as damage can be done to joints, causing pain and injury to residents.

Lifting, moving and handling

Some residents are unable to assist with washing and dressing. Ensure that you are aware of the mobility and abilities of the resident. They may not have a good sitting balance, and may not remember that they have a paralysed arm or leg. Safe moving and handling can prevent injuries and falls. *If there is a need for two assistants to wash and dress a resident, never undertake these procedures alone.*

Ensure all carers know how to move a resident who requires hoisting and that appropriate seating for the needs of the residents are used at all times (see Chapter 6.2).

Carers must ensure safe lifting, moving and handling of residents and must also be responsible for their own health and safety. This includes the situation in which a resident becomes uncooperative or aggressive (see Chapter 3.3).

Occasionally, residents may claim physical or sexual abuse. If there are any concerns, ensure that solo carers are not used and any comments and/or complaints are recorded, investigated and the care plans amended (see Chapter 4.3).

Further reading

Cohen-Mansfield J, Creedon M, Malone T, et al. 2006. Dressing of the cognitively impaired nursing home residents: description and analysis. *Gerontologist* 46: 88–96.

Beck C, Heacock P, Mercer SO, et al. 1997. Improving dressing behaviour in cognitively impaired nursing home residents. *Nursing Resources* 46: 126–132.

Section D

Common Clinical Conditions

Chapter 6

Mobility and Falls

6.1 Exercise and mobility

Miranda Jacobs and Marianne van Iersel

Radboud University, Nijmegen Medical Centre, The Netherlands

Key points

- Impaired mobility is one of the major issues in elderly care.
- It often has many causes and it is important to determine the reasons for poor mobility.
- Correct positioning is vital and may require the skills of a physiotherapist.
- Passive movements are not effective.
- Active movements should be encouraged wherever possible – exercise such as walking, dancing and Tai Chi could be considered.
- Try to organise individual exercise programmes – ideally, encouraging residents to exercise for 30 minutes, five days a week.

Impaired mobility

Mobility problems can impair many activities in daily life; from the basics, such as transfers in and out of a bed or chair and getting to the toilet, to being able to participate in leisure activities and visit friends and family.

- Sometimes a decrease in mobility has a single reason, such as a stroke or a broken hip. More often it is multifactorial.
- When there are more debilitating factors than compensating mechanisms, a resident can find him/herself in a downwards spiral.
- The good thing is that with the appropriate treatment, improvement is possible in many residents.

For causes of a sudden loss of mobility, please see the list printed in bold in Figure 6.1.1 *and inform a physician.*

Impaired mobility: what to assess and discuss in the multidisciplinary team as a nurse

- Level of mobility, for example: bedbound, transfer with one person, use of a walking aid.

- Pain (at rest and with movement): location, intensity, aggravating and relieving factors.
- Unsafe situations/risk of falling.
- Motivation/behaviour.
- Signs of complications: pressure sores? Constipation? Incontinence? Fear of falling?

Positioning

In the case that a resident is poorly mobile, their positioning in a chair and in bed becomes more and more important.

The aim is to maintain as much function as possible.

The ideal position is highly individual and depends on the resident's abilities and limitations.

It should aim to:

- Provide a comfortable sitting position, without leaning forwards or sideways.
- Keep residents as independent as possible, for example in wheeling their own wheelchair, eating, or reading.
- Prevent pressure sores, contractures and increases in muscle tension.

Often a physiotherapist and occupational therapist will be involved in choosing the appropriate tools/equipment and adjusting them. Examples of equipment are

The Care Home Handbook, First Edition. Edited by Graham Mulley, Clive Bowman, Michal Boyd and Sarah Stowe.
© 2015 John Wiley & Sons, Ltd. Published 2015 by John Wiley & Sons, Ltd.

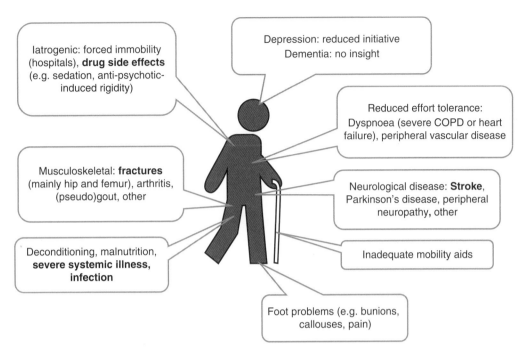

Iatrogenic: forced immobility (hospitals), **drug side effects** (e.g. sedation, anti-psychotic-induced rigidity)

Depression: reduced initiative
Dementia: no insight

Reduced effort tolerance: Dyspnoea (severe COPD or heart failure), peripheral vascular disease

Musculoskeletal: **fractures** (mainly hip and femur), arthritis, (pseudo)gout, other

Neurological disease: **Stroke**, Parkinson's disease, peripheral neuropathy**, other**

Deconditioning, malnutrition, **severe systemic illness, infection**

Inadequate mobility aids

Foot problems (e.g. bunions, callouses, pain)

Figure 6.1.1 Causes of impaired mobility.

different types of wheelchairs, seats, cushions and the type of mattress.

Outdated treatment

Passive movement therapy, previously recommended for prevention of contractures and muscle spasms, has no beneficial effects.

Exercise

'Use it or lose it', some key facts:

- Spending 10 days in bed equals 15 years of muscle ageing (decline in muscle mass and strength).
- Average physical activity in nursing home patients: a mean of 98.5 minutes/day as registered with questionnaires, but only 5.3 minutes/day as measured with an accelerometer (a device that measures actual movements of the limbs).

Why exercise?

A low level of physical activity is an important risk factor for ADL disability, immobility, diabetes, cardiovascular diseases and obesity. One way to improve physical fitness is exercise.

Exercise can also help to prevent the complications of immobility, such as muscle wasting and contractures, osteoporosis, constipation, incontinence, pressure sores, depression and social isolation.

How much exercise is enough?

To improve (note that this also applies to nursing home residents)

- Health in general: 30 minutes daily, 5 times a week.
- Strength, endurance, balance and functional performance: progressive resistance training 3 times a week, minimum of 45–60 minutes per session for 3 months.

How to achieve this?

- Walking on a treadmill and exercising on a home trainer.
- Functional training of walking and activities of daily living.
- Tai Chi and dancing, which improve balance, endurance and quality of life.
- Adopting a more physically active lifestyle.

Why older adults do or do not want to exercise

Over 80% of the adults have at least some resistance to exercise.

What can you do as a nurse to stimulate physical activities and prevent mobility loss?

Some tips:

- Make a daily programme with activities that involve movement/walking/exercise.
- Stimulate the resident to do as many of the ADL tasks themselves as possible and to walk all functional distances, if necessary with rests in between.
- Stimulate family and friends to walk with the resident, both indoors and (if possible) outside.
- In case of cognitive impairment: practise transfers or walking with an aid over and over again until it becomes automatic.
- In cases of acute illness: encourage the resident to get up into a chair again, for example initially three times daily before meals, to prevent pneumonia and deconditioning as far as possible.
- Do not be too concerned about the risk of falls (Chapter 6.6).

Barriers:

- Health problems and pain.
- Difficult access to exercise facilities.
- No physician recommendation or only general advice 'to be more physically active'.
- Cognitive impairment: forgetting advice.
- Perceive sweating and muscle aches as 'not good' or not 'lady like'.

What motivates exercise

- Recommending physical activities as a 'geriatric drug' and making it fun!
- Setting realistic goals to sustain the behaviour.

When to ask a physiotherapist for help

Signs of …

1. Deconditioning: quick exhaustion, dyspnoea on exertion
2. Instability: dangerous transfers, falling, fear of falling and moving
3. Immobility: being bedbound, needing a lot of assistance during transfers, stiffness, inactivity
4. Functional decline: acute or chronic diseases of the musculoskeletal system (for example osteoarthritis, intermittent claudication, vertebral and hip fractures, orthopaedic surgery) and chronic pulmonary or cardiac diseases

Further reading

Chen Y-M. 2010. Perceived barriers to physical activity among older adults residing in long-term care institutions. *Journal of Clinical Nursing* 19: 432–439.

Hobbelen JSM, Tan FES, Verhey FRJ, Koopmans TCM, de Bie RA. 2011. Passive movement therapy in severe paratonia: a multicenter randomized clinical trial. *International Psychogeriatrics*, onlineDOI:10.1017/S1041610211002468.

Opdenacker J, Delecluse C, Boen F. 2011. A 2-year follow-up of a lifestyle physical activity versus a structured exercise intervention in older adults. *Journal of the American Geriatric Society* 59: 1602–1611.

Rand D, Miller WC, Yiu J, Eng JJ. 2011. Tai Chi: Interventions for addressing low balance confidence in older adults: a systematic review and meta-analysis. *Age and Ageing* 40: 297–306.

Schutzer MG, Graves BS. 2004. Barriers and motivations to exercise in older adults. *Preventative Medicine* 39: 1056–1061.

Weening-Dijksterhuis E, de Greef M, Scherder E, Slaets J, van der Schans C. 2011. Frail institutionalized older persons: A comprehensive review on physical exercise, physical fitness, activities of daily living and quality of life. *American Journal of Physical Medical Rehabilitation* 90: 156–168.

6.2 Transferring: bed, chair, moving and handling

Audrey Redshaw and Michael Vassallo

Royal Bournemouth and Christchurch NHS Foundation Trust, Bournemouth, UK

Key points

- Correct moving and handling is essential to maintain the safety and dignity of residents.
- Incorrect moving and handling can cause injury to both residents and staff.
- The manual handling of residents requires careful preparation.
- A range of equipment is available to facilitate safe transfers – training must be undertaken before use.

In this chapter the correct techniques of transferring are explained and illustrated.

Incorrect moving and handling can cause distress and possible injury to residents. The correct approach, techniques and equipment can help to reduce these problems.

Musculoskeletal injuries to care givers can also result from inappropriate moving and handling. As well as back pain of the care giver, there could be problems with trauma, safety and comfort to the resident.

Back injuries are the most common cause of work-related sickness in care givers.

Receiving instruction in the correct techniques of moving and handling is therefore of paramount importance. Recourse should be sought from your manual handling trainers as they are the experts in safe handling techniques.

Risk assessment

An appropriate patient risk assessment should precede all manual handling tasks.

STILE

When faced with a manual handling task, it is essential to risk assess the situation under five headings using the acronym STILE.

- **S**ubject: many care home residents who require help with moving and handling will be frail and have complex needs. Person-centred care is central to optimum manual handling and a detailed awareness of the resident's medical conditions (stroke, arthritis, dementia, etc.) and of the individual are most important.
- **T**ask: refers to the evaluation of the task ahead, including the movements required and duration of effort.
- **I**ndividual capacity: do you have the experience and competence to undertake the task?
- **L**oad: evaluating features such as the resident's weight and size and their ability to assist.
- **E**nvironment: evaluating the space, lighting and flooring where the task has to be performed.

The 'sit to stand' transfer

Transferring means helping a resident to move from bed to chair; chair to bed, wheelchair, or other chair; chair or bed to a standing position.

If the resident is able to participate safely in a sit to stand transfer, then this should be encouraged. This manoeuvre can promote independence and maintains current mobility levels, as well as assisting care givers with the provision of personal care, bed linen changes and other activities.

Examples of handling equipment to facilitate sit to stand transfers include:

- Riser recliner chairs.
- 'Mangar' cushions (light, portable cushions which, by using low air pressure, gently lift even very heavy seated residents and enable them to stand from sitting more easily.
- Grab rails.

The Care Home Handbook, First Edition. Edited by Graham Mulley, Clive Bowman, Michal Boyd and Sarah Stowe.
© 2015 John Wiley & Sons, Ltd. Published 2015 by John Wiley & Sons, Ltd.

- Hand blocks or bed levers if getting up from a bed.
- Rotastand (a standing aid combined with turn assist).
- Standing aid hoist for mechanical assisted stand.

'Resident ability' criteria for safe sit to stand transfers

Before attempting a transfer, assess the resident's receptiveness to the idea of being moved in this way. Consider their dignity. Establish whether they need pain killers before the procedure.

The resident must be able to:

- Move from chair sitting to edge of chair/bed/plinth sitting.
- Maintain sitting balance.
- Place and maintain feet firmly on the floor.
- Achieve sit to stand – have the ability to take their own weight through their legs.
- Maintain a midline position when standing and sit upright unsupported.
- Be able to flex forward.
- Push-up off the bed or arms of the chair.
- Understand instructions.

The optimum start position:

- Resident is sitting in a chair or at the side of a bed/plinth.
- The handler is standing on the (weaker) side.
- The resident is wearing appropriate footwear.

Instructions to enable the resident to assist with the sit-to-stand manoeuvre (see Figure 6.2.1):

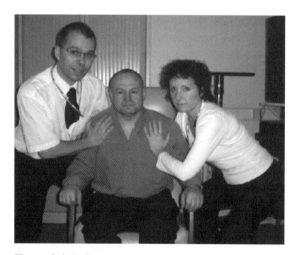

Figure 6.2.1 Correct sit to stand technique.

- Lean forward so that their back is away from the back of the chair.
- Shuffle their bottom towards the front of the chair/edge of the bed/plinth.
- Place their feet flat on the floor (weaker one slightly in front).
- Place their hands on the arms of the chair (or on the mattress, or just above their knees).
- They should lean forward so that their chin is over their knees, keep their head up, and look ahead not at the floor.
- Explain that when you say 'ready, steady, *stand*', you would like them to '*stand*': *push* with their hands and stand up.
- Say 'Is that OK?' (and wait for agreement/consent).
- 'Ready, steady, *stand*'.
- A gentle rocking motion can be used as the instructions 'ready, steady' are given.
- On the instruction '*stand*' the handler and the resident move together in the direction of movement – first forward and then upwards.
- The handler transfers their body weight from the back foot to the front foot or steps forward with the back foot.
- Stand next to the person for a moment – making sure they are not feeling dizzy before asking him/her to move.

Sit to stand transfer (Smith, 2011)

Preparation of the environment/equipment:

- Ensure brakes are on if standing up from a wheeled item of furniture.
- Ensure the area is free from trip hazards.
- If standing up from a high/low bed, it may assist if the bed is raised slightly.

Preparation of the handler:

- Stand beside the resident, facing the direction of movement.
- Adopt a stable base with feet slightly apart and the outer foot ahead.
- Flex hips and knees to lower position.
- If the resident does not meet the criteria, further assessment is required so a safe transfer can be completed.

Completion

Check that the resident is comfortable and free from distress:

- Ensure the resident is balanced and safe in the final sitting position, with correct body and limb alignment.

Standing a resident who is unable to take their own weight through their legs is highly likely to cause injury to the resident and handlers – therefore the drag lift, bear hug or pivot transfer techniques are unacceptable and are not justified (see Figure 6.2.2).

Reference

Smith, J (ed.) 2011. *The Guide to Handling of People: A Systems Approach*. 6th edn. Backcare, Middlesex.

Further reading

Cornish J, Jones A. 2012. Factors affecting compliance with moving and handling policy: student nurses' views and experiences *Nurse Educational Practice* 10: 96–100.

Tofts, D, Arnold M. 2012. Moving and handling in the community: update on legislation and best practice *British Journal of Community Nursing* 17(50): 52, 54–57.

Useful web site

www.backcare.org.uk [Accessed October 2013].

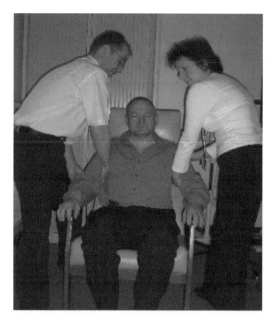

Figure 6.2.2 Poor and unsafe sit-to-stand technique.

- Ensure that their limbs are appropriately supported and that their moving and breathing are not restricted.
- Ensure their feet are firmly placed on the floor.

Risks and controversial techniques

Risk of injury in helping a person stand increases when consideration is not given to their skin condition – there must be no gripping of the resident, as this can bruise soft tissue.

6.3 Using a hoist

Michael Vassallo and Audrey Redshaw

Royal Bournemouth and Christchurch NHS Foundation Trust, Bournemouth, UK

Key points

- All care homes should have a moving and handling policy.
- Hoists can help avoid manual lifting and can reduce the incidence of injuries to staff and residents.
- The correct use of hoists is essential and all staff must be trained in their correct use.
- Make sure that you are familiar with lifting equipment before using a hoist.
- Two care givers should work together when using a hoist.
- Do not apply the brakes when hoisting (unless hoisting on a slope) and do not use the hoist for transporting residents.

A hoist is used to facilitate the mobilisation of poorly mobile residents. There are various designs available depending on the manufacturer, but there are three main types.

All hoists are used in combination with a sling to support the patient.

- Mobile hoists (full hoist): are used for residents requiring maximum support who are unable to stand.
- Standing hoists: are designed to enable a resident to transfer in a standing position and require the resident to be able to bear weight through their legs and have cognitive ability.
- Ceiling track and gantry hoists: are designed for use in limited space. The resident is transported along a rail track and repositioned and transferred accordingly.

Maintaining safety

Maintaining resident safety is paramount when using hoists. The following points are important:

1. Staff must have appropriate training before using the equipment and they must follow manufacturers' instructions to ensure safe use. One important principle that applies to all is that *inappropriate use can result in significant harm to residents for which one is likely to be held responsible*. It is incumbent on the user to be familiar with the instructions and be well trained in using the equipment.
2. Not every hoist is appropriate for every resident. Note the safe working load of the hoist and the sling. This is clearly marked and the resident's weight should never exceed this safe working load. Bariatric residents may need to be hoisted using specially designed slings with a suitable hoist.
3. It is considered safe practice to have a minimum of two carers using the mobile hoist. This is to avoid injury to both the resident and carers.
4. Using a hoist can be part of a resident's regular care. A care plan should be developed, with the resident where possible, following risk assessment, The care plan should include the resident's weight, specific details of the type of hoist and sling to use, fixing clips or loops and the number of carers needed to safely facilitate the move.
5. All equipment, including slings, has a unique serial number to identify the equipment and its service history from an equipment database.
6. Whenever possible, explain what you are doing and, when appropriate, obtain consent. Respect the resident's dignity and privacy. Reassure the resident throughout the move. The resident's wishes must be accommodated and safety must not be compromised.

The Care Home Handbook, First Edition. Edited by Graham Mulley, Clive Bowman, Michal Boyd and Sarah Stowe.
© 2015 John Wiley & Sons, Ltd. Published 2015 by John Wiley & Sons, Ltd.

Operating the hoist

A few general points apply:

1. Be vigilant in observing the position of the resident's head in relation to the overhead spreader bar (the bar to which the sling is attached), especially if the resident has any medical items *in situ*, such as naso-gastric tubes, Hickman catheters and so on.
2. When moving a hoist, maintain a good posture and push rather than pull, if possible. *The brakes must never be used when hoisting – unless hoisting on a slope*. Although there is no specific guidance on what distance a hoist may be moved with a resident in the sling, they are designed as a means of transfer, *not* transport. Always consider the resident's comfort and dignity.
3. Ensure that electric hoists (whichever model) are fully charged before use. Keep on charge when not in use.
4. All hoists need to be maintained regularly and are subject to lifting operations and equipment regulations (LOLER). Maintenance and repair is a specialised task and requires a competent engineer. Equipment that has not been serviced should not be used.

Training

Your care home must have a moving and handling policy. A competent qualified trainer is required to instruct staff hoists. Training delivered to informal carers in the resident's care plan must be signed by both parties to confirm that training has been given and that the trainee feels confident to use the equipment.

Infection control

Best practice would indicate that slings should be allocated to specific individuals (single resident use). They must be laundered (as per manufacturer's instructions) frequently. Consider using disposable slings for residents with known infections or incontinence. A sling that has been used on a resident with a known infection and/or has been contaminated with blood and/or body fluids must undergo thermal decontamination before being used on another resident. The home should have a hoist and sling cleaning schedule in place.

Compatibility of hoist and sling

Irrespective of the manufacturer, ensure that the hoist/sling interface is compatible, and that the sling is securely attached to the header bar. Ensure that the safe working load of the sling is the same or greater than that of the hoist.

Inappropriate or incorrect usage of a hoist can result in a resident's injury and even death.

It is imperative that staff are competent in equipment use before using a hoist to transfer residents.

Further reading

Stanav S, Bailer J, Straker JK, Mehdizadeh S, Park RM, Li H. 2012. Worker injuries and safety equipment in Ohio nursing homes. *Journal of Gerontology Nursing* 38: 47–56.

Waters, K. 1988. Hoists. *British Medical Journal* 296: 1114–1117.

6.4 Examining a walking aid and wheelchair

Steven Parke[1] and Baldeep Sagu[2]

[1]*Leeds Teaching Hospitals NHS Trust, Leeds, UK*
[2]*Riverside GP Vocational Training Scheme, London, UK*

Key points

- Walking aids can improve balance, mobility, safety and confidence, and can help to relieve pain.
- Physiotherapists can advise on the need for a walking aid, the most suitable type, and details such as the correct length and style of handle.
- Occupational therapists can advise on the need for a wheelchair, as well as the most appropriate model for a resident.
- All mobility aids must be examined frequently to ensure that they are safe to use.

Walking aids

Residents with poor or deteriorating mobility will often benefit from assessment by a physiotherapist, who may be able to develop a treatment plan to improve muscle strength and posture. In many cases, particularly when an individual's balance is affected or they remain unsteady when mobilising, the therapist may recommend the use of a walking aid. These can also be of benefit if a resident has a painful gait, for example as a result of osteoarthritis.

There are many different kinds of walking aid (Figure 6.4.1), though the most common are sticks and walking frames. In deciding on the most appropriate type for a resident, a physiotherapist will consider whether they need mild or moderate assistance, and whether the aim is to increase safety or achieve independence when mobilising.

Walking sticks

Walking sticks are generally made out of either wood or metal (Figure 6.4.2). It is extremely important that they are adjusted to the correct height for a resident. If the stick is too low or too high, it will fail to provide the required support and, worryingly, will also promote poor posture by causing the person to lean to one side.

In order to determine the most appropriate height for a walking stick, the resident should stand upright, wearing their regular footwear, and hold their arms slightly flexed by their sides. A measurement should then be taken from the ground to their ulnar styloid process. Wooden walking sticks should subsequently be cut to the correct length, though one must account for the ferrule, which is the rubber tip applied to the bottom end (Figure 6.4.3). Most metal sticks are adjustable – they normally have a telescopic design with a clip or spring-loaded ball mechanism to secure them at the desired height.

The choice of walking stick is generally down to availability and individual preference, though adjustable designs typically have a lower weight limit and may feel less solid when used.

Several different shaped handles are available (examples given in Figure 6.4.4). Each type has specific characteristics and will be suitable for some residents but not others; it is therefore important that handles are tried for size and comfort.

Walking frames

Walking frames are extremely stable and ideal for someone who has problems with balance. They are made of a lightweight material to aid ease of movement.

Some frames have two wheels attached at the front and static legs at the back; these are sometimes called 'rollators' or wheeled walking frames. However, the

The Care Home Handbook, First Edition. Edited by Graham Mulley, Clive Bowman, Michal Boyd and Sarah Stowe.
© 2015 John Wiley & Sons, Ltd. Published 2015 by John Wiley & Sons, Ltd.

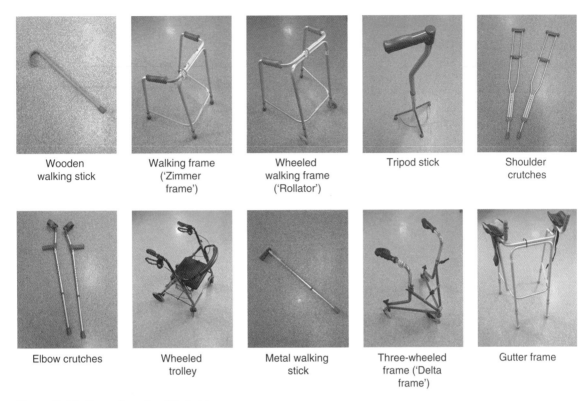

Wooden walking stick

Walking frame ('Zimmer frame')

Wheeled walking frame ('Rollator')

Tripod stick

Shoulder crutches

Elbow crutches

Wheeled trolley

Metal walking stick

Three-wheeled frame ('Delta frame')

Gutter frame

Figure 6.4.1 Examples of walking aids.

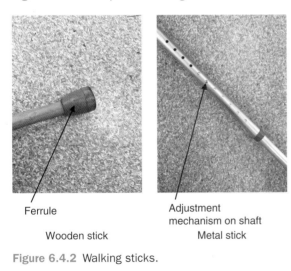

Ferrule

Wooden stick

Adjustment mechanism on shaft

Metal stick

Figure 6.4.2 Walking sticks.

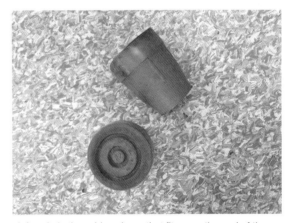

A ferrule is the rubber dome that fits over the end of the walking stick which is in contact with the ground. They wear surprisingly quickly, and should be checked regularly and replaced promptly.

Figure 6.4.3 Walking stick ferrules.

terminology is inconsistent and different names are used in different countries. Rollators allow an individual to walk at a faster pace, though cannot be used by everyone as they can easily roll away. This can be a problem in some Parkinsonian residents.

As with a walking stick, a walking frame must be of the correct height (Figure 6.4.5). If too high, the person using the frame will struggle to straighten their elbows and therefore find it difficult to put their weight through it. Frames that are too low should also generally be avoided because they will cause the resident to stoop down and adopt a poor posture;

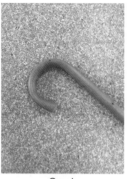

- Traditional design.
- Easily hung-up when not in use.
- Can be difficult to grasp.
- Generally not recommended if a resident puts a lot of weight through their stick.

Crook

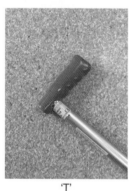

- Common.
- Suitable for many people.

'T'

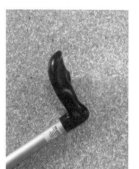

- A specially moulded plastic handle.
- Spreads the resident's weight across the palm, thereby reducing pain on the pressure points of the hand.
- Useful if a resident places a lot of weight on their stick, or has arthritis of the hands.
- Right- or left-handed version needed depending on which side the stick is to be used.

Fischer

Figure 6.4.4 Some types of walking stick handle.

physiotherapists may deliberately set the frame low, however, if an individual is at risk of falling backwards.

Other aids

Tripods and quadropods are metallic walking sticks with three or four feet, respectively. They are designed to give increased stability and are often used for people who require assistance with walking following a stroke.

Three- and four-wheeled walkers are also available. They should only be provided after a physiotherapy assessment, but can be useful because they can be used with a range of accessories, including trays for carrying food and drinks and seats for taking a rest.

Safe use of a walking aid

While walking aids undoubtedly help to keep people mobile and reduce their risk of falling, they must be

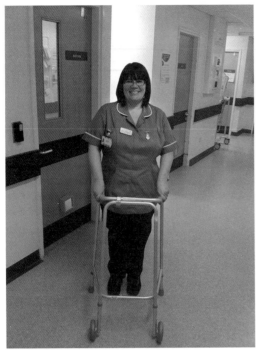
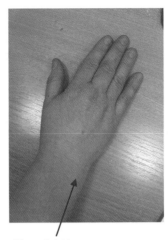

Ulnar styloid process

- The resident should stand in front of the walking frame wearing their regular footwear.
- Their arms should be held by their sides, but slightly flexed at the elbows (to approximately 15 degrees).
- The rubber handgrips on the frame should reach the ulnar styloid process at their wrists.
- Most metal frames have adjustable legs by virtue of a clip or spring-loaded ball mechanism – these should be lengthened or shortened appropriately.

Figure 6.4.5 How to measure and adjust the height of a walking frame.

used appropriately and with safety in mind. It is important to ensure that:

- Aids are kept within easy reaching distance of the resident to reduce the risk of falls as they get up/start mobilising.
- Equipment does not obstruct walkways and corridors – remember sticks and frames can themselves represent a falls hazard, particularly to other people.
- There are no obstructions such as rugs and cables – wet floors should also be avoided.
- Lighting is adequate.
- Comfortable and well-fitting footwear is worn.
- Aids are regularly inspected for signs of wear and tear or other damage, and where necessary repaired or replaced.

Wheelchairs

Unfortunately, some individuals have such severe disability that they are unable to walk or remain unsafe to do so even with the use of a walking aid. For these people, wheelchairs can provide a means of mobilising.

As with walking aids, there are many different types of wheelchair. In general, however, those with two large wheels at the back are used by individuals who are able to push themselves. A transit wheelchair has smaller wheels, and is appropriate if the person using it will be pushed by an attendant (Figure 6.4.6).

In order to choose the correct wheelchair design, an occupational therapist would generally be asked to make an assessment based on the resident's

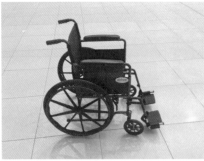

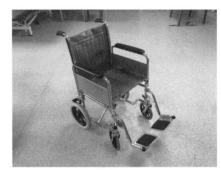

Propelled by occupant   Transit

Figure 6.4.6 Types of wheelchair.

Box 6.4.1 A wheelchair safety checklist

Wheels and castors
✓ Tyres properly inflated
✓ Metal rim attached tightly and undamaged
✓ Running freely

Frame
✓ Clean
✓ Intact and undamaged

Footrests
✓ Open correctly
✓ Undamaged
✓ At the correct height for the resident

Brakes
✓ Fully functioning

Seat
✓ Clean
✓ Intact and undamaged
✓ Cushioning and bouncy but supportive
✓ Lap straps (if any) undamaged

Back canvas
✓ Clean
✓ Intact and undamaged

Armrests
✓ Clean
✓ Intact and undamaged
✓ Cushioning and bouncy but supportive

condition, daily activities and other special requirements. They also need to consider posture support and the use of cushions.

Wheelchairs have many components, and it is important to check at regular intervals that none of these have become worn or damaged. To continue using a wheelchair that has developed faults risks causing injury to both the occupant and attendant. Completing a simple checklist at regular intervals, and ensuring deficiencies are repaired promptly, should help to ensure a wheelchair can continue to be used both safely and comfortably (Box 6.4.1).

Further reading

Mulley GP. 1989. Walking sticks. In: *Everyday Aids and Appliances*. BMJ Books, pp. 35–39.
Mulley GP. 1991. Walking frames. In: *More Everyday Aids and Appliances*. BMJ Books, pp. 174–182.
Young JB. 1989. Wheelchairs. In: *Everyday Aids and Appliances*. BMJ Books, pp. 40–44.

6.5 Seating

Tharani Thirugnanachandran and Helen Brooks

Leeds Teaching Hospitals NHS Trust, Leeds, UK

Key points

- Providing a chair that maintains mobility, activity and independence is of paramount importance.
- Nursing staff need to be able to identify a good basic seating position and have an understanding of the function of seating.
- Further advice on correct seating can be sought from occupational therapists or physiotherapists.

The ideal sitting position

- Weight is evenly distributed through the pelvis and thighs, with the trunk in the midline and a 90-degree angle of flexion at the hips, knees and ankles (Figure 6.5.1). This encourges a larger base of support and reduces the pressure on bony prominences. Pressure-relieving cushions can further reduce the risk of damage.
- The size of the user needs to match the internal dimensions of the chair – seat height, width and depth and backrest height.

- The chair must be:
  - *high enough* to allow a person's feet to rest on the floor, to facilitate getting up from the chair and maintaining a stable posture;
  - *wide enough* to accommodate the person's hips plus a clenched fist either side, to allow room for the resident to change position;
  - *deep enough* to comfortably support the full length of the thighs without having to lean back to support the shoulders. The backrest should also provide full support for the back and head.

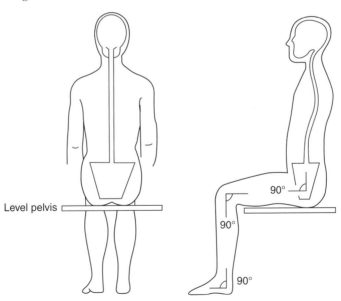

Figure 6.5.1 The ideal sitting position. Reproduced from Thirugnanachandran and Bateson (2012) with permission from Elsevier.

The Care Home Handbook, First Edition. Edited by Graham Mulley, Clive Bowman, Michal Boyd and Sarah Stowe.
© 2015 John Wiley & Sons, Ltd. Published 2015 by John Wiley & Sons, Ltd.

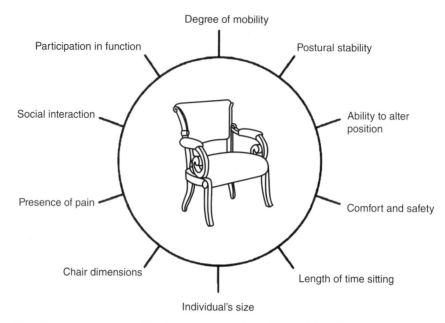

Figure 6.5.2 Considerations to account for in choosing a chair. Adapted from Thirugnanachandran and Bateson (2012) with permission from Elsevier.

Goals of seating

- Promotion of mobility – a chair that is easy to get in and out of helps to maintain mobility.
- Maintaining postural stability and control – adequate postural support can help to prevent or reduce pain and the development of postural deformities and enhance functional activity.
- Improving respiratory function – good postural support and an upright position can maximise respiratory function.
- Providing safe oral intake – sitting upright for eating and drinking can reduce the risk of aspiration in those with swallowing problems.
- Reducing the development of pressure sores – seating, which distributes weight evenly and increases surface area support, can reduce excessive pressures and maintain skin integrity (Chapter 5.6).
- Providing comfort – this can improve sitting tolerance and compliance – which is especially important to help reduce agitation in patients with dementia.

- Encouraging social interaction and communication through an upright position.

Important factors to consider when choosing a chair are highlighted in Figure 6.5.2.

Reference

Thirugnanachandran T, Bateson A. 2012. Seating for improving function in older people. *European Geriatric Medicine* 3(1): 67–72.

Further reading

Edlich RF, Heather CL, Galumbeck MH. 2003. Recent advances in adaptive seating systems for the elderly and persons with disabilities. *Long Term Effective Medical Implants* 13: 31–39.

Miller WC, Miller F, Trenholm K, Grant D, Goodman K. 2004. Development and preliminary assessment of the measurement properties of the Seating Identification Tool. *Clinical Rehabilitation* 18: 317–325.

6.6 Falls

Shona McIntosh

Retired Geriatrician, Leeds, UK

Key points
- All residents are at risk of falling and half of them will fall in a year.
- About a third of falls result in injury.
- Most falls occur while doing everyday activities.
- Not all falls are preventable.
- Consider risk factors, particularly blackouts, medications and falls in blood pressure in all those who fall.
- Residents who injure their face in a fall may have had a blackout (syncope).
- Suspect a hip fracture if the resident has hip pain, is unable to weight-bear, or if the leg is shortened and rotated outwards.
- Avoid restraints.

Falls are a common reason for residents being admitted to care homes or hospital.

Which residents fall?

- Falls are more common with age when balance (Figure 6.6.1) is challenged by *ageing*, *diseases* (such as strokes) and *medications*.
- Falls can still occur in those who are unable to walk but the risk factors here may be different (e.g. transfers and moving and handling equipment may be implicated).
- *All residents should be considered as being at high risk of falls.*

Why do they fall?

- Falls often occur during everyday activities.
- Falls are most frequent at staff handover times.
- Falls often occur in the resident's room and while standing up or toileting.
- Most falls are due to a combination of risk factors and the likelihood of falling becomes greater as the number of these increases.

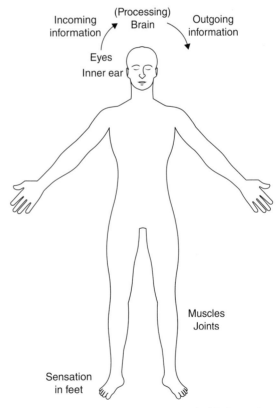

Figure 6.6.1 What keeps us upright and balanced.

The Care Home Handbook, First Edition. Edited by Graham Mulley, Clive Bowman, Michal Boyd and Sarah Stowe.
© 2015 John Wiley & Sons, Ltd. Published 2015 by John Wiley & Sons, Ltd.

Facts and figures

- About 50% of residents fall each year, with many doing so more than once.
- Residents are up to three times more likely to fall than those who live at home and those with memory problems are at particularly high risk.
- About 30% of falls in care homes result in injury and 3–5% in a fracture.

What are the effects of falls?

- The most feared complications are serious injuries, such as hip fracture and head injury. About a third of hip fracture patients die within one year and, of those who survive, many are left more dependent. Hip fractures are 10 times more common in residents than in old people at home, which probably reflects raised risk, but also emphasises the need for an active approach to safety.
- Falls may result in litigation.
- They can have a negative impact on staff morale.

How can falls be prevented?

- Not all falls can be prevented and a home with no falls is probably either not reporting properly or inappropriately restricting residents' movements.
- There has been little research on falls in care homes but addressing recognised risk factors for falls is worthwhile.
- Just giving information is not effective in preventing falls.

How to manage falls

Management is based on limited evidence and common sense.

First, establish the individual's risk factors. In care homes, risk factors include:

- Gait and balance problems.
- Memory problems with wandering.
- Use of medicines which affect the brain (e.g. sleeping tablets).
- Urinary symptoms.
- Visual problems.
- A history of falls.

Do try to ascertain if the individual has had a blackout. The number of falls due to blackouts is underestimated, as older people often cannot recall the event and these are often unwitnessed. (The latter does not indicate poor care, as even when falls are witnessed it can be difficult to stop them.)

Suspect a blackout if:

- the individual does not have significant falls risk factors, or
- they have sustained a facial injury (suggesting that they were unable to protect themselves when falling)

Blackouts in older people may be due to heart disease and require medical assessment (Chapter 9.4).

There are several falls risk scores which aim to identify people at high risk of a fall. None of these scores is perfect. They may not identify all those who are likely to fall. Checking for risk factors and intervening on these as part of the care plan is a more realistic approach (see Table 6.6.1).

Assess the appropriateness of exercise on an individual basis to avoid any increase in falls. It is possible that exercise may enable a previously immobile person to stand unsafely (see Chapter 6.1).

Avoid restraints. Using restraints actually increases injuries (see Chapter 4.2). Allowing autonomy will always entail risk. The aims of falls management are to reduce this risk and probably to reduce the number of falls per person rather than the number of people who fall.

It can be difficult to make beneficial intervention into routine practice.

Other measures to consider:

- Treat urinary symptoms (although the effectiveness of this is not known).
- Ensure that the bed height is appropriate (ultra-low beds and bedrails should only be used in accordance with local guidelines and never as restraints).
- Check walking aids (see Chapter 6.4).
- Ensure appropriate supervision of mobility.
- Educate staff on falls management.

Be aware that falls prevention programmes might deflect staff from other duties.

As yet there is little evidence that falls can be prevented in individuals with dementia. These individuals may walk too quickly for their ability. Residents with dementia should not be excluded from assessment but interventions need to be planned with care. A common modifiable risk factor is postural hypotension.

Table 6.6.1 Some modifiable fall risk factors and interventions.

Risk factor	Possible interventions
Single interventions	
Certain medications or multiple medications	Review by pharmacist or GP. Withdraw unnecessary medications acting on brain (e.g. sleeping tablets) and review any medications which lower blood pressure (e.g. diuretics). Monitor carefully after starting any new drug.
Vitamin D deficiency	Many residents will be deficient and supplements can reduce falls. When combined with calcium, supplements also reduce fractures.
To be used as part of a multifactorial approach	
Gait, balance or mobility problem	Individually tailored exercises, if appropriate, from falls team member but only as part of a multifactorial falls intervention programme. Most evidence is for exercise which challenges balance – not seated exercise.
Eyesight problem	Clean glasses. Use correct glasses for activity. Regular eye tests. Cataract surgery. Bifocals and multifocals can cause falls but changing lenses only helps if going outdoors regularly. May need time to adapt to new glasses.
Fear of falling	A very common psychological problem which follows falls. Causes individuals to restrict their activity, which makes them less fit and actually more likely to fall. Refer to falls team.
Environment	Review by occupational therapist of trip hazards, adequate space to mobilise, lighting, non-slip flooring, hand rails, distances to toilet or dining room, call bell within reach etc.
Feet and footwear	Refer to podiatry if foot pain. Exercises for reduced ankle movement. Low heeled shoes. Try to avoid slippers.
Dizziness or blackouts	Check for postural hypotension. Record blood pressure (ideally first thing in the morning) after resident has been lying down for at least 5 minutes and repeat on standing up. Medical review for cardiac problems.

What to do if an individual falls

- Resuscitate them if necessary.
- Assess them for injury (see Chapter 9.4).
- Consider the possibility of hip fracture, spinal injury or intracranial bleed (particularly if the resident is on warfarin) as rapid treatment of these conditions is important. The key signs of a hip fracture are pain and inability to weight bear. If the resident is lying on their back, the fractured leg may look shorter and be rotated outwards.

If the resident is going to hospital, useful information to send might include:

- A witness account of the event, if available.
- Any recent new symptoms and any observations taken since the fall.
- A history of falls.
- A summary of previous medical problems, usual physical and mental function, medications and allergies.

- Information on next of kin and GP, together with any advance directive (see Chapter 17.4).

What to do after a fall

- Care home staff should very carefully consider whether there is any issue that they can remedy, for example, loose footwear, rugs, clothing that makes toileting difficult, the need for a walking aid or accompanied walking.
- Ideally, all individuals should be assessed by healthcare professionals trained in falls to identify risk factors – unless it is clear that this was an accident. Such assessments may modify medicines and consider specific treatments, for example for bone health. Referral should certainly be considered if the resident is unsteady, if there has been an injury or if there have been other falls in the past year.
- Older people respond better if the focus is on the positive objectives of interventions. Falls can be

associated with a loss of confidence, and a plan to maintain independence rather than placing the emphasis on preventing falls is likely to be more positively received.

- Falls may, unfortunately, continue in a small number of individuals. Here it is best to involve both health and social care professionals in drawing up a person-centred management plan. Trials of different approaches may be needed.
- Hip protectors (pads worn within special undergarments) do not prevent falls but might reduce hip fractures in residents at high risk, particularly if there are no easily correctable risk factors. They are not without problems – particularly in people with confusion, where they may increase the risk of falls during toileting. The main problem is that people do not keep them on reliably.

Falls audits

It is good practice to maintain records of falls in a home and to audit the actions taken to prevent falls. These might include the percentage of residents screened for falls risk factors and whether these have been addressed.

National audits of falls and bone health highlight that care home staff are not always aware of which falls services are available locally, and so it is good practice to understand what local health services provide.

Unanswered questions

We do not know:

- Which aspects of the multifactorial approach work best.
- Which interventions are cost-effective.

- The benefits of alarms, telehealth, balance training using games consoles, changing the type of flooring, staff training and increasing supervision of residents. Further research is required before these interventions can be recommended.

Further reading

Cameron ID, Gillespie LD, Robertson MC, Murray GR, Hill KD, Cumming RG, Kerse N. 2010. Interventions for preventing falls in older people in nursing care facilities and hospitals. *Cochrane Database of Systematic Reviews*. Issue 1.

NICE. 2004. Falls. The assessment and prevention of falls in older people. London: NICE (update in progress and will include information on care homes).

Oliver D, Connelly JB, Victor CR, Shaw FE, Whitehead A, Genc Y. 2007. Strategies to prevent falls and fractures in hospitals and care homes and effect of cognitive impairment: systematic review and meta-analysis. *British Medical Journal* 334: 82–85.

RCN. 2004. Clinical practice guideline for the assessment and prevention of falls in older people. London: Royal College of Nursing.

Useful web site

Managing falls and fractures in care homes for older people. Good practice self assessment resource. Communications. Social Care and Social Work Improvement Scotland 2011. www.careinspectorate.com (in 'Professionals' section of web site) [Accessed October 2013].

Chapter 7

Vision, Hearing and Foot Care

7.1 Eye care

Mary Shaw[1], Heather Waterman[1] and Paul Diggory[2]

[1] *University of Manchester, Manchester, UK*
[2] *Croydon University Hospital, Croydon, UK*

Key points

- Good vision helps avoid falls and reduces confusion, especially in those with cognitive impairment.
- Spectacles and low vision aids need to be kept clean, in a good state of repair and to hand. Remember both reading (used when eating) and distance glasses (used to watch TV) may be needed. A small colour-coded tag can identify the type of spectacles and a nametag reduces the likelihood of losing a reading aid. People with confusion may need help and reminding which glasses to use.
- *Elderly people should have eye checks by opticians about every other year.* Many opticians will visit residents in care homes.
- *Things to watch out for:*
  - New visual symptom – you may have to ask the resident and not rely on them volunteering this information.
  - Look for conjunctival redness: are the eyelashes clean and the pupils round and reactive to light? Is the cornea clear? Are eye movements full, is there a squint?
  - Does the upper eyelid droop (ptosis)?
  - Does the lower eyelid turn out (ectropion)?
  - *Seek medical review for new visual loss or facial weakness.*

Visual assessment

- Ensure good lighting, head positioning and appropriate glasses. Assess visual acuity in both eyes.
- A Snellen chart, read at 6 m with distance glasses, gives a measure. Alternatively acuity may be recorded as:

  1. 'Large newsprint'
  2. 'Small newsprint'
  3. 'Finger counting'
  4. 'Hand movements'
  5. 'Perception of light'
  6. 'No perception of light'

- Visual field loss is common with glaucoma and stroke. It may mean a person does not notice people or objects to one or other side despite good acuity when looking straight ahead (see Chapter 8.1).
- The commonest cause of visual loss in old age are (i) age-related macular degeneration (with loss of central vision); (ii) cataract (usually treatable) and (iii) glaucoma (loss of peripheral vision, a potentially preventable cause of blindness)

Low vision aids are available from eye units, optometrists, hospital departments and the Royal National Institute for the Blind. In the UK, local authorities have teams who will assess visual impairment in care homes.

Procedures

Eye procedures are often distressing, especially for those with cognitive impairment. Reassurance, a relaxed, well-lit environment, without disturbance, and a familiar face, can all help.

Eye care

Infection easily passes between eyes. Use a clean, rather than an aseptic, technique, with hand washing between each task and non-sterile, powder free gloves for procedures.

The Care Home Handbook, First Edition. Edited by Graham Mulley, Clive Bowman, Michal Boyd and Sarah Stowe.
© 2015 John Wiley & Sons, Ltd. Published 2015 by John Wiley & Sons, Ltd.

Eye drops and ointment

- Eye drops are commonly prescribed for chronic conditions, such as glaucoma or dry eyes, as well as temporarily for infection and after eye surgery. Adherence to treatment should be promoted. It is preferable that residents administer their own drops, but arthritis and stroke may make it difficult.
- A number of aids are available to help self-administration. The International Glaucoma Association can advise on this.
- Those with significant cognitive impairment may be unable to self-administer drops.
- Observe a resident's instillation technique, help them with any difficulties but administer the drops if residents cannot manage this themselves.

To administer an eye drop the resident should:

1. Tilt their head back.
2. Form a small pocket by pulling down the lower lid.
3. Hold the dropper vertically.
4. Without touching, instill a drop into the pocket.
5. Keep eye closed for 30 seconds.
6. Allow two-minutes before instilling a second drop.

See Figure 7.1.1.

Ointments have the advantage of being longer acting and are often more soothing. A similar technique to eye drop instillation is used to apply a 20 mm squeeze of ointment to the junction of the lower lid pocket and cornea, starting nasally and moving laterally.

Instill drops before ointment. Residents commonly have different drops or ointment for each eye and care needs to be taken to ensure the correct drugs are given daily and on time. Hands should be washed between administrations; each eye should have a separate bottle/tube.

Eye drops may cause allergy and should be stopped if a red eye develops, and a medical review obtained. The drops

(a)

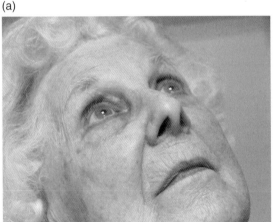

(b)

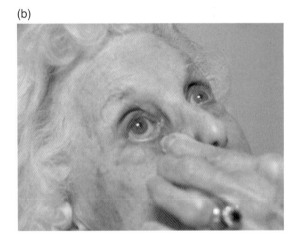

(c)

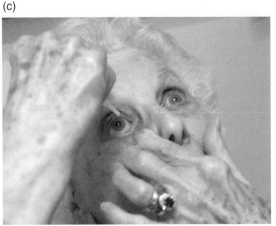

(d)

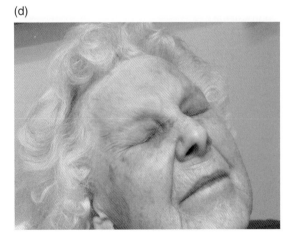

Figure 7.1.1 (a–d) Instillation of eye drops.

or ointment often need to be stored in a fridge: look at the manufacturer's leaflet.

Eye swabs

These may be used to remove foreign bodies from the surface of eye or eyelid or to obtain a bacterial sample. To clean an eyelid, moisten (use sterile water) gauze and wipe over the closed eye, from the nose outward.

Sore red eye(s)

These need a medical review.

Tear problems

Tear quality declines with age and the eye may become gritty and mildly inflamed. Medical review is needed so that artificial tears can be prescribed.

Blepharitis

- A common cause of itchy, red, often watery eyes. Often confused with conjunctivitis because of conjunctival injection.
- Caused by blockage of glands around the eyelashes, which become encrusted. The tear film dries out causing irritation.
- More common in elderly people as tear production declines with age. Paradoxically, reflex increased tear production can lead to watery eyes. Treatment is a twice daily eyelash cleaning with cotton wool/gauze soaked in saline of dilute bicarbonate of soda. Dilute baby shampoo, which does not sting the eyes, is an alternative. Occasionally, topical antibiotics and tear film supplements are needed. *Seek a medical review if there has been no improvement within a week.*

Conjunctivitis

- Usually bilateral and due to infections.
- Eyes are very red with irritation/pain and often discharge.
- Treatment is local care, as for blepharitis
- *Seek a medical review if pain is a major feature and/or if the pain and redness do not settle in a week.*

Artificial eye care

Most artificial eyes are removable and *should be removed and washed monthly*, in contact lens solution.

- Pull down gently on the lower lid; press inward so the edge of the prosthesis comes forward so it can be removed.
- The socket is cleaned using a moistened swab and irrigation with sterile water.

Contact lenses (hard and soft)

Hard lenses are plastic and are generally worn for no more than 12–18 hours (lenses used after surgery may be worn for longer periods). Soft lenses are flexible and may be worn, with weekly cleaning, for up to thirty days. Disposable lenses are worn for a week only. The lenses are stored in containers with cleaning/storage according to the manufacturer's instructions.

To remove hard lenses:

- Separate the eyelids and gently push on the upper (cranial) edge of the lens.
- Lever it off from the lower edge.

To remove soft lenses:

- Separate the eyelids with the fingers of one hand.
- Ask the resident to look up, move the lens down and pinch it between thumb and index finger and remove.

Further reading

Khaw PT, Shah P, Elkington AR. 2004. *ABC of Eyes*. British Medical Association, London.

Useful web sites

RNIB http://www.rnib.org.uk [Accessed October 2013]
The International Glaucoma Association http://www.glaucoma-association.com/ [Accessed October 2013]

7.2 Hearing impairment

Evelyn Tan

Leeds Teaching Hospitals NHS Trust, Leeds, UK

Key points

- Hearing loss is the commonest sensory impairment in care home residents.
- It can result in reduced exchange of information, communication difficulties, frustration, loneliness and depression.
- If there is sudden loss of hearing or ear discharge, refer the resident urgently to a doctor.
- Staff should learn how to communicate with deaf residents and how to assess and care for hearing aids.

Recognising deafness

Deafness is defined by the World Health Organization (WHO) as a complete loss of hearing ability in one or both ears, whereas *hearing impairment* refers to both complete and partial loss of the ability to hear (Table 7.2.1).

Hearing deteriorates as one gets older. This is called presbycusis and is the single biggest cause of deafness. Other common causes of deafness are listed in Table 7.2.2.

Table 7.2.2 Common causes of deafness.

Conductive	Sensorineural
Wax build up	Excessive noise exposure
Infection in the ear canal or middle ear	Ototoxic drugs
Fluid in the middle ear	Diabetes
Otosclerosis	Stroke
Perforation or scarring of the eardrum	Meniere's disease

Table 7.2.1 WHO grades of hearing impairment.

Grade of impairment	Impairment description
0 (no impairment)	No or very slight hearing problems. Able to hear whispers
1 (slight impairment)	Able to hear and repeat words spoken in normal voice at 1 metre
2 (moderate impairment)	Able to hear and repeat words in raised voice at 1 metre
3 (severe impairment)	Able to hear some words when shouted into better ear
4 (profound impairment including deafness)	Unable to hear and understand even a shouted voice

Recognising deafness is important. There is a higher prevalence of depression, anxiety and stress found in people with hearing loss. Other consequences of hearing loss include loss of independence, as there is a need to rely on others to acquire information, and withdrawal from social activities. Hearing impairment is also a risk factor for delirium.

Box 7.2.1 illustrates a questionnaire useful in assessing whether someone may be having hearing loss and needs assessment of their hearing.

Communicating with a deaf person

Communicating with someone who is deaf can take time but doesn't have to be difficult. It is worth checking with the individual how they would like to communicate. While some may prefer using writing to communicate, others may prefer using speech.

The Care Home Handbook, First Edition. Edited by Graham Mulley, Clive Bowman, Michal Boyd and Sarah Stowe.
© 2015 John Wiley & Sons, Ltd. Published 2015 by John Wiley & Sons, Ltd.

Box 7.2.1   Questions to assess whether someone may be having hearing loss and needs assessment of their hearing

1. Do you have a problem hearing over the telephone?
2. Do you have trouble following the conversation when two or more people are talking at the same time?
3. Do people complain that you turn the TV volume up too high?
4. Do you have to strain to understand conversation?
5. Do you have trouble hearing in a noisy background?
6. Do you find yourself asking people to repeat themselves?
7. Do many people you talk to seem to mumble (or not speak clearly)?
8. Do you misunderstand what others are saying and respond inappropriately?
9. Do you have trouble understanding the speech of women and children?
10. Do people get annoyed because you misunderstand what they say?

If the answer is yes to three or more of the questions, then a hearing assessment may be needed.

For those who want to use speech, remember that not everyone can lip read and, even if an individual is wearing a hearing aid, it does not mean they can hear perfectly. If there is an interpreter present, speak to the person and not the interpreter (Boxes 7.2.2 and 7.2.3).

Hearing aids and how to care for them

There are several types of hearing aids available nowadays. All hearing aids, however, work in a similar way, which is to make sounds louder so that hearing can be improved. Behind the ear (BTE) hearing aids have a mould which fits snugly in the ear while the rest of it rests behind the ear. They are commonly used, as are in the ear (ITE) hearing aids which fit entirely in the ear. Tips on how to care for BTE and ITE aids can be found on Boxes 7.2.4 and 7.2.5.

Box 7.2.2   Tips on talking with a deaf person

- Make sure you can be seen by the person you are talking to and there are no shadows or glare from light on your face, which makes it hard for the person to lip read.
- Avoid covering your lips as you speak.
- Ensure that the place where you are conversing has as little noise and distraction as possible.
- Get the listener's attention before you start speaking and use natural facial expressions and gestures.
- Speak clearly and do not exaggerate lip movements.
- Do not shout as this can be uncomfortable if the listener has a hearing aid and can look aggressive.
- If what you have said is not understood, do not keep repeating it but try saying it in a different way.
- Check that the listener is able to follow the conversation and do not waffle or use jargon.

Box 7.2.3   Tips for those who prefer to use writing to communicate

- Keep the message short and simple.
- It is not necessary to write out every word.
- Using diagrams or pictures may be useful if trying to explain something technical or specific.
- Face the person after writing the message so you can see each other's facial expression.

Box 7.2.4   Tips on how to care for BTE aids

- Only the ear mould and tubing is water resistant and not the hearing aid itself. Therefore, disconnect the ear mould and tubing from the hearing aid before washing them.
- Ideally, the ear mould and tubing needs to be washed in warm soapy water and dried with a soft, dry cloth or tissue daily. However, once a week is fine.
- Do not reattach the ear mould and tubing until dry.
- The tubing needs to be changed every 3 to 6 months before it hardens, splits or causes problems.

Box 7.2.5   Tips on how to care for ITE aids

- There is no ear mould or tubing to detach.
- Do not let the aid come into contact with liquid. Instead, clean it with a dry cloth.
- If there is ear wax, use a wax pick to remove it from the opening at the end of the aid.

Ear wax (cerumen)

Excessive or impacted ear wax is present in about 1 in 3 older adults. Ear wax consists of secretions from the glands in the ear canal, skin cells, normal skin bacteria and occasionally hair. This is usually cleared from the ear canal by the outward movement of the skin lining the ear canal. In elderly subjects, the ear wax is harder and drier and moves more slowly, leading to accumulation in the ear canal.

Ear wax does not need removal unless it is symptomatic, for example causing hearing loss, pain or itchiness. If wax is causing symptoms, consult the resident's GP about the best way of removing the wax.

Ask the GP to ascertain if there is perforation or infection *and do not syringe the ear until this is known.*

Contacting audiology

An audiologist is able to assess hearing loss and recommend and provide appropriate management for it. If a resident appears to have hearing loss, they may benefit from an assessment by an audiologist (see Chapter 17.11).

Do not refer to audiology if there is ear discharge, sudden onset or rapidly progressing deafness, or unilateral deafness. Such symptoms are suggestive of an acute problem and should be referred to the GP, A&E or the ENT specialist.

Further reading

Anand JK, Court J. 1989. Hearing loss leading to impaired ability to communicate in residents of homes for the elderly. *British Medical Journal* 27: 1429–1430.

Sprinzl GM, Riechelman H. 2010. Current trends in treating hearing loss in elderly people: a review of the technical and treatment options – a mini-review *Gerontology* 56: 351–358.

Useful web sites

http://www.actiononhearingloss.org.uk/ [Accessed October 2013]

http://www.deafnessresearch.org.uk/ [Accessed October 2013]

http://www.nhs.uk/Conditions/Hearing-impairment/Pages/Introduction.aspx [Accessed October 2013]

7.3 Everyday foot care and footwear

Pauline Bailey

Newcastle University Medicine, Johor, Malaysia

Key points

- Good foot care is essential for older people.
- Healthy feet are vital if mobility is to be preserved.
- Poor foot care can lead to pain, discomfort, reduced mobility and falls.
- Foot problems (see Table 7.3.1) are common in older people due to arthritic changes in the bones of the feet, soft tissue changes and the legacy left from previous poorly fitting shoes.

Foot care

It is hard for older people to care for their own feet for a variety of reasons: poor vision, reduced manual dexterity, limited flexibility and fitness often lead to neglect of basic foot care.

Basic foot care should be carried out at least on alternate days. This should follow a basic regime of washing, drying and dressing.

Daily foot care

- Washing – clean feet thoroughly in warm water.
- Drying – pat feet dry with a soft, clean towel, paying particular attention to the spaces between the toes.
- If feet tend to be sweaty or moist, apply a small amount of talc.
- If feet tend to be dry, use an emollient cream, but avoid using this between the toes as this can lead to dampness and fungal infection.
- Clean socks or stockings should be applied daily.

Once a week the feet should be inspected and the toenails tended.

Weekly foot care

- Inspection – check thoroughly for abrasions, blisters, colour changes and swelling or lesions.
- Toenails – soak feet, if toenails are hard, soften them before cutting. The nail should be cut with a pair of nail clippers and cut straight to avoid any sharp edges. Any edges that are left should be filed.

Footwear

Appropriate footwear is important (see Figure 7.3.1), as ill-fitting shoes can cause crowding of the toes, foot blisters and ulcers and lead to pain. These can result in reduced mobility and possibly falls.

It is important that older people are encouraged to wear shoes and not go barefoot, as this can lead to injury. The wearing of slippers should also be discouraged, as often they do not provide adequate support or protection to the feet. The shoes should have a low heel, as a high heeled shoe can be detrimental to posture, balance and gait. The sole should be thin and hard to optimise foot position. There should be a tread on the sole of the shoe and the heel to provide grip and prevent slipping. It is important that the shoes are of the correct width and length.

Older feet tend to widen as the bones in the feet splay. Adequate arch support is important to encourage good posture and joint positioning.

The upper part of the shoe should be made of either fabric or leather, bearing in mind that leather can be heavy for frail older people.

The shoes should fasten securely to provide support and stability, but if possible should use a mechanism that the older person can operate themselves to promote independence.

Specialised foot care

See Table 7.3.1 for common conditions and their management.

The Care Home Handbook, First Edition. Edited by Graham Mulley, Clive Bowman, Michal Boyd and Sarah Stowe.
© 2015 John Wiley & Sons, Ltd. Published 2015 by John Wiley & Sons, Ltd.

Table 7.3.1 Common problems in older feet.

Condition	Description	Management
Corns	Thickened and hardened dead tissue over bony prominences	Warm water soak and gentle rubbing with pumice stone. Assess footwear, as may be rubbing on foot
Callouses	Dead, compacted tissue on soles or heel of feet	Warm water soak and gentle rubbing with pumice stone. Apply emollient cream and use soft insoles in shoes
Bunion	Bony protuberance on the side of the great toe – angulation of the big toe laterally	Appropriate shoes – soft leather or fabric, wide fitting and flat. May need surgery
Hammer toe	Claw-like appearance of toe	Properly fitting non-constrictive shoe, orthotic support or surgery
Toenails	Thickening	Soak nails before cutting, may need chiropody
	Infection (discolouration)	Topical anti-fungal agents

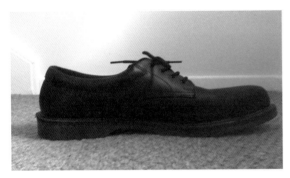

Figure 7.3.1 Example of appropriate footwear.

The diabetic foot

The feet of residents with diabetes merit special attention, as circulatory and sensory problems associated with the disease can lead to serious problems (see Chapter 8.4).

Poor circulation in the feet can lead to skin changes that in turn mean injuries to the feet take longer to heal and are more prone to infection. Reduction in sensation in the feet can lead to unknown injuries, and a lack of pain sensation results in failure to protect the wound or painful joint. This exacerbates the problem and leads to further slowing of the healing process. Therefore preventative measures are extremely important.

Daily care:
- Inspect – look for blisters, breaks in the skin, callouses and bruises.
- Wash with warm water and use a pumice stone if there are callouses or corns.
- Use emollient cream if skin is dry or there are callouses.

- Inspect the inside of shoes for foreign bodies and ensure socks are free from holes before putting them on. Flatten out wrinkles in socks before putting on shoes.

General notes:
- Avoid putting feet near heat sources (hot water bottles, fires, electric blankets).
- Avoid constrictive garments (tight socks, shoes).
- Always wear shoes to prevent injury.
- Cut toenails straight and file edges.

Specialised footwear

Special footwear may be required where a deformity of the foot is present. This is in order to relieve pain and/or improve mobility.

The commonest reasons for special footwear in older people is to accommodate deformities due to bunions, hammer toes and rheumatoid arthritis. It can also be used to correct for unequal leg length or provide extra support. Ideally, the older person's own shoe should be adapted to accommodate the deformity or provide extra support or cushioning. Possible modifications include raises or orthotic supports. When necessary, custom made footwear may be required.

Specialised footwear is provided through an orthotic service; these are usually based in hospital and a referral is required from a healthcare professional. Once the person has accessed the service, they can contact the department directly for further advice, adaptations or products.

Podiatrists can also provide and manufacture some orthotic devices.

Further reading

Blainey C, Filipick S.1993. High-risk pathophysiology in the elderly: medical and nursing management. In: Carnevali DL, Patrick M (eds.) *Nursing Management for the Elderly*. 3rd Edn. Pennsylvania, Lippincott Williams and Wilkins, pp. 452–478.

Ebersole P, Hess P. 1988. *Towards Healthy Aging*. 5th Edn. Missouri, Mosby.

Meiner S. 2011. *Gerontologic Nursing*. 4th Edn. Missouri, Elsevier.

Menant JC, Steele JR, Menz HB, Munro BJ, Lord SR. 2008. Optimising footwear for older people at risk of falls. *Journal of Rehabilitation Research and Development* 45: 1167–1182.

Orchard S, Ahearn DJ, Bhat S, Baker P. 2011. What to expect from a general podiatry service. *CME Journal Geriatric Medicine* 13: 54–57.

Chapter 8

Major Medical Problems

8.1 Stroke

David Cohen[1] and Fiona Cristol[2]

[1]*Northwick Park Hospital, Harrow, UK*
[2]*Northwood Nursing and Care Services Ltd, Northwood, UK*

Key points

- Many care home residents who have had a stroke have complex disabilities.
- Stroke care requires a practical knowledge of the effects and complications of stroke: motor weakness, loss of balance, apraxia, sensory impairment, perceptual problems, speech and language difficulties, swallowing difficulties, drooling, visual impairment and cognitive problems.
- Depression is easily overlooked and can be misdiagnosed in those with emotional lability.
- Correct positioning, support and movement are important in optimising recovery and preventing complications. Physiotherapists have a key role in stroke care.
- Stroke rehabilitation is best achieved by the input of all members of the interdisciplinary team.

Stroke is a condition when the blood supply to the brain is interrupted and the brain is damaged. After the injury, the brain recovers because undamaged areas 'learn' how to take over from the damaged area. This may take weeks or months and is usually not complete. Many stroke patients have some permanent damage causing disability. About a third of people who have a stroke die, a third are left significantly disabled and a third have minor or no disability.

Care homes will tend to look after people with a major disability. Stroke can affect any part of the brain's function: controlling movement, feelings, speech, vision, thinking and emotions.

Causes and consequences

Stroke can be caused either by *bleeding* in to the brain or *blockage* of an artery to the brain. In the United Kingdom, 85% of strokes are *ischemic* due to a blockage and only 15% are *haemorrhagic* due to bleeding.

In both cases, blood supply is cut off to part of the brain and that part is damaged. The brain can only manage without blood for a few minutes. If a blockage lasts more than this time, damage to the brain is permanent. There may be an area around the permanently damaged brain which is *stunned* and recovers with time, but this recovery may take days or weeks.

Damage can cause different problems depending on which part of the brain is affected.

- A resident who has had a stroke often shows signs of *weakness* and this is what people usually notice first. Weakness may be mild or severe. In stroke, weakness usually affects one side of the body. This is because the nerves that control movement are arranged this way. Damage on one side of the brain usually causes symptoms on the other side of the body.
- Many people have *loss of feeling* in a limb. People say this is like an injection at the dentist, sometimes with pins and needles as well.
- A stroke affecting the back part of the brain may cause *loss of vision*. Usually one half of vision is affected: it may look as if only half of a TV picture or newspaper is visible (see Chapter 7.1).
  - The resident may only eat the food on one side of their plate; remember to turn the plate round after half the meal has been eaten.
  - They may not be able to see someone standing on the affected side *so always stand directly in front of a person with suspected stroke.*
- Strokes affecting the right side of the body often affect *communication*. Sometimes people can understand but not speak. Sometimes they can speak but not understand. These are *dysphasias*. Most often both expression and understanding are affected. People may look as if they understand

The Care Home Handbook, First Edition. Edited by Graham Mulley, Clive Bowman, Michal Boyd and Sarah Stowe.
© 2015 John Wiley & Sons, Ltd. Published 2015 by John Wiley & Sons, Ltd.

but do not: families often make this mistake. To check, you can do some simple tests.

If a resident does not understand, you need to keep communication very simple and use gestures. People can often make choices; they just are unable to tell you. So, if you want to know whether they want water or tea, give them both and let them choose. You can do this with clothes, jewellery or food as well. This is important for their dignity and self-respect.

- Strokes often cause problems with *complex functions* such as *attention, thinking and concentration*. *Dyspraxia* is when someone cannot do a complex action like putting on their glasses – even though their arms are not weak. This may affect their ability to do things for themselves. It is different from dementia, as stroke patients may be able to do some things perfectly well. No two strokes are the same so people need close attention to understand how to treat them as individuals.
- Sometimes stroke patients have *perceptual problems*. This is when they do not understand where their body is in space. This ability may be lost in stroke, especially when the left side of the body is affected so that affected residents do not 'know' where their left side is.

  They may even not know it has been affected by a stroke. It can be very hard to look after residents like this: for example, they may constantly let their arm fall off the armrest of a chair and you have to keep reminding them to 'pick it up'.
- Stroke patients often have difficulty swallowing safely. This is called *dysphagia*. It can lead to food going down the windpipe and causing infections. Each person should have guidelines for what is and is not safe for them. If you notice a resident choke or cough after food or drink, alert a doctor. Swallowing assessment is dealt with in full in another section (see Chapters 5.2 and 8.2).

- *Drooling* may occur because of difficulty controlling the lips and mouth. Good nursing care involves making sure there is no un-swallowed food in the mouth, ensuring good oral hygiene and making sure the patient has access to tissues.
- *Spasticity and contractures* happen when a limb has been paralysed. The muscles tighten up, and tendons contract. This often happens many months after stroke and can be reduced by gently moving limbs through their full range as often as possible.
- Over time residents can have a number of strokes. This is called multi-infarct disease. The more strokes there are the worse the recovery each time. Residents may end up with a form of dementia (vascular dementia).

Therapy

Therapy is when specialists treat different problems caused by a stroke. Therapists may try to improve walking, activities of daily living or speech. In the early days following a stroke, therapy and practice are really important.

After about three months, most people have made most of the improvement they are going to, although some continue to get a little better. It is important for stroke patients to try to do things for themselves as this is the best type of therapy. *Always encourage them and try not to do things for them if they can do them themselves.* Formal therapy usually stops when people stop improving but sometimes more therapy is needed if people get worse later on.

Physiotherapy is important as exercise stimulates the brain to make new connections. This leads to return of function in the limb.

Carers can help by encouraging residents to do prescribed exercises and to try to do as much for themselves as possible. Any movement of a limb or attempt to talk stimulates the brain and is good.

People with a paralysed arm can easily develop *shoulder pain*. This is because the weak shoulder muscles let the arm drop out of the shoulder socket. The arm should always be supported on a pillow (see Figure 8.1.1).

It is important to position stroke patients properly. Healthy people move about all the time to prevent

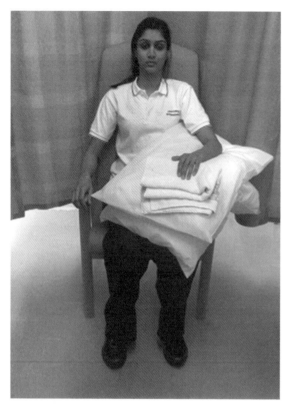

Figure 8.1.1 How to support the weak left arm of a stroke patient sitting in a chair.

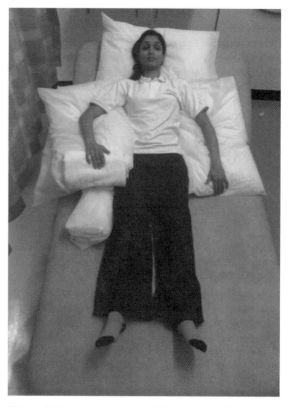

Figure 8.1.2 How to support the weak right arm of a stroke patient lying down.

pressure on one spot or 'cramping' of a limb. Residents with stroke cannot do this so carers have to do it for them. Sometimes a sling may be prescribed by a physiotherapist.

Poor positioning can lead to:

- aspiration of secretions
- pressure sores
- contractures
- poor recovery
- neck and back pain.

Figure 8.1.2 shows how to position a stroke patient whose right arm is paralysed when they are lying on their back:

1. The patient's back and neck are supported at a comfortable angle so she can see what is going on.
2. The paralysed (right) arm is supported on a pillow.
3. To eat or drink she would have to sit up (see previous picture).

Figure 8.1.3 shows how to position a stroke patient whose left arm is paralysed when they are lying on their side.

When lying down:

1. The non-paralysed (right) arm is comfortably bent.
2. The paralysed (left) arm is supported on a pillow.
3. The top leg is slightly bent so that knees and ankles do not rub, and the leg is supported by a pillow.

Stroke patients often move about and need repositioning regularly. This can be frustrating both for the resident, who gets uncomfortable, and for the staff who need to check and reposition them often. *Remember that these residents may not notice where their limbs are because of inattention. Drawing attention to this and repositioning the limb gently is good nursing and good therapy too.*

Secondary prevention

Secondary prevention is treatment designed to reduce the chance of another stroke. People often ask what their chance of another stroke is. It depends on many things and is very hard to quantify. The important thing is for residents to understand what they need to

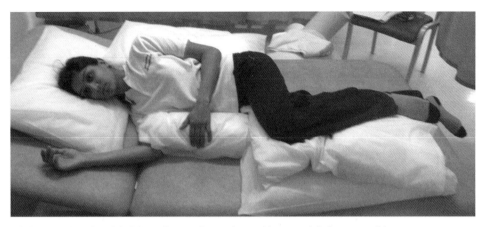

Figure 8.1.3 Positioning for side-lying of a stroke patient with a weak left arm and leg.

Secondary prevention

Lifestyle changes:
- Stop smoking
- Take regular exercise
- Reduce alcohol
- Lose weight
- Reduce fat and salt in food.

Medical treatment:
- Aspirin or warfarin
- Treatment of high blood pressure
- Treatment of high cholesterol.

do (lifestyle changes) and what the medical team need to do (medical treatment). It is not useful to worry about risks that no one can change.

Mood changes

About one in six people with stroke get depressed. This is important because it can be treated (see Chapter 10.3). *If you feel a resident has low mood or depression, please tell a doctor.* Sometimes stroke leads to inappropriate crying.

The resident may cry uncontrollably for no obvious reason. This is called emotional lability or emotionalism. Try to find out if there is a reason for the crying and comfort the resident, but if it happens often, tell a doctor. Emotional lability can be precipitated by *sadness, sentimentality (such as the visit of a grandchild) or symptom discussion (people asking why they are upset)*. It is helpful to change the topic of conversation to something neutral. Remember to tell the family that weepiness after stroke is common and that it usually does not mean that the resident is deeply distressed. Relatives are understandably upset by this emotionalism and might wrongly believe that their loved one is being treated badly in the care home.

What to do if you think someone is having a stroke

Emergency treatment may be possible for a stroke occurring in someone who was well beforehand. This treatment is not usually appropriate for someone who is either mentally or physically disabled. If a care home resident develops symptoms of a stroke, always first discuss whether emergency admission and treatment is really in their best interests. This should be done with a manager, trained nurse or doctor.

Further reading

Horgan DL, McGee H, Hickey A et al. 2011. From prevention to nursing home care: a comprehensive national audit of stroke care. *Cerebrovascular Disease* 32: 385–392.

Kumlein S, Alexsson K. 2000. The nursing care of stroke patients in nursing homes. Nurses' descriptions and experiences relating to cognition and mood. *Journal of Clinical Nursing* 9: 489–497.

Smith LN, Craig LE, Weir CJ, McAlpine CH. 2008. The evidence base for stroke education in care homes. *Nurse Education Today* 28: 829–840.

8.2 Speech and language difficulties after a stroke

Marissa Minns[1] and Stephanie Verity[2]

[1]*Leeds Teaching Hospitals NHS Trust, Leeds, UK*
[2]*Friarage Hospital, Northallerton, UK*

Key points

- There are several speech and language problems that can be the result of stroke: dysarthria, dysphasia and dyspraxia of speech.
- The speech and language therapist has a role in assessing these difficulties, providing therapy and supervising nurses and other care workers as well as the resident's family.
- There are some simple tips that will help in improving communication with residents whose speech and language are affected by stroke.

Communication difficulties following a stroke can vary depending on the part of the brain affected. Strokes may affect a person's ability to talk, write or understand spoken/written languages, while sometimes leaving other cognitive abilities intact.

How a person's language can be affected by a stroke

Problems with language are known as *dysphasias* (from the Greek for 'speechlessness') and can affect:

- an individual's ability to express themselves (an *expressive* dysphasia) or
- their capacity to understand and respond to communication with other people (a *receptive* dysphasia). Whether someone develops a particular type of dysphasia or language problem depends on which part of the brain has been affected by their stroke.

Table 8.2.1 shows examples of what you might encounter when communicating with dysphasic residents.

Once we have decided what it is we wish to say/express, we also need our facial, oral and respiratory muscles to work normally to produce sounds/words. When these 'mechanics' of speech are affected by a stroke, residents can develop several different speech problems, two common examples of which are shown in Figure 8.2.1.

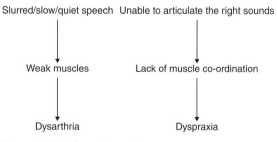

Figure 8.2.1 Speech problems.

Table 8.2.1 Types of speech problems

Problem	Mild	Severe
Receptive	• Struggle to follow busy conversation • Difficulty understanding humour • Problems understanding complex grammar or longer/lesser known words	• Unable to understand SINGLE spoken or written words • Cannot follow even basic instructions
Expressive	• Word finding difficulties – feels like the word is 'on the tip of their tongue'	• Only able to produce single words • Incoherent speech

The Care Home Handbook, First Edition. Edited by Graham Mulley, Clive Bowman, Michal Boyd and Sarah Stowe.
© 2015 John Wiley & Sons, Ltd. Published 2015 by John Wiley & Sons, Ltd.

How to support a resident's communication

Dysphasia/language problems

- Only one person should talk at a time to help the person concentrate and understand what is being said.
- Long sentences should be broken down into smaller chunks. Try not to give too much information in one go.
- Think about different ways of communicating, encourage the use of gesture, facial expression, drawing, writing (if able) or pictures/objects that the person can point to. Non-verbal communication is an important part of understanding a conversation.
- Consider the person's environment. Turn off any background noise. Sit in front of them.
- Give them time. If you still cannot understand the message, perhaps take a break but remember to go back and try again. Imagine how you would feel if you were unable to tell someone an important piece of information.
- If the person cannot think of a word, encourage them to try and think of other ways:
    - What does the object look like?
    - What is its function?
    - What does the word start with?
    - Is there a similar word that they can say, such as clock instead of watch?

Speech/motor disorders

- Turn off any background noise to make it easier to hear.
- Encourage the person to speak slowly and pace their speech. *Saying less on each breath can improve intelligibility.*
- Encourage over-articulation. Ask the person to over-pronounce their words to improve their clarity.
- Taking a relaxed deep breath before speaking can help reduce speech rate and help pacing.
- If you do not understand what the person is saying, let them know, and try asking yes/no questions to get the message.

The role of the speech and language therapist

The speech and language therapist (SLT) will carry out a comprehensive assessment of the person's communication to determine the nature of the difficulty and its severity. Intervention is then aimed at maximising communicative potential through individual or group therapy, supporting the person's communicative partners and working alongside other professionals.

Further reading

Kelly H, Brady MC, Enderby P. 2012. Speech and language therapy for aphasia following stroke *Cochrane Database System Review* 5: CD000425.

Rudd AS, Wolfe CD. 2012. Is early speech and language therapy after stroke a waste? *British Medical Journal* 345: e4870.

8.3 Parkinson's disease

Katie Athorn

Hull and East Yorkshire Hospitals NHS Trust, Hull, UK

Key points

- Parkinson's disease is a progressive motor disorder which may cause a number of non-motor problems.
- Cognitive, speech, swallowing, urinary and bowel problems, falls and hypotension require full assessment.
- Good management requires the input of an interdisciplinary team, ideally including a nurse who is a specialist in this disorder.
- Medication is not curative but is usually life-long and should not be stopped abruptly. Correct timing of drug administration is most important.

Parkinson's disease (PD) is a progressive degenerative condition affecting the basal ganglia in the brain.

It is a motor or movement disorder causing:

1. bradykinesia – slowness of movement
2. rigidity – stiffness
3. tremor – involuntary shaking, trembling or quivering
4. postural hypotension – fall in blood pressure on standing which can cause balance problems and falls.

It also causes other problems such as:

1. urinary and bowel disturbance
2. anxiety, depression, dementia
3. speech and swallowing problems
4. sleep disturbance
5. pain.

It is important to involve the entire multi-disciplinary team in the treatment of residents with PD. This should include nurses, doctors, physiotherapists, occupational therapists (OTs), speech and language therapists (SLTs) and dieticians. If you have Parkinson's disease specialist nurses (PDNS) in your area, they can be invaluable in coordinating all aspects of care and providing information and support for everyone.

Medications

Education and support is the most important treatment. Medication is usually used for the rest of the resident's life, as stopping it will result in the return of troublesome symptoms. Medication only treats symptoms, it does not stop or slow down the underlying disease.

Most common medications used are listed in Table 8.3.1, but sometimes other rarer medications may be used – your PDNS can provide information and help with these.

The timing of drugs is vital to achieve optimal treatment with minimal movement side effects. If the routine is disrupted, for example if the resident is vomiting, or admitted to hospital (where medication timing is different), it can take a long time for the patient to stabilise again. In the meantime, they may be less mobile, fall, be more confused, and their swallowing may be affected. Levo-dopa must be taken at least 30 min before or 60 min after food, as the protein or fat in food can stop the drug from being absorbed.

Bowel dysfunction

Constipation is very common. Faecal incontinence is usually due to overflow around faecal impaction (see Chapter 5.5) (see Table 8.3.2).

The Care Home Handbook, First Edition. Edited by Graham Mulley, Clive Bowman, Michal Boyd and Sarah Stowe.
© 2015 John Wiley & Sons, Ltd. Published 2015 by John Wiley & Sons, Ltd.

Table 8.3.1 Common medications used.

Medication	Trade name	Advantages	Disadvantages
Levo-dopa (+ substance to reduce effects away from the brain)	Madopar, Sinemet, Duodopa (via tube straight into gut)	Most effective treatment	Dyskinesia (involuntary movements), Movement fluctuations (e.g. freezing), Confusion, falls
L-Dopa/Carbidopa/ Entacapone	Stalevo		
Pramipexole, Ropinirole, Rotigotine	Mirapexin, Requip, Neupro (patch)	Longer duration of action, fewer side effects	Nausea and vomiting, Drowsiness, Visual hallucinations, behaviour changes (e.g. gambling, hypersexuality)
Apomorphine (rarely used)	APO-go (subcutaneous injection or infusion)	Rapid response, treats movement complications	Hallucinations, behaviour changes, confusion, falls, skin nodules, anaemia
Selegiline, Rasagiline	Eldepryl, Zelapar (buccal), Azilect	Fewer side effects, help with movement complications	Can act as a stimulant, can interact with anti-depressants (SSRIs)
Entacapone	Comtess	Increases levo-dopa action	Movement complications, nausea, hallucinations, falls, diarrhoea
Procyclidine	Kemadrin, Arpicolin	Useful for treating tremor	Dry mouth, blurred vision, constipation
Amantadine	Symmetril (tablet and syrup)	Can improve movement complications	Short acting, confusion, hallucinations, leg oedema

Dieticians and continence nurses can also be helpful for review and advice.

Bladder dysfunction

- Urinary problems include nocturia, frequency, urgency and urge incontinence.
- You must exclude urinary tract infections and diabetes (see Chapters 13.9 and 8.4) if urinary symptoms develop or worsen.
- Bladder scanning helps guide treatment options (see Chapter 5.4).

Management options

- Aim for a fluid intake of 1.5–2l per day (remember that concentrated urine irritates the bladder).
- Bladder training if post-void residual is less than 150 ml.

- Keep a bladder diary of frequency of urination, then help the resident to try and suppress urge and lengthen times between toilet visits.
- Ensure easy access to the toilet, bottles or a commode, and clothes may need to be adapted (e.g. Velcro instead of zips).
- Intermittent catheterisation if post-void residual greater than 150 ml. The resident may not be able to do this themselves (if not mobile enough, or confused).
- Permanent catheterisation (urethral or suprapubic) (see Chapter 5.4). This may need continence nurse or district nurse involvement for monitoring and changing.
- Convenes (condom catheter) and pads can help maintain skin health if the resident is incontinent.
- Continence nurses can be helpful for review and advice.
- If you are unsure, involving a continence nurse, a GP or a urologist may be required.

Table 8.3.2 Causes, treatment and management of bowel dysfunction.

Causes	Treatment and management
Gut failure due to changes in the bowel wall	Adequate dopamine therapy – ask the doctor/PDNS to review
Reduced physical mobility	Encouragement and opportunity to move and exercise as much as possible
Inadequate fluid and fibre intake because of chewing and swallowing problems	Encouragement and provision of at least 8 glasses of water and day and a diet with plenty of fibre/roughage
Weak abdominal muscles stopping adequate straining	Exercise and good positioning on the toilet – sitting with upper body slightly forward, forearms resting on thighs and knees above the hips
Medications such as anti-cholinergics, analgesics, iron	Ask the doctor/PDNS to review
Reluctance to open bowels, especially if uncomfortable	Encourage regular toileting

Mobility

See Figure 8.3.1.

Helpful hints to avoid falls (see Chapter 6.6):

- Visual cues – stepping over white strips of tape on the floor.
- Auditory cues – metronomes, singing.
- Proprioceptive cues – step back before starting to walk.

Physiotherapy can help with gait, balance, posture and strength. OTs can help with cueing and decluttering the environment.

If postural hypotension is a problem, try:

- Avoiding rapid postural changes – encourage residents to take their time.
- Avoiding straining at micturition and defaecation.
- Avoiding large amounts of alcohol.
- Increasing diet salt and fluid intake (seek GP advice first).
- Elevating the head of the bed to 30–40 degrees.
- Compression stockings.

Mental dysfunction

Dementia and depression are common and can overlap. They can both cause high levels of stress and anxiety for the resident and family. It is useful to talk to the resident and family about how they are feeling, and how memory and mood are changing over time. Some treatments are helpful but need specialist input, for example from a memory clinic, psychiatrist or neurologist.

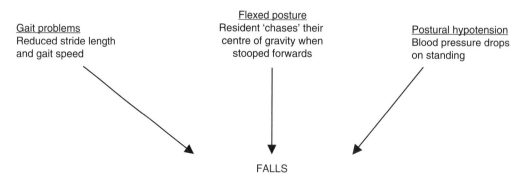

Figure 8.3.1 Reasons for falls.

Communication problems

Common speech problems are:

- monotonous voice
- quiet voice
- difficulty in initiating speech
- variable rate.

These may be the results of:

- rigidity of the respiratory and throat muscles
- stuttering speech pattern
- slow movement of the tongue and lips
- depression and dementia.

Do	Do not
Give them time and be patient	Force them to speak clearly if they are struggling
Ensure medication is given on time	Talk for them
Ask for early referral to speech and language therapy	Interrupt them
Encourage exercises (e.g. improving facial expression or breathing control)	Get annoyed with them
Use aids such as word charts or picture boards	Ignore or isolate them

Writing can also be affected – it commonly becomes small, spidery and shaky. An OT can help and advise on techniques and tools to help.

Swallowing problems

Clues to a poor/inadequate swallow:

- drooling
- weight loss
- fear and avoidance of swallowing
- 'gurgly' or 'wet' voice
- coughing before, during or after swallowing
- recurrent chest infections.

Key professionals to involve

Speech and Language Therapy	Dietician
Assessment, sometimes with video fluoroscopy	Advice on supplements
Advice on oro-facial exercises	Advice on strategies, e.g. little and often, snacking
Advice on swallowing manoeuvres	Advice if alternative feeding considered, e.g. nasogastric tube, PEG
Advice on modification of food (e.g. pureed)	

If the resident cannot maintain their weight and health with oral feeding, it is important to ascertain their views on nasogastric (in the short term) or percutaneous gastrostomy feeding (PEG). Risks and benefits would need to be fully discussed (see Chapter 14.1).

Further reading

Gage H, Storey L. 2004. Rehabilitation for Parkinson's disease: a systematic review of available evidence. *Clinical Rehabilitation* 18: 463–482.

Buchanan RJ, Way S, Huang C, Simpson P, Manyam BV. 2002. Analysis of nursing home residents with Parkinson's disease using the minimum data set. *Parkinsonism Related Disorders* 8: 368–380.

Thanvi BR, Muashi SK, Vijaykumar N, Lo TC. 2003. Neuropsychiatric non-motor aspects of Parkinson's disease. *Postgraduate Medical Journal* 79: 561–565.

Thomas S, MacMahon D. 2002. Managing Parkinson's disease in long term care. *Nursing Older People* 14: 23–30.

Useful web sites

Bladder and Bowel Foundation www.bladderandbowel foundation.org [Accessed October 2013]

National Association for continence www.nafc.org [Accessed October 2013]

The Parkinson's Disease Society www.parkinsons.org.uk [Accessed October 2013]

The Royal College of Nursing www.rcn.org.uk [Accessed October 2013]

8.4 Diabetes

Ahmed Abdelhafiz[1] and Alan Sinclair[2]

[1]*Rotherham General Hospital, Rotherham, UK*
[2]*Bedfordshire and Hertfordshire Postgraduate Medical School, University of Bedfordshire, Luton, UK*

Key points

- The prevalence of diabetes in residents with complex comorbidities in care homes is increasing.
- Quality of life should always be the focus for individual care.
- Control of blood pressure is more important than tight control of blood glucose.
- It is vital to recognise and treat hypoglycaemia, which can present in different ways.
- Residents with diabetes should have optimum foot and eye care.
- Diabetes increases the risk of nursing home admission three fold.
- Older people with diabetes living in care homes tend to have more comorbidities, disability and cognitive dysfunction than non-diabetic residents.
- Type 2 diabetes affects about 25% of nursing home residents.

Complications

In addition to traditional vascular complications, diabetes in older people is also associated with cognitive disorders, physical disability, falls, fractures and incontinence.

Care home residents with diabetes have more cardiovascular disease, visual problems, pressure sores, limb amputations and kidney failure than residents without diabetes.

Guidelines for the management of diabetes in care homes do not have the same evidence base as those for younger diabetic populations because of the exclusion of frail older people from clinical trials.

Currently, there is no evidence to suggest that tight blood glucose (glycaemic) control improves outcomes relevant to older people. In fact, low HbA1c (<7%) (a measure of blood glucose over the preceding three months) has been shown to increase the risk of falls.

In older patients with type 2 diabetes, intensive blood pressure control has a larger benefit than glucose control. Therefore, guidelines generally recommend strict glucose control in healthier older patients and a less rigorous approach in frail ones with multiple comorbidities and a high risk of hypoglycaemia.

Diabetes management

Diabetes management of older people in care homes should take into account their frail condition and complex needs and should achieve targets relevant to them – particularly quality of life. The European Diabetes Working Party for Older People (EDWPOP) clinical guidelines provides a comprehensive review of evidence to enhance quality of diabetes care (Box 8.4.1)

Hypoglycaemia

Setting glycaemic targets and hypoglycaemia risk: A relaxed target for HbA1c around 8% or 8.5% is recommended:

- Tight glycaemic control is not necessarily the sole reason for hypoglycaemia in nursing home residents with diabetes.
- The occurrence of hypoglycaemia is likely to be related to overall health condition and associated multiple comorbidities.
- Training of staff to recognise symptoms and risks of hypoglycaemia is important (Box 8.4.2).
- Providing a list of the risk factors for hypoglycaemia that is available to the staff is recommended.

Box 8.4.1 European Diabetes Working Party for Older People 2011 recommendations for care homes

On admission to care home:

- Each resident should be screened for the presence of diabetes.
- Each resident with diabetes should have assessment for functional loss and interventions in place to delay disability.

During their stay at care home:

- Residents on insulin-secreting medications and/or insulin should be regularly reviewed for the presence of hypoglycaemic symptoms.
- Resident with diabetes should have optimal blood pressure and blood glucose regulation to help maintain cognitive and physical performance.

Good clinical practice in care homes:

- All residents should have an annual screen for diabetes.
- Each resident with diabetes should have an individualised diabetes care plan.
- Care homes with diabetes residents should have an agreed diabetes care policy or protocol which is regularly audited.
- Diabetes education and training courses should be available to care home staff.
- Adoption of risk–benefit approach in the management of residents with diabetes in terms of medications, metabolic targets and extent of performing investigations, with a focus on enhancing quality of life, maintaining functional status and avoiding hospital admission for diabetes-related complications.

- Medications should be reviewed to switch residents taking longer acting drugs (sulfonylureas) who experience recurrent hypoglycaemia to shorter acting agents.
- In insulin treated residents, the new class of long acting insulin analogues may be a good option, as they reduce the risk of hypoglycaemia and can be conveniently injected once daily.

Box 8.4.2 Common symptoms of hypoglycaemia in old people

Pallor	Visual disturbances
Sweating	Slurring of speech
Dizziness	Tiredness
Trembling	Falls
Poor coordination	Sleepiness
Weakness	Faintness
Inappropriate behaviour	Seizure
Visual disturbances	Confusion
Drowsiness	Coma

- Residents who have erratic eating patterns and unpredictable caloric intake could be managed with short acting insulin preparations administered only after meals, thus preventing insulin-induced hypoglycaemia if a meal is missed or only partly consumed (Box 8.4.3).

Hyperglycaemia

Avoidance of *hyperglycaemia* is as important as avoidance of *hypoglycaemia* to prevent hyperosmolar states, infections and other complications. Maintaining a random blood glucose of more than 4 but less than 15 mmol/l is a reasonable target as blood glucose outside this range is likely to be symptomatic and cause cognitive changes. Therefore, HbA1c is reasonably used for short-term monitoring rather than for long-term complication prevention.

Care plans

Care homes should have a policy for diabetes care, including:

Box 8.4.3 Insulin use in care homes

Requirements

- Ability of residents and/or care staff to administer insulin and to recognise and manage hypoglycaemia.
- Availability of community nursing to administer insulin when self-injection is not possible, for example for residents with severe cognitive, physical or behavioural problems.

Blood glucose monitoring

- A defined person responsible for blood glucose monitoring.
- Staff training on using the glucose meter, interpretation of readings, how to act on them as well as up keeping and quality control checks of the meter and storage of test strips.
- Aseptic technique for finger stick lancing use and good infection control practices to avoid outbreaks of infections such as hepatitis B.
- Safe disposal of the needles from syringes, insulin pen devices, and lancets from finger-pricking devices.
- Glycaemic goals of fasting blood glucose >7–8.5 mmol/l and a random glucose <12 mmol/l are reasonable to avoid hypoglycaemia and the osmotic symptoms and lethargy of hyperglycaemia.
- Actions to be taken effectively if blood glucose is outside the above ranges and in the event of illness.

Insulin prescription

- Clear prescription of insulin dose and frequency to avoid drug errors and risks of severe hypoglycaemia, as well as appropriate documentation of blood glucose readings which should be standardised on a local basis.
- Insulin regimen will vary between residents, but for those with erratic dietary intakes, bolus injections of analogue short-acting insulin may be very useful, as they can be given at the same time as (or immediately after) the resident eats their meal, decreasing the risk of hypoglycaemia.

- Diabetes screening for residents on admission and periodically thereafter.
- An audit tool to ensure policy implementation.
- Individualised care plans for residents.

Care plans should be tailored to residents' needs, which take into consideration the individual's values, preferences, their life expectancy, comorbidities and the impact of diabetes management (polypharmacy, glucose monitoring) on quality of life. For example, many residents with diabetes are on multiple medications for prevention of cardiovascular disease. which may be inappropriate in this population with limited life expectancy.

Screening for complications relevant to older people, such as cognition, physical function and depression, should be included in their annual review (Figure 8.4.1).

Quality of life

Tight glycaemic control (including dietary restriction, frequent blood testing, insulin injections and polypharmacy) may be a burden. For example:

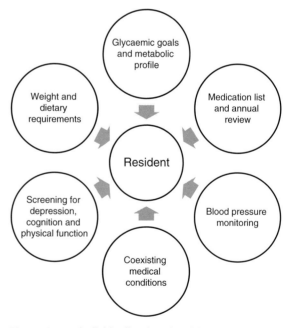

Figure 8.4.1 Individualised and resident-centred care plan.

Box 8.4.4 Roles of the podiatrist and community-based optometrist in the management of residents with diabetes

Podiatrist:

* To assess pre-existing foot pathologies, physical deformity, callous formation, infection, ulceration, vascular status, toenail pathologies and suitability of current footwear.
* To actively treat diabetic foot disease.
* To educate residents and care staff about foot care, correct toenail cutting, heel protection.

Optometrists:

* Screening for diabetic eye disease.
* Visual acuity measurement and evaluation of uncorrected refractive errors.
* Assess for cataract formation and diabetic retinopathy.
* Intra-ocular pressure measurement to screen for glaucoma.
* Prescription for new glasses, where appropriate.
* Referral for specialist ophthalmological input, where necessary.

---

* Dietary restriction may cause weight loss.
* Frequent finger sticks and insulin injections may lead to agitation (especially in cognitively impaired residents).
* Polypharmacy may increase the risk of falls (see Chapter 6.6).

Nutrition

Nutritional guidelines should not be too restrictive but tailored to be healthy and to reflect personal preferences. Individuals are free to exercise personal choice with respect to food selection. Diabetes treatment is then adjusted accordingly. The aims of nutritional choices for elderly residents with diabetes include:

* Maintenance of healthy body weight and avoidance of malnutrition.
* Coordinated nutritional needs with glycaemic targets and adjustment of diabetes medication, especially if food intake is variable.
* Maintenance of hydration.

Foot care and eye screening

Foot ulcers and infection are common in patients with diabetes. Residents with diabetes should have an annual comprehensive foot examination to identify risk factors for ulcers and amputations. The foot examination should include inspection, assessment of foot pulses, and testing for loss of protective sensation such as the pinprick sensation. Podiatry input should be available regularly (see Chapter 7.3).

Glaucoma, cataract, refractive errors and retinopathy occur frequently in people with diabetes. Diabetic retinopathy is a vascular complication, strongly related to duration of diabetes, and is the most frequent cause of blindness in these patients. Residents with diabetes should have an initial comprehensive eye examination by an ophthalmologist or optometrist and further examinations annually thereafter (see Chapter 7.1). Examinations will be required more frequently if retinopathy is progressing. Domiciliary optometric services may be an option for residents who are not able to travel to optometric practice (Box 8.4.4) (see Chapter 17.10).

Future perspectives

* Introducing advanced nurse practitioners in care homes has a positive impact in improving staff confidence and in reducing hospital admissions.
* Expansion of the nurse practitioner role will have the potential to improve care for diabetic residents.
* Healthcare assistants or support workers could act as a lead or a link person to liaise with other healthcare professionals (such as district nurses) and to take responsibility for disseminating information and sharing good practice within the care home. The competencies required and the main focus of the roles are summarised in Box 8.4.5.

Diabetes education is an integral part of diabetes care. However, existing educational programmes are not specific to the needs of older people with diabetes. Development of such educational programmes adapted to older people with cognitive and physical dysfunctions – as well as regular exposure of care home staff to education and training – would provide the means to better knowledge and care.

Box 8.4.5 Competencies and role of healthcare assistant

Key competencies required:

- Blood glucose monitoring skills.
- Skills in administering insulin injections.
- Recognition of hypoglycaemia symptoms.
- Recognition of diabetes complications.
- Good knowledge of diabetes care as a whole.

Key role:

- Insulin administration (in some cases up to twice daily) to residents with diabetes, who are unable to self-administer insulin because of physical or cognitive disability or behavioural disturbance.
- A source of information for diabetes care to the staff and families of residents with diabetes.
- To ensure that residents are receiving a regular healthy diet and that staff have confidence with regard to what people with diabetes can eat.
- To ensure that blood glucose testing is carried out appropriately based on individual residents' needs.
- A link with other healthcare professionals, such as general practitioners or district nurses, to ensure that all care home residents with diabetes have their regular structured care in place, such as annual review, feet checks and retinal screening.
- To ensure that the results of the above checks are fed back to the relevant staff within the care home.
- To keep accurate documentation and medical records of each resident with diabetes and to ensure that all relevant investigations are available when required by a healthcare professional.

Further reading

Abdelhafiz AH, Sinclair AJ. 2009. Hypoglycemia in residential care homes. *British Journal of General Practice* 59: 49–50.

American Diabetes Association. 2010. Executive summary: standards of medical care in diabetes-2010. *Diabetes Care* 33: S4–S10.

Aspray TJ, Nesbit K, Cassidy TP, et al. 2006. Diabetes in British nursing and residential homes: a pragmatic screening study. *Diabetes Care* 29: 707–708.

Childs BP, Clark NG, Cox DJ, et al. 2005. Defining and Reporting Hypoglycaemia in Diabetes: A report from the American Diabetes Association Workgroup on Hypoglycaemia. *Diabetes Care* 28: 1245–1250.

Diabetes UK. 2010. Good Clinical Practice Guidelines for Care Home Residents with Diabetes. London: Diabetes UK, 2010. Available at: http://www.diabetes.org.uk [Accessed October 2013]

Nelson JM, Dufraux K, Cook PF. 2007. The relationship between glycaemic control and falls in older adults. *Journal of the American Geriatric Society* 55: 2041–2044.

Sinclair AJ, Aspray T. 2009. Diabetes in care homes. In: Diabetes in Old Age. Sinclair AJ, (ed.) Chichester, UK, John Wiley and Sons, pp. 311–324.

Sinclair AJ, Paolisso G, Castro M, et al. 2011. European Diabetes Working Party for Older People 2011 Clinical Guidelines for Type 2 Diabetes Mellitus (EDWPOP). *Diabetes & Metabolism* 37: S27–S38.

8.5 Heart failure

Tajammal Zahoor[1] and Amanda Foster[2]

[1] Edinburgh Royal Infirmary, Edinburgh, UK
[2] Calderdale and Huddersfield NHS Trust, Huddersfield, UK

Key points

- Heart failure is characterised by breathlessness, oedema and lethargy.
- It is often associated with other chronic conditions and the heart failure may not be recognised.
- Treatment includes lifestyle changes, drugs and devices.
- Drug therapy can greatly improve symptoms and quality of life.
- Palliative care should be considered in the last year of life.

Introduction

Heart failure is a common and complex syndrome, which is not always recognised or adequately treated.

Heart failure is caused by structural or functional abnormalities, which prevent the heart from being able to (i) fill with enough blood or (ii) pump with enough force – or (iii) both of these.

Heart failure is a syndrome that is initially diagnosed by its symptoms and physical findings. Most definitions emphasise both the presence of symptoms of heart failure and the physical signs of fluid retention. Heart failure can affect the left side, the right side, or both sides of the heart. Most cases involve the left side where the heart cannot pump enough oxygen-rich blood to the rest of the body. With right-sided failure, the heart cannot effectively pump blood to the lungs where the blood picks up oxygen.

Heart failure in elderly and care home residents

Diagnosis of heart failure nursing home residents is often delayed because of atypical presentation.

Older patients with heart failure commonly have other chronic diseases, such as hypertension, obstructive lung disease, diabetes and stroke. These diseases may show signs and symptoms similar to those of heart failure and thus may be difficult to interpret.

Early diagnosis and treatment aim to delay the progression of heart failure and improve symptoms and quality of life.

What causes heart failure?

The leading causes of heart failure include:

- Coronary artery disease.
- High blood pressure.
- Diabetes.
- Cardiomyopathy (a disease of the heart muscle).
- Diseases of the heart valves.
- Abnormal heartbeats (arrhythmias or dysrhythmias).
- Congenital heart disease.

Other conditions that may injure the heart muscle and lead to heart failure include:

- Treatments for cancer, such as radiation and chemotherapy.
- Thyroid disorders.
- Alcohol abuse.
- HIV/AIDS.
- Cocaine and other illegal drugs.

Signs and symptoms of heart failure

The most common signs and symptoms of heart failure are:

- Shortness of breath.
- Swelling of the ankles, legs and sometimes the abdomen.
- Tiredness.
- Cough.

The Care Home Handbook, First Edition. Edited by Graham Mulley, Clive Bowman, Michal Boyd and Sarah Stowe.
© 2015 John Wiley & Sons, Ltd. Published 2015 by John Wiley & Sons, Ltd.

Shortness of breath is the result of the inefficiency of the left side of the heart to pump blood into the arteries. This causes 'back pressure,' which causes fluid to collect in the air spaces of the lungs and sometimes around the lung (pleural effusions).

Individuals may begin to feel short of breath and tired after simple daily activities. Breathlessness when lying flat (orthopnoea) may occur and, in advanced stages of heart failure, breathlessness may occur at rest.

Fluid build-up in the lungs can also cause a cough. Coughing is generally worse at night and when lying down. Crackles can often be heard in the bases of the lung.

Excessive fluid in the lungs can cause a life-threatening condition called acute *pulmonary oedema*. This condition presents with sudden onset of profound breathlessness and requires emergency treatment (see Chapter 9.6).

Swelling of the ankles and legs (oedema) is generally linked to right-sided heart failure. Because of poor perfusion of the kidneys, the body retains fluid and salt, which results in fluid build-up in the systemic circulation.

Tiredness and loss of energy is often troublesome. Tiredness can be linked to severity of breathlessness and reduction in blood flow to muscles.

Investigations

Heart failure is initially diagnosed clinically by obtaining a detailed history and conducting a comprehensive physical examination.

While several tests (including electrocardiograms, blood tests and chest x-rays) assist in the diagnosis and management of heart failure, echocardiograms are most useful as they can reveal details of the function of the heart chambers and valves. Echocardiograms confirm the presence and type of heart failure.

Management of heart failure

Drug therapy

Treatments predominantly aim to improve symptoms and prognosis. The following medications are the most common in treating heart failure and should be used as directed by the specialist team.

- *ACE inhibitor/ARB* – First-line treatment that aims to reduce the workload of the heart. An ARB (angiotensin receptor blocker) should be used in those intolerant of ACE-Is.
- *Beta-blockers* – First-line treatment which increases the efficiency of the heart contraction by decreasing the heart rate.

- *Loop diuretics* – Loop diuretics (such as Furosemide) work by increasing the amount of sodium and water excreted in the urine to reduce the amount of excess fluid in the lung bases and peripheries.
- *Aldosterone antagonists (also known as potassium-sparing diuretics)* – A diuretic used as a second line treatment. Used in combination with a loop diuretic in those who have persisting signs and symptoms of heart failure.
- Most residents with heart failure will be on Aspirin and some will also be prescribed digoxin and statins.

Devices

Specific individuals with heart failure may benefit from technical devices as below:

- *Cardiac resynchronisation therapy* (CRT) – A type of pacemaker used to help coordinate the contractions between the pumping chambers of the heart (ventricles). CRT can improve cardiac muscle function and symptoms of heart failure.
- *Implantable cardioverter defibrillator* (ICD) – Used in individuals who are thought to be at risk of developing abnormal heart rhythms which could be life threatening. ICDs are designed to identify such life-threatening events and deliver a 'shock' to restore a normal heart rhythm.

Lifestyle modification

Lifestyle factors that are considered important are general health measures which include:

- Stopping smoking – even in the very elderly.
- Eating a balanced diet – for those who are overweight, weight loss should be advised.
- Eating a diet with no added salt – high levels of salt can increase blood pressure and make the body retain water and sodium.
- Alcohol intake – in those in whom alcohol is the cause of heart failure, abstinence is advised.
- Taking exercise – regular exercise can improve heart failure symptoms. Exercise should be individualised but can be useful even in disabled residents (see Chapter 6.1).

Progression of heart failure

Heart failure is often associated with debilitating symptoms of breathlessness, oedema and lethargy. Acute episodes of worsening symptoms require hospitalisation. While treatments frequently improve symptoms, acute exacerbations can be life-threatening and could result in death. It means that life expectancy is difficult to predict.

Individuals who have peripheral oedema should be weighed daily and at the same time of day. A gain in weight of 1–2 kg over two or more consecutive days can indicate early signs of fluid build-up and should therefore be reported to the' GP or heart failure nurse.

As heart failure progresses, periods of instability may become more frequent, symptoms are difficult to manage and function decreases. Heart failure nurses can play a key role in the management of symptoms at this stage and are also able to offer advice and support.

Despite optimising therapies, progressive pump failure eventually leads to increasingly severe chronic symptoms at rest or during very minimal exertion.

When conventional therapies are unable to realistically offer any gain, prognosis is poor and end of life care should be considered (see Chapter 16.4). This might include withdrawal of life-lengthening treatments and the reprogramming of cardiac devices.

Consideration to palliative care (Heart Foundation New Zealand, 2009)

Palliative care should be considered for patients with the strong possibility of death within 12 months and who have advanced symptoms, for example NYHA Class IV (Box 8.5.1), a poor quality of life, and who are resistant to optimal pharmacological and non-pharmacological therapies. Strong markers of impending mortality include:

- Advanced age.
- Recurrent hospitalisation for decompensated heart failure and/or related diagnosis.
- NYHA Class IV symptoms.
- Poor renal function.
- Cardiac cachexia (weight loss).
- Low sodium concentration (hyponatraemia).
- Hypotension necessitating withdrawal of medical therapy.

References

The Criteria Committee of the New York Heart Association. 1994. *Nomenclature and Criteria for Diagnosis of Diseases of the Heart and Great Vessels*. 9th Edn. Boston, Mass, Little, Brown & Co, pp. 253–256.

Heart Foundation New Zealand. 2009. Guideline for management of chronic heart failure, 2009 update. Available at:

Box 8.5.1 New York Heart Association functional classification system for congestive heart failure severity

(From The Criteria Committee of the New York Heart Association. Nomenclature and Criteria for Diagnosis of Diseases of the Heart and Great Vessels. 9th edn. Boston, Mass: Little, Brown & Co; 1994:253–256.)

Class I

No limitations. Ordinary physical activity does not cause undue fatigue, dyspnoea or palpitations

Class II

Slight limitation of physical activity. Ordinary physical activity results in fatigue, palpitations, dyspnoea or angina pectoris (mild CHF)

Class III

Marked limitation of physical activity. Less than ordinary physical activity leads to symptoms (moderate CHF)

Class IV

Unable to carry on any physical activity without discomfort. Symptoms of CHF present at rest (severe CHF)

Reproduced with kind permission from the American Heart Association.

http://www.heartfoundation.org.nz/uploads/Guideline-Management-Chronic-Heart-Failure-5.pdf [Accessed October 2013].

Further reading

British Heart Foundation. 2011. Living with heart failure [online] Available at: http://www.bhf.org.uk/publications [Accessed October 2013]

Daamen MA, Schols JM, Jaarsma T, Hamers JP. 2010. Prevalence of heart failure in nursing homes: a systematic literature review. *Scandinavian Journal of Caring Science* 24: 202–208.

Dickstein K, Cohen-Solal A, Filippatos G, McMurray JJ, et al. 2008. ESC Guidelines for the diagnosis and treatment of acute and chronic heart failure *European Heart Journal* 29: 2388–2442.

Gaulden L. 2003. Diagnosis and management of heart failure in the long term care setting. *Director* 11: 177–181.

The Gold Standards Framework 2009. GSF Factsheet 2 [online]. Available at: http://www.goldstandardsframework.org.uk/ [Accessed October 2013].

Lewis EF. 2011. End of life care in advanced heart failure. *Current Treatment Options in Cardiovascular Medicine* 13: 79–89.

NICE. 2010. Guidelines August 2010 Management of chronic heart failure in adults in primary and secondary care. London, NICE.

Tresch DD. 2000. Clinical manifestations, diagnostic assessment, and etiology of heart failure in elderly patients. *Clinical Geriatric Medicine* 16: 445–456.

8.6 Pain

Desmond O'Neill[1] and Martin Mulroy[2]

[1]Trinity College Dublin, Dublin, Ireland
[2]Our Lady of Lourdes Hospital, Drogheda, Co. Lough, Ireland

Key points

- More than half of care home residents will experience pain.
- Pain can be overlooked, and all staff should look for signs and symptoms of pain.
- Ask residents if they have pain and listen carefully to family and other team members, who may have noticed signs of distress.
- Ensure that you have a pain scale that everyone involved can use. Use a pain chart and report pain to the doctor.
- Familiarise yourself with the different drugs used for pain relief and be aware of their side-effects.
- Remember to give laxatives to those on opioids.

- Pain is common, under-recognised, under-measured and under-treated: in addition, care home residents with dementia and stroke may not be able to signal their suffering through direct and clear speech.
- You should develop a practice of regularly seeking out pain – to understand ways of detecting and measuring it in those with language and memory difficulties, and also to consider that *pain may be a cause of restlessness and disturbed behaviour.*
- *Please, please, please* agree on a common pain scale in your care home, as well as a chart for assessing pain and response to treatment – this allows residents, families, care assistants, nurses and doctors to sing from the same sheet.

How common is pain and why does it matter in care home residents?

Pain occurs in *at least* every second resident in your home: studies suggest levels ranging between 49–83%, more than twice that reported in the community, and similar to levels in older people in hospitals.

Pain reduces activities of daily living and quality of life, and adequate pain relief can make a big difference to your resident's life.

Who is best placed to diagnose pain in care home residents?

- Do not fall into the trap of thinking: 'he/she has dementia, and cannot tell me'. Babies cannot verbalise, yet we use our clinical observations, as well as what the parents tell us (the collateral history), to work out whether the baby is in pain and what the underlying cause may be.
- If you do not ask, you will not know! Start with the resident – he or she is best placed to help guide you to the presence of pain and the underlying cause. Clearly, this is more challenging for those with an underlying learning disability, dementia or communicative difficulties from stroke.
- This is when the collateral history and observations of staff are vital. It may be the physiotherapist who has observed that the resident is unable to stand because of pain, or the household staff may have noted that the resident is unable to use cutlery because of a swollen joint. The resident's family or carer, who will always know the individual better than we do, may recognise subtle changes that may assist nursing and medical staff.

How should I record whether pain is present?

Empower your patient. Residents usually wish to participate in this process when asked so, if possible, provide a diary for them to record where the pain may be and how it may differ each day.

The standard nursing observations recorded include blood pressure, pulse rate, temperature and respiratory rate.

The fifth, unrecorded 'vital sign' should be PAIN. You need a *pain scale* to assess the severity of the pain, and a *pain chart* to record this over time, and these should be used consistently in your care home. The British Geriatrics Society and the Royal College of Physicians of London have published a very concise guide to good practice in assessing pain in older people. Helpful illustrations of pain scales include the Numeric Rating Scale and Abbey pain scales – are all readily available (see Appendix 1, 1.3).

The measurements recorded in the pain chart need to be discussed with, and reviewed, by the resident's doctor: you may need to be *appropriately assertive* in ensuring that the doctor takes note of your observations. If you are concerned that the pain measurements are not getting the attention that they deserve, discuss this with the Director of Nursing in your care home.

Most pain is chronic, so ongoing attention to effectiveness of pain relief is *very* important.

What measures can be used by care home residents to treat pain?

A team approach is important, as attention to appropriate seating (occupational therapy) (see Chapter 6.5) and treatment of musculoskeletal pain by physiotherapy can be effective.

In addition, pain can be magnified by depression or boredom, and appropriate attention to relieving both of these is worthwhile (see Chapter 10.3).

We can also use a range of medications, and familiarity with these is important.

Non-opioids

Paracetamol:

- Safe, tried and trusted for pyrexia and indicated for musculoskeletal pain.
- Well tolerated without any sedative or major adverse side-effects.
- Maximum dose 1 g orally, 4 times a day. Eight tablets can be a lot of medication for older residents to take, so consider a suspension or rectal route if the oral route is not possible.

Non-steroidal Anti-Inflammatory Agents (NSAIDs):

- Avoid these wherever possible: only use them if there is no readily available alternative – especially where there has been a history of gastro-intestinal bleeding.
- A good choice for acute bone fractures or bony metastasis, however; prescribe a short course of treatment.
- For an acute gouty flare, consider colchicine or a steroid as an alternative. If an NSAID is unavoidable, the doctor will often prescribe a medication to protect the stomach lining.
- NSAIDs can increase fluid retention, so avoid in patients with heart failure. Also, try to avoid these drugs (and aspirin) in those with diabetes and advanced renal disease.
- Start with the lowest dose, review how effective it is, and stop if there is no objective improvement in symptoms.

Opioids

- The old wives' tale of over-using opioids, resulting in respiratory depression, has been a barrier to prescribing adequate pain relief.
- The opioids are very effective analgesics.
- In general, for chronic pain, we start with low doses of long-acting opiate (such as MST) and doses of short-acting opiates for breakthrough pain. If a resident requires greater than two breakthrough doses of morphine over 24 hours, then the longer-acting preparation can be increased.
- Prescribe a laxative in all patients with opioids, and pre-emptive bowel care is very important. Constipation is more common than respiratory depression.

Pain modifying agents

- Some anti-depressants (e.g. amitriptyline) and anti-epileptic agents (e.g. gabapentin, pregabalin) can modify pain, particularly if coming from the nerves (neuropathic) and can also be helpful in chronic pain.
- Sedation and constipation/urinary retention may limit their efficacy.

Reference

Herman AD, Johnson TM, Richie C et al. 2009. Pain management interventions in the nursing home: a structured review of the literature. *Journal of the American Geriatric Society* 57: 1258–1267.

Chapter 9

Medical Emergencies

9.1 Anaphylaxis

Soma Kar and Maureen Whittaker

Hull and East Yorkshire Hospitals NHS Trust, Hull, UK

Key points

- Anaphylaxis is a life threatening medical emergency.
- Early recognition and prompt action could save someone's life.
- Adrenalin is the mainstay of treatment.
- Awareness is important, clear protocol including doses of adrenalin must be available.
- **Remember the 3 A's:**
  - A- **A**wareness of anaphylaxis
  - A- **A**voidance of triggers
  - A- early **A**ction.

Anaphylaxis is a severe systemic allergic reaction characterised by rapidly developing life-threatening airway and/or breathing and/or circulation problems, usually associated with skin or mucosal changes. It usually happens on exposure to foreign bodies (allergens) commonly foods, medications or insect stings.

It is a medical emergency and can lead to death if untreated.

How anaphylaxis happens

It typically occurs due to release of chemical mediators from mast cells (a class of white blood cell) by immunoglobulin E (IgE), which are proteins produced in the body on exposure to a specific allergen (Figure 9.1.1).

There are many triggers for anaphylaxis. Some common causes are shown in Figure 9.1.2.

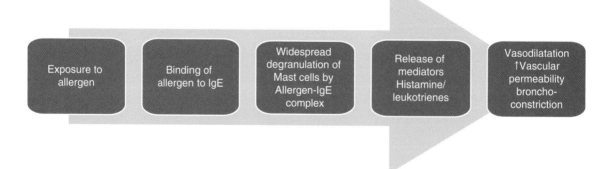

Figure 9.1.1 How anaphylaxis happens.

The Care Home Handbook, First Edition. Edited by Graham Mulley, Clive Bowman, Michal Boyd and Sarah Stowe.
© 2015 John Wiley & Sons, Ltd. Published 2015 by John Wiley & Sons, Ltd.

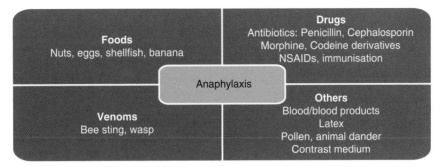

Figure 9.1.2 Common causes of anaphylaxis.

Box 9.1.1   Signs and symptoms of anaphylaxis

Airway: stridor (high pitched inspiratory noise caused by airway obstruction), laryngeal oedema (airway swelling), hoarseness of voice
Breathing: dyspnoea, wheeze, respiratory arrest
Circulation: hypotension, chest pain, collapse, cardiac arrest
Skin: wheals, urticaria, angio-oedema (swelling of lips and eyelids)
Gastrointestinal: abdominal pain, vomiting, diarrhoea
Others: rhinitis, conjunctivitis

Suspect anaphylaxis when all of the following three criteria are met:

- Sudden onset rapidly progressing symptoms
- Life-threatening Airway, Breathing, Circulation problems
- Skin/mucosal changes

Supporting criterion:
Exposure to a known allergen for the residents

Clinical features

Anaphylaxis usually manifests immediately with variable severity. It may progress rapidly causing life-threatening airway, breathing and circulation problems (Box 9.1.1).

What you must do

Managing anaphylaxis in a community is different from an acute setting depending on training and skills of rescuers, number of responders and types of equipment and drugs available.

Patients having an anaphylactic reaction in any setting require the following:

1. Recognition of anaphylaxis by staff.
2. Early call for help.
3. Remove suspected triggers.
4. Assess and treat based on the Airway, Breathing, Circulation, Disability and Exposure approach.
5. *Protect airway* by using oropharyngeal or naso-pharyngeal airways.
6. Give 100% oxygen, where available.
7. Rapid infusion of intravenous crystalloid (500–1000 ml of 0.9% normal saline) if blood pressure systolic ≤ 90 mmHg and/or diastolic ≤60 mmHg.
8. Salbutamol nebuliser, if wheezy.
9. Start CPR, if appropriate, according to basic life support guidelines.
10. Early administration of adrenalin.

See Figure 9.1.3.

Adult dose of intramuscular (IM) adrenalin in anaphylaxis

1,1000 Adrenalin 0.5 mg (=500 microgram = 0.5 ml). Repeat in 5 minutes if no better.
Do not give intravenous adrenalin unless patient is severely ill with poor circulation.

Adrenalin auto-injectors

Patients at risk of anaphylaxis are often prescribed auto-injectors, a pre-filled syringe with 0.3 mg or 0.15 mg adrenalin, for their own use.
Healthcare professionals should use auto-injectors in anaphylaxis if it is the only preparation available.

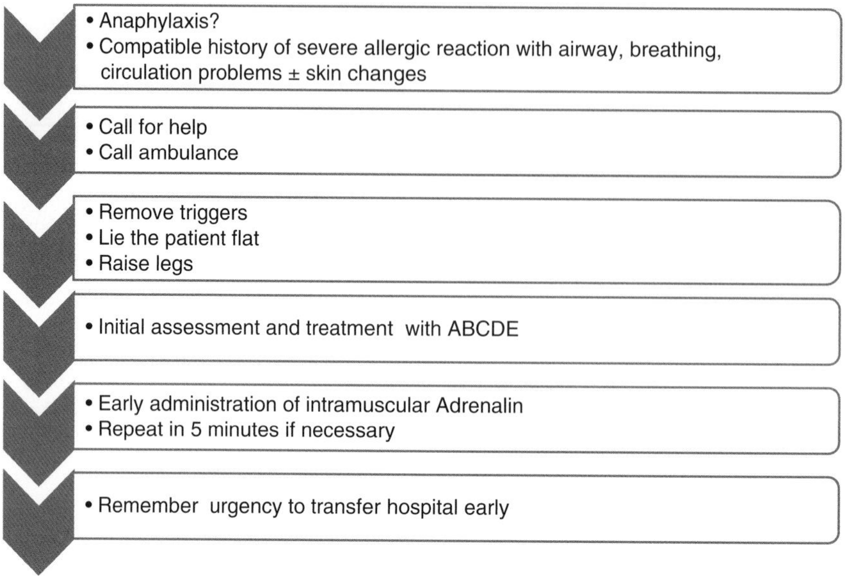

- Anaphylaxis?
- Compatible history of severe allergic reaction with airway, breathing, circulation problems ± skin changes

- Call for help
- Call ambulance

- Remove triggers
- Lie the patient flat
- Raise legs

- Initial assessment and treatment with ABCDE

- Early administration of intramuscular Adrenalin
- Repeat in 5 minutes if necessary

- Remember urgency to transfer hospital early

Figure 9.1.3 Anaphylaxis management algorithm. Based on the Resuscitation Council UK, Anaphylaxis algorithm in *Emergency Treatment of Anaphylatic Reactions: Guidelines for healthcare providers*, Resuscitation Council, UK 2008. www.resus.org.uk/pages/reaction.pdf

Reference

Resuscitation Council, UK (2008). Emergency Treatment of Anaphylatic Reactions: Guidelines for healthcare providers. www.resus.org.uk/pages/reaction.pdf

Further reading

Pham TS, Rudner EJ. 2000. Peanut allergy. *Cutis* 65(5): 285–289.

9.2 Asthma

Laura Cook

Leeds Teaching Hospitals NHS Trust, Leeds, UK

Key points

- Chronic lung diseases (including asthma and COPD) are common.
- Symptoms include: breathlessness, wheeze, cough and chest tightness.
- Use the Airway, Breathing and Circulation approach to assess someone who is unwell.
- Try to keep calm.
- Call an ambulance if there are worrying features, such as noisy or rapid breathing, severe wheeze, or cyanosis.
- Be familiar with common treatments, such as different preventer and reliever inhalers.
- Try to give some 'reliever' medication, if available.

Asthma is a common problem, affecting 5.4 million people in the UK where there are 700,000 people aged over 65 being treated for asthma.

People with asthma are prone to narrowing of the small airways in their lungs, which causes recurrent 'attacks'.

Asthma can be diagnosed for the first time in late life. However, it is more difficult to diagnose in old age and there is often some overlap with other types of chronic lung disease, such as Chronic Obstructive Pulmonary Disease (COPD).

The best way to diagnose asthma (as opposed to COPD) is by lung function tests, but these are not always practical to perform in frail, elderly people. For this reason, there are no reliable statistics on the rates of asthma compared to other breathing problems in care home residents.

'True' asthma is more likely in people who:

- have never smoked/passively smoked
- suffer from eczema and hay fever
- have a strong family history of asthma, eczema or hay fever
- suffer obvious attacks that respond quickly to reliever inhalers
- can identify specific triggers to the attacks
- have had chest problems since childhood or young adulthood.

People with asthma usually take one or more medicines via an inhaler.

There are two main types of inhalers:

1. **'Preventers'**

   These are taken regularly, for example one or two times a day, to help prevent an attack from happening. They contain either an inhaled steroid, or other long-acting medication, or a combination of both, to help keep the airways open.

   Examples include:
   - beclomethasone (e.g. QVAR, Clenil Modulite)
   - budesonide (e.g. Pulmicort)
   - fluticasone (Flixotide)
   - salmeterol (Serevent)
   - salmeterol and fluticasone (Seretide)
   - formeterol and budesonide (Symbicort)
   - tiotropium (Spiriva).

2. **'Relievers'**

   These are used to ease the symptoms when they occur. They act quickly (in minutes) but also wear off quickly.

   Examples include:
   - salbutamol (e.g. Ventolin, Salamol)
   - terbutaline (e.g. Bricanyl)
   - ipratropium bromide (e.g. Atrovent).

The Care Home Handbook, First Edition. Edited by Graham Mulley, Clive Bowman, Michal Boyd and Sarah Stowe.
© 2015 John Wiley & Sons, Ltd. Published 2015 by John Wiley & Sons, Ltd.

Symptoms suggesting an attack

- Wheezing
- Chest tightness
- Difficulty in breathing
- Cough

In practice, the emergency assessment and treatment of a person with difficulty in breathing is the same for asthma and COPD.

The following pathway would also identify an unwell person if they had another cause of difficulty in breathing (e.g. heart failure, chest infection, pulmonary embolus), and would appropriately prompt you to call the GP or ambulance, depending on the presence of worrying symptoms and signs:

Airway, Breathing, Circulation (or 'ABC') approach

A – Airway

- Can they *speak normally*?
- Can you hear:
  - *Wheezing*? A musical sound, usually when breathing out (suggesting a narrowing of the small airways).
  - *Stridor*? A high pitched rasp when breathing in (suggesting a narrowing of the windpipe or larger airways).

B – Breathing

- Are they *struggling for breath*, for example using *accessory muscles*?
- Are they *breathing very quickly*? How many breaths do they take in a minute?
- Can the resident *complete a sentence* without stopping to breathe?

C – Circulation

- What do they look like? For example, cyanosed (blue), pale, grey or clammy.
- What is their *pulse rate*? (In beats per minute, felt at the wrist or neck – or use a stethoscope and count their heart rate.)
- What is their *blood pressure*? (If this can be recorded.)
- If you are trained to do so, check their capillary refill time.

Decide if there are any worrying features and refer to the following flow chart:

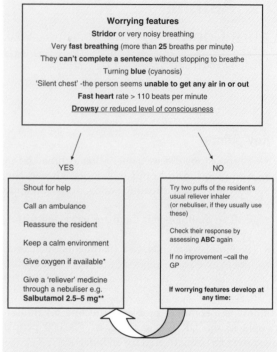

*Some people living in care homes use oxygen. They can be given their usual amount or, if this is not known, as much oxygen as can be delivered through their mask or nasal cannulae.

**If a nebuliser is unavailable, try repeated puffs of a reliever inhaler, through a spacer device if possible.

If at any point the resident becomes unconscious or has stopped breathing, start cardiopulmonary resuscitation (CPR) (see Chapter 9.7).

Further reading

British National Formulary. 2012.*63rd Edition*, March 2012 Available at www.bnf.org [Accessed October 2013]

The British Thoracic Society and Scottish Intercollegiate Guidelines Network. 2011. 'British Guideline on the Management of Asthma' 2011.Available at www.brit-thoracic.org.uk [Accessed October 2013]

NICE. 2010. Guideline: Chronic Obstructive Pulmonary Disease (CG101) Available at http://guidance.nice.org.uk/CG101 [Accessed October 2013]

Resuscitation Council (UK). 2011. *Advanced Life Support*. 6th Edn. Available at: www.resus.org.uk [Accessed October 2013]

Useful web site

Asthma UK web site: www.asthma.org.uk [Accessed October 2013]

9.3 Bleeding

Steven Parke and Beverley Brown

Leeds Teaching Hospitals NHS Trust, Leeds, UK

Key points

- Always take bleeding seriously.
- Consider the possibility of internal bleeding after a fall or trauma – this can be difficult to detect.
- Take particular care if an individual is on medication that can exacerbate bleeding – especially warfarin.
- Monitor bleeding individuals closely – deterioration can be rapid.
- Dial an emergency service if there are signs of hypovolaemia – do not wait for shock to develop.

Bleeding can occur as the result of trauma, an underlying medical disorder or a combination of the two. Any body organ can be injured and bleed, and blood loss can be either internal or external (Figure 9.3.1):

- *Internal* blood loss is not usually readily apparent. For example, the liver, spleen and kidneys may bleed into the abdominal cavity.
- *External* bleeding is easily identified, since blood leaves the body through either a break in the skin or a natural orifice such as the mouth, anus or vagina.

If left untreated, bleeding can eventually lead to hypovolaemic shock and ultimately death.

Diagnosis of bleeding

The presence of bleeding is obvious when external blood loss is detected, although blood may often be seen on clothing, bed sheets or toilet tissue after wiping rather than coming directly from an orifice. Internal bleeding can be harder to diagnose and calls for close clinical assessment – especially after any trauma. Pointers to the presence of blood loss include:

- Symptoms at the site of any injury such as severe pain.
- Symptoms related to the bleeding itself, for example limb weakness or speech disturbance following intracerebral haemorrhage (see Chapter 8.1)
- Signs of hypovolaemia (Box 9.3.1).

Box 9.3.1 Signs suggesting the presence of hypovolaemia.

- Low blood pressure (or blood pressure that is lower than an individual's norm) (see Chapter 15.2).
- Increased heart and/or respiratory rate.
- Cool, sweaty skin.
- Increased capillary refill time.
- Reduced urine output.

Hypovolaemia is defined as an abnormal decrease in the volume of circulating blood in the body. It can lead to shock, an emergency condition in which the heart is unable to pump enough blood and oxygen around the body to keep the vital organs functioning correctly.

Hypovolaemic shock

Most individuals tolerate mild bleeding well and there is typically no change in vital signs. As blood loss becomes more severe, however, the heart rate becomes more rapid, the blood pressure begins to fall and the skin starts to become pale and cold as a result of peripheral vasoconstriction. Later, as less and less oxygen reaches the brain, a person's mental state will alter, ranging from slight behavioural change to agitation/confusion and eventually reduced consciousness (Table 9.3.1). Eventually, unless action

The Care Home Handbook, First Edition. Edited by Graham Mulley, Clive Bowman, Michal Boyd and Sarah Stowe.
© 2015 John Wiley & Sons, Ltd. Published 2015 by John Wiley & Sons, Ltd.

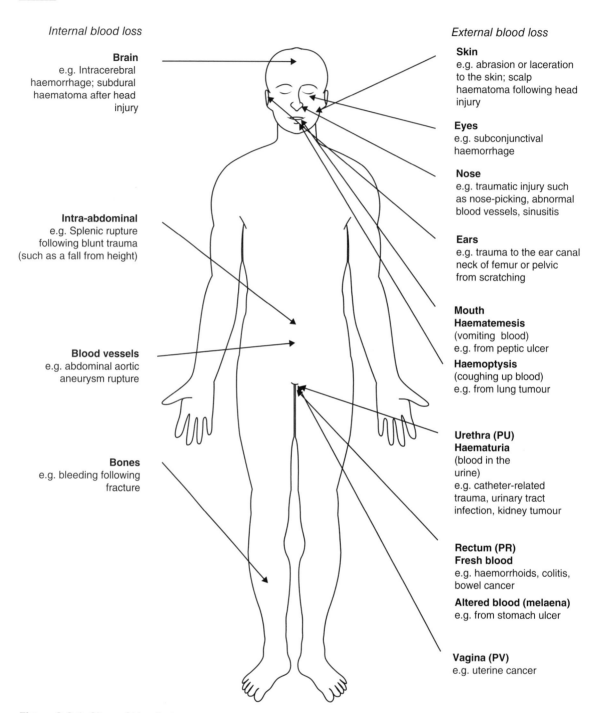

Internal blood loss

Brain
e.g. Intracerebral
haemorrhage; subdural
haematoma after head
injury

Intra-abdominal
e.g. Splenic rupture
following blunt trauma
(such as a fall from height)

Blood vessels
e.g. abdominal aortic
aneurysm rupture

Bones
e.g. bleeding following
fracture

External blood loss

Skin
e.g. abrasion or laceration
to the skin; scalp
haematoma following head
injury

Eyes
e.g. subconjunctival
haemorrhage

Nose
e.g. traumatic injury such
as nose-picking, abnormal
blood vessels, sinusitis

Ears
e.g. trauma to the ear canal
neck of femur or pelvic
from scratching

Mouth
Haematemesis
(vomiting blood)
e.g. from peptic ulcer
Haemoptysis
(coughing up blood)
e.g. from lung tumour

Urethra (PU)
Haematuria
(blood in the
urine)
e.g. catheter-related
trauma, urinary tract
infection, kidney tumour

Rectum (PR)
Fresh blood
e.g. haemorrhoids, colitis,
bowel cancer

Altered blood (melaena)
e.g. from stomach ulcer

Vagina (PV)
e.g. uterine cancer

Figure 9.3.1 Sites of bleeding.

is taken to stem the bleeding and support the circulation with intravenous fluids and/or blood transfusion, cardio-respiratory arrest will occur.

Although a healthy 70 kg adult has about 5 litres of blood and can lose around 10 to 15% of their total blood volume without serious consequences, elderly

Table 9.3.1 Classification of hypovolaemia and hypovolaemic shock.

| | | Worsening shock ——————→ Death | | |
	Compensated	Mild	Moderate	Severe
Degree of blood loss	10–15%	15–30%	30–40%	>40%
Heart rate (bpm)	<100	>100	>120	>140
Blood pressure	Normal	Postural drop	Marked fall (< 90 mmHg systolic)	Profound fall
Capillary refill	Normal	May be delayed	Usually delayed	Always delayed
Respiration	Normal	Mild increase	Moderate tachypnoea	Marked tachypnoea
Mental state	Normal or agitated	Agitated	Confused	Drowsy, obtunded

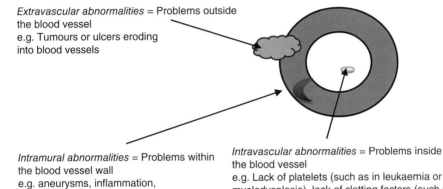

Extravascular abnormalities = Problems outside the blood vessel
e.g. Tumours or ulcers eroding into blood vessels

Intramural abnormalities = Problems within the blood vessel wall
e.g. aneurysms, inflammation, arterio-venous malformations

Intravascular abnormalities = Problems inside the blood vessel
e.g. Lack of platelets (such as in leukaemia or myelodysplasia), lack of clotting factors (such as in haemophilia), medication effects

Figure 9.3.2 Causes of bleeding.

individuals, and particularly those with multiple comorbidities, often:

- Have less physiological reserve to compensate.
- Take medications, such as anti-hypertensives and beta-blockers, which can potentially blunt their cardiovascular response.
- Take drugs that impair blood clotting.

They may therefore have less tolerance of blood loss and can deteriorate rapidly; close care must be taken in their assessment and monitoring.

Causes

Apart from direct trauma to blood vessels, bleeding can also occur due to extravascular, intramural and intravascular changes (Figure 9.3.2).

Several medications work by impairing the body's natural clotting mechanisms making bleeding more likely after relatively minor trauma and exacerbating

Box 9.3.2 Drugs which can exacerbate bleeding

- Given by mouth
  - Aspirin
  - Clopidogrel
  - Dipyridamole
  - Ticagrelor
  - Warfarin
  - Dabigatran
  - Rivaroxaban
  - Apixaban
- Given by injection
  - Low molecular weight heparin, e.g. Dalteparin, Enoxaparin, Tinzaparin
  - Fondaparinux

any that does occur (Box 9.3.2). Some, such as aspirin, can also irritate the upper gastrointestinal tract, predisposing to inflammation and ulcers that can be a cause of blood loss.

Particular attention should be given to individuals on warfarin; the effect of this drug can vary, especially as a result of interactions with other medication such as antibiotics, and must therefore be closely monitored with regular blood tests.

Nursing assessment

After noticing any external blood loss, or following a fall or other trauma, it is important to perform baseline observations – including pulse rate, blood pressure, respiratory rate and capillary refill time – and then to monitor closely. Any abnormality, deviation from the individual's norm or subsequent deterioration should trigger a request for medical advice. This should be an emergency call (999 in the UK) if there are any signs of hypovolaemia.

Unexplained bleeding should never be ignored, as it may indicate a serious underlying illness, though routine medical review via a GP can be sought if the resident is otherwise well.

For bleeding following traumatic injury, basic first aid rules should be followed:

- Firm, direct pressure should be applied to the bleeding point.
- The affected body part should be elevated, if possible.
- The resident should be nursed in a lying position with their legs raised if blood loss is heavy or if there are concerns about hypovolaemia.

Reference

Copland M, Walker ID, Tait RC. 2001. Oral anticoagulants and hemorrhagic complications in an elderly population with atrial fibrillation. *Archives of Internal Medicine* 161: 2125–2128.

Gurwitz JK, Field TS, Radford MJ, et al. 2007. The safety of warfarin therapy in the nursing home setting. *American Journal of Medicine* 120: 539–544.

Suatengco R, Posner GL, Marsh F, Jr. 1995. The significance and work-up of minor gastrointestinal bleeding in hospitalised nursing home patients. *Journal of the National Medical Association* 87: 749–750.

9.4 Collapse
Steven Parke and Elaine Carr

Leeds Teaching Hospitals NHS Trust, Leeds, UK

Key points

- Collapses in elderly residents are common and, though many have a benign cause, some signal underlying pathology.
- A simple faint (vasovagal syncope) can mimic seizures.
- A thorough assessment is important, and should adopt an 'ABC' approach.
- Postural blood pressure measurements should always be performed where possible to look for orthostatic hypotension.
- Hypoglycaemia is a cause of collapse that should not be missed.
- Medical advice should always be sought – especially to conduct a medication review.

Collapse

A collapse is a sudden loss of postural tone. Collapses are frequently unannounced and often accompanied by loss of consciousness. They are extremely common and have numerous causes – ranging from the benign to the serious – and often provoke significant anxiety in individuals and their carers.

Collapses occur more frequently in elderly individuals because of:

- Age-related physiological changes.
- An increased incidence of chronic health conditions, such as ischaemic heart disease, diabetes, congestive cardiac failure and strokes.
- An increased likelihood of polypharmacy (the use of multiple medications), often including sedatives, diuretics and anti-hypertensives.

Syncope

Syncope is a collapse associated with brief loss of consciousness following a temporary reduction in the amount of blood and therefore oxygen reaching the brain (see Chapter 6.6).

Syncopal episodes typically:

- Develop rapidly.
- Are of short duration (unconsciousness usually lasting no more than 30 seconds).
- Conclude with an almost spontaneous and complete recovery (there may be marked fatigue, however, especially in older individuals).

Causes

There are many causes of collapse, including:

- Neurally-mediated syncope (due to abnormal nerve activity):
  - common faint (also known as vasovagal syncope);
  - situational syncope (after coughing, sneezing, micturition or gastrointestinal stimulation, such as swallowing or opening one's bowels);
  - carotid sinus hypersensitivity (see Chapter 6.6).
- Postural, or orthostatic hypotension (triggered by a fall in blood pressure on standing or remaining upright for a prolonged period):
  - (over judicious) use of anti-hypertensive and other medications (Box 9.4.1);

The Care Home Handbook, First Edition. Edited by Graham Mulley, Clive Bowman, Michal Boyd and Sarah Stowe.
© 2015 John Wiley & Sons, Ltd. Published 2015 by John Wiley & Sons, Ltd.

Box 9.4.1 Drugs are often a contributing factor in collapses in elderly residents. Common culprits are:

- vasodilators:
  - nitrates – e.g. isosorbide mononitrate, GTN
  - calcium channel blockers – e.g. diltiazem, nifedipine
  - ACE inhibitors – e.g. ramipril, perindopril
  - hydralazine.
- anti-hypertensives – e.g. calcium channel blockers, beta-blockers.
- diuretics – e.g. furosemide, bumetanide.
- sedatives and antidepressants – e.g. citalopram, amitriptyline.

  - hypovolaemia due to blood loss, vomiting or diarrhoea;
  - damage to the autonomic nervous system, for example in diabetes or Parkinson's disease.
- Post-prandial syncope (a fall in blood pressure after a meal).
- Cardiac:
  - arrhythmias (abnormal heartbeat rhythms);
  - valvular heart disease (narrowed or leaky heart valves);
  - heart attack.
- Pulmonary embolism.
- Epileptic seizures.
- Metabolic disorders – particularly hypoglycaemia.
- Substance abuse, including alcohol intoxication.
- Anxiety/panic attacks/hyperventilation.
- Strokes (collapse associated with focal neurological problems, such as weakness).
- Narcolepsy and cataplexy (disorders of sleep).

Nursing assessment

After witnessing a collapse, or discovering a resident who appears to have collapsed, it is important to perform a rapid and thorough assessment. This should initially involve an 'ABC' (Airway, Breathing, Circulation) approach to confirm signs of life. Assuming these are present, the resident should be made as safe as possible, for example by placing them in the recovery position or, in the event of a seizure, removing furniture that could potentially cause injury (see Chapter 9.5). Basic life support/cardiopulmonary resuscitation should be commenced immediately if a pulse cannot be felt or respiratory effort is absent.

Box 9.4.2 Assessing a resident following a collapse

- Baseline observations:
  - Pulse
  - Blood pressure
  - Respiratory rate
  - Pulse oximetry (if available)
  - Capillary blood glucose
  - Neurological observations/Glasgow coma score.
- Subsequent observations:
  - Continue monitoring
  - Postural blood pressure (Figure 9.4.1).
- Assess for injury – particularly to head, neck, hips.
- Assess possible causes (Box 9.4.3):
  - Obtain a history from the resident and any witnesses if possible.
  - Look for evidence of bleeding.
  - Consider medications.

When it is safe to do so, a full set of baseline observations should be performed (Box 9.4.2). It is important not to forget to undertake a capillary blood glucose reading to exclude hypoglycaemia. If present, this should be treated initially with GlucoGel® (or similar), and subsequently sugary drinks/food when the individual is able to swallow safely.

After a collapse, the resident should be nursed in the lying position and monitored regularly until their conscious level has improved. At this point, the carer should look for signs of any injuries, particularly to the head, neck and hips, and for evidence of any precipitating cause for the collapse (e.g. bleeding). If and when it is possible to move the resident, a set of postural blood pressure recordings should be undertaken (Figure 9.4.1).

Learning point

- Orthostatic hypotension is diagnosed when postural blood pressure readings demonstrate a reduction of at least 20 mmHg in systolic blood pressure or 10 mmHg in diastolic blood pressure within 3 minutes after standing.
- The diagnosis of this condition is extremely important, since it is responsible for symptoms such as recurrent dizziness, light-headedness and syncope.

(a)

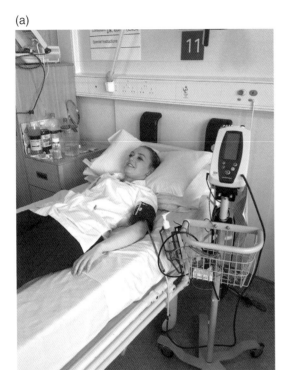

1. Ask the resident to relax whilst lying down for at least five minutes.

2. Remove any tight clothing from around their arm, which should be supported at the level of the heart.

3. Select an appropriately sized sphygmomano-meter cuff and place this around the resident's arm.

4. Measure their systolic and diastolic blood pressure.

5. Leave the cuff in place and ask the resident to stand up, ensuring their safety.

6. Measure their blood pressure **immediately** after standing, and at **1 and 3 minutes** thereafter.

7. Help the resident to sit or lie down, and document all readings.

(b)

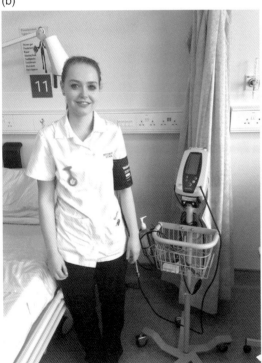

Figure 9.4.1 How to perform postural blood pressure measurements.

Seizure or syncope?

Both epileptic seizures and syncopal episodes can cause abnormal limb movements/shaking, the latter being due to abnormal nerve cell activity in the brain as a result of transient hypoxia. In syncope, however, the movements are typically short-lived uncoordinated jerks/twitches, and tend to occur after the onset of unconsciousness. In seizures, long-lasting generalised tonic-clonic movements are more common, and these episodes are much more likely to be associated with tongue biting and urinary incontinence. Furthermore, subsequent disorientation is common.

> **Learning point**
>
> • A simple faint (vasovagal syncope) may mimic seizures.

Medical assessment

Any collapse should be seen as a trigger for medical review.

The main tool used to determine the cause of a collapse is a careful history of the events before, during and after the episode, from the resident as well as from any bystanders (Box 9.4.3). It is therefore vitally important that this is well-documented as

> **Box 9.4.3** Important features to record about a collapse
>
> • Possible precipitants including painful stimuli, sudden bad news, postural change, meals, pain, cough, micturition, defaecation, swallowing, neck movement and exercise.
> • Mode of onset, including individual's skin colour/general appearance and body position, and preceding symptoms (e.g. dizziness, nausea, flashing lights).
> • Subsequent progression of event.
> • Depth and duration of altered consciousness.
> • Rate of recovery of consciousness.
> • Associated symptoms such as palpitations, chest pain and breathlessness.
> • A full drug history, including recent medication changes.

soon as possible and, if A&E attendance is arranged, that a carer capable of providing a witness account accompanies the resident concerned.

A collapse does not always require an immediate emergency call (999 in the UK) and hospital admission, particularly if a witnessed episode and subsequent observations are consistent with either a simple faint, situational syncope or postural hypotension (Box 9.4.4).

Whether or not to call for urgent medical advice is clearly a matter for professional judgement, but if an individual recovers quickly, is otherwise well and has none of the features listed in Box 9.4.5, advice from a GP during normal working hours, particularly for medication review, is usually sufficient.

> **Box 9.4.4** Features of collapse due to fainting, postural hypotension or situational syncope
>
> • Onset during or immediately after:
>   ◦ Fear, pain, emotional distress or sudden unexpected unpleasant sensory stimulation.
>   ◦ Rapid movement from seated/lying position to standing or prolonged standing, especially in crowded/hot places.
>   ◦ During or shortly after coughing, vomiting, swallowing, sneezing, opening bowels or passing water.
> • Preceding sensation of dizziness and/or nausea.
> • Resident appears pale/grey and/or clammy before collapse.
> • Loss of consciousness lasts no more than 30 seconds, recovery is rapid and there is no prolonged disorientation after the event.
> • Short-lived uncoordinated jerking movements of the limbs may occur but there is no tongue biting.
> • The individual may be subject to polypharmacy, particularly involving several anti-hypertensive medications; drugs may have been recently started or increased in dosage.
> • There may have been recent fluid loss (e.g. diarrhoea and vomiting).
> • A postural blood pressure drop is identifiable on lying/standing readings.

Box 9.4.5 Reasons to consider urgent hospital review following a collapse

- Worrying symptoms before or after the collapse, especially chest pain and shortness of breath.
- Probable seizure causing collapse.
- Abnormal observations, particularly if these fail to improve as consciousness recovers, for example bradycardia or persistently low blood pressure (or lower than the individual's norm).
- Hypoglycaemia not improving despite Gluco Gel® (or similar) and/or sugary drinks/foods, or occurring in residents taking sulphonylureas (e.g. Gliclazide) or insulin.
- Incomplete recovery after the event, such as persisting new or increased confusion.
- Concerns about possible bony or other injury.
- Resident taking warfarin or other anti-coagulant, especially if they have suffered a head injury.
- Recurrent episodes.

Further reading

Aronow WS, Ahn C. 1994. Postprandial hypotension in 499 elderly persons in a long-term care facility. *Journal of the American Geriatrics Society* 42: 930–932.

Lipsitz LA, Pluchino FC, Wei JY, Rowe JW. 1986. Syncope in institutionalised elderly: the impact of multiple pathological conditions and situational stress. *Journal of Chronic Diseases* 39: 619–630.

9.5 Seizures

Lauren Ralston

Bradford Teaching Hospital Foundation Trust, Bradford, UK

Key points

- Epilepsy is more common with advancing years.
- It is helpful to be aware of the types of seizure, what triggers them and how they can be treated.
- Ensure you observe the seizure closely and that no one aggravates the problem by potentially harmful interventions, such as forcing something into the resident's mouth.
- Get urgent medical help if the seizure lasts more than five minutes or if there are multiple seizures or serious injury.

What is epilepsy?

- Seizures are the result of an abnormal burst of electrical activity within the brain, and epilepsy is the tendency to have recurrent unprovoked seizures.
- Over the age of 80, the diagnosis of new onset epilepsy is likely to be related to stroke and dementia.
- The diagnosis of epilepsy in an older person may still be associated with the stigma of years ago when it was perceived to be a mental health problem. Carers who have an understanding of epilepsy may therefore be reassuring to residents with epilepsy.

Seizures – general points

There are many different types of seizures ranging from minor absences to major fits (see Table 9.5.1).

- Diagnosis can be very difficult, particularly of minor episodes and where the individual may have memory of cognitive impairment.

Your witness account will be very important to the medical team. Do make a note of what actually happened to include if at all possible what the individual was doing before the seizure, the sequence of events, how long they lasted and how quickly they recovered.

Table 9.5.1 Types of seizure.

Simple partial seizure	• No loss of awareness • One or more of: twitching, dizziness, lip smacking, numbness, repetitive movement • Lasts a few seconds, may progress to other seizure types
Complex partial seizure	• Some loss of awareness • May display automatisms, e.g. lip smacking, plucking at clothes, swallowing repetitively or wandering around as if drunk • May progress to tonic-clonic seizures
Tonic-clonic seizure	• Loss of consciousness • **Tonic phase**: Forceful contractions of large muscle groups (body stiffens) followed by • **Clonic phase**: Uncontrollable jerking. May be associated with tongue biting, incontinence or cyanosis (blue discolouration due to lack of oxygen) • **Postictal phase (common)**: muscles relax, decreased conscious level

Box 9.5.1 outlines the questions you may be asked.

The Care Home Handbook, First Edition. Edited by Graham Mulley, Clive Bowman, Michal Boyd and Sarah Stowe.
© 2015 John Wiley & Sons, Ltd. Published 2015 by John Wiley & Sons, Ltd.

Box 9.5.1 Questions to ask about a resident who might be having a fit

(from '6 key questions to ask the witness'. Epilepsy in later life: A guide for clinicians dealing with older people. Epilepsy Action, 2011)

1. What was the person doing at the time?
2. Did you notice anything, or did the person complain of anything before it happened? For example, changes in skin colour, altered speech, sweating, nausea, vomiting or confusion?
3. Did they lose consciousness, become unresponsive, or seem unaware that you were there? How long for?
4. Were they still, or did they twitch, jerk or move around?
5. What happened after the event? Were they confused, nauseated or aggressive? Was their speech altered? Were there any other more specific complaints from the resident?
6. Did anyone try to take the resident's pulse?

Box 9.5.2 Factors which may increase the risk of a seizure

- Infection
- Medication changes/missed doses
- Alcohol
- Missed meals – hypoglycaemia
- Photosensitivity – flickering TV
- Boredom/stress
- Dehydration and other metabolic upsets

Thinking about these or writing down answers as soon as possible after the event could be extremely useful.

If this is not the first occasion and there are recurrent seizures, consider possible triggers listed in Box 9.5.2.

First aid and when to call for help

- During a tonic-clonic seizure, first aid can prevent a person experiencing a seizure coming to harm. Box 9.5.3 outlines the approach.
- Most seizures last from a few seconds to a few minutes and terminate without the need for medication.

Seizures lasting more than 30 minutes are termed status epilepticus; this is a medical emergency and requires urgent transfer to hospital.

Table 9.5.2 Some of the common anti-epileptic drugs used in older people.

Drug	Side effects
Lamotrigine	Insomnia
	Rash
Leveriacetam	Sedation
	Mood disturbance
	Dizziness
	Tremor
Oxcarbazepine	Electrolyte disturbance – low sodium
	Dizziness
	Drowsiness
Pregabalin	Dizziness
	Weight gain
Sodium Valproate	Drowsiness
	Weight gain
	Tremor
	Parkinsonism
Tiagabine	Dizziness
	Impaired concentration
	Tremor
Zonisamide	Increased temperature
	Mood disturbance
	Weight loss

A doctor may prescribe sedative drugs for patients known to develop status to calm the brain and terminate the seizure. Choices include:

- Rectal diazepam.
- Buccal midazolam given into the buccal cavity between cheek and gum.

These drugs may cause respiratory depression, so the resident should therefore be closely observed until fully recovered.

Specialist training to give such drugs is required and a protocol should be devised detailing the circumstances in which these drugs should be used.

Starting treatment

Decisions to start treatment should be made by a specialist in secondary care. The risks of further seizures are weighed against the potential side-effects of long-term medication, which together with drug interactions are more common in older people.

An awareness of some of the common side-effects can alert you to problems with medication.

Box 9.5.3 Do's and don'ts in a tonic-clonic seizure

✓ During a tonic-clonic seizure bystanders SHOULD	✓ During a tonic-clonic seizure bystanders SHOULD NOT
• Time the seizure • Allow space around the person • Support their head and neck, for example with a pillow • Position the person on one side to help breathing and aid drainage of secretions • Stay until the seizure has stopped or help has arrived	• Move the person – unless they are at risk of further injury • Try to restrain or lift the person • Place anything in the person's mouth

Monitoring epilepsy

Individual care plans for epilepsy should be made and agreed between residents (where possible), families/carers, and primary and secondary care providers. They should include medication and lifestyle details. An example of a care plan can be found on the Epilepsy Action web site.

All residents should have an annual review of their epilepsy by their GP, or more frequently if drug changes have been made.

Box 9.5.4 When to get urgent medical help

Call the emergency paramedic or ambulance if:

- The seizure lasts > 5 minutes
- Multiple seizures (>3 in an hour)
- The resident has injured themselves badly
- The resident has trouble breathing after the seizure has stopped

Decisions on management should be recorded in the resident's notes.

Acknowledgement

The author wishes to thank Lynda Dorsey for helpful advice in the preparation of this chapter.

Reference

Epilepsy action. 2011. Epilepsy in later life: A guide for clinicians dealing with older people. www.epilepsy.org.uk [Accessed October 2013]

Useful web sites

The following websites are excellent resources for further information on epilepsy, patient leaflets, epilepsy posters and details of future training events:

Epilepsy Action www.epilepsy.org.uk [Accessed October 2013]
The National Society for Epilepsy www.epilepsysociety.org.uk [Accessed October 2013]

9.6 Dyspnoea

Daniel Harman and Lisa Wickens

Hull and East Yorkshire Hospitals NHS Trust, Hull, UK

Key points

- Dyspnoea is the subjective sensation of shortness of breath.
- It is a normal symptom of heavy exertion, but is abnormal if it occurs in unexpected situations, such as at rest or on minimal exertion.
- The decision to seek help is based on clinical judgement with the assistance of the Modified Early Warning Score.
- Dyspnoea may represent the 'end stage' of a chronic illness and therefore require palliative care.

Causes

Care home residents can experience *acute* dyspnoea as a result of a variety of clinical conditions (see Table 9.6.1):

Persistent or chronic dyspnoea may also be seen in residents with long-term conditions such as Congestive Cardiac Failure (CCF, Chronic Obstructive Pulmonary Disease (COPD) or Pulmonary Fibrosis).

Assessment

The initial approach begins by assessment of the airway, breathing and circulation (ABC) followed by a medical history and physical examination.

Medical history

By definition, a person's airway must be patent in order to provide a history. If it is not, this MUST be addressed before any further assessment

Specific questions that may help identify the diagnosis of airways obstruction include:

- Onset and duration of dyspnoea (is this an acute/chronic problem)?
- Associated symptoms (see Table 9.6.2).
- Existing medical conditions: asthma, COPD, pulmonary fibrosis, congestive cardiac failure (CCF).
- Exposure to allergens or new medications.

Seek emergency medical help if the airway is compromised.

Examination

The Modified Early Warning Score (MEWS) (Chapter 15.8) should be used when assessing *all* patients with dyspnoea. It will assist in assessing the severity of the illness of the patient.

Respiratory rate is the most sensitive marker of acute illness and yet it is rarely measured.

The competent practitioner should then examine the resident to identify and exclude any immediate life-threatening causes of breathlessness. A systematic approach will avoid missing important clinical signs (see Table 9.6.3).

Investigations

Pulse oximeters allow for a simple assessment of oxygenation. Pulse oximetry should be available in all locations where emergency oxygen is used (see Chapter 15.3).

Treatment

Treatment of the underlying clinical condition is essential in order to resolve the dyspnoea. For example, antibiotics will be required to treat an underlying pneumonia.

Oxygen, if available, may be indicated.

The Care Home Handbook, First Edition. Edited by Graham Mulley, Clive Bowman, Michal Boyd and Sarah Stowe.
© 2015 John Wiley & Sons, Ltd. Published 2015 by John Wiley & Sons, Ltd.

Table 9.6.1 Causes of acute dyspnoea.

Airway	Breathing	Circulation	Other
• Airway obstruction, e.g. foreign body, mucus	• Lower respiratory tract infection • Pneumonia • Pneumothorax • Acute exacerbation of asthma • Acute exacerbation of COPD	• Acute pulomnary oedema • Pulmonary embolus • Shock	Metabolic acidosis, e.g. DKA, acute kidney injury Neurological, e.g. stroke Psychogenic, e.g. panic attacks

COPD, chronic obstructive pulmonary disease; DKA, diabetic keto-acidosis.

Table 9.6.2 Associated symptoms.

Associated symptom	Possible diagnosis
Sputum production with colour	Lower respiratory tract infection Pneumonia
Chest pain	Acute coronary syndrome Pulmonary embolus
Wheeze	Asthma Acute pulmonary oedema
Haemoptysis (bloody sputum)	Pulmonary embolus Infection
Stridor (inspiratory wheeze)	Airway obstruction

Table 9.6.3 Important clinical signs.

Look	Feel	Listen
Colour	Tracheal position (central/deviated to one side)	Breath sounds
Sweating	Chest expansion	Added sounds (e.g. crepitations or crackles)
Distress +/ Exhaustion Respiratory rate Chest wall movement	Percussion	Stridor

Indications for oxygen therapy include:

- Any critically ill resident (clinical judgement and MEWS).
- Tachypnoea (respiratory rate ≥20 breaths/minute).
- Maintenance of O_2 saturations to 94–98%.

Patients with COPD known to retain CO_2 – maintain O_2 sats at 88–92% (see Chapter 15.3).

When to seek help or admit

The decision to seek help or acutely admit a resident to hospital will be based on clinical judgement with the assistance of the MEWS.

Indications to seek help/admit a resident include:

- hypotension
- hypoxia
- stridor
- tracheal deviation
- altered conscious level

- cyanosis
- absent breath sounds.

Consider palliation

Occasionally, dyspnoea may represent the 'end stage' of a chronic illness. Establishing this fact early and advanced care planning regarding 'end of life' care may prevent the resident receiving unwanted and or futile treatment.

Further reading

Caprio AJ Hanson LC, Munn JC, Williams CS, et al. 2008. Pain, dyspnoea, and the quality of dying in long-term care. *Journal of the American Geriatrics Society* 56: 683–688.

Forman CD, Rayner AV, Tobin EP. 2004. Pneumonia in older residents of long-term care facilities. *American Family Physician* 70: 1495–1500.

Waldrop DP, Kirkendall AM. 2009. Comfort measures: a qualitative study of nursing home-based end-of-life care. *Journal of Palliative Care* 12: 719–724.

9.7 Canadiac arrest

Laura Cook

Leeds Teaching Hospitals NHS Trust, Leeds, UK

Key points

- If unsure about resuscitation status in a collapsed adult, the presumption should be to start basic life support.
- Call for help promptly if a resident is unresponsive.
- Open the airway.
- Check for breathing and pulse.
- If in doubt, start CPR.
- Continue until you are relieved by another person capable of performing CPR, or the resident regains consciousness.
- Remember to ask someone to call an ambulance.

Decisions about resuscitation

Those living in care homes are usually frail, older people, often with multiple medical problems (ONS, 2010). Many will remain living in a care home until the end of their life. Those working within care homes need to be able to identify when a death of a resident is anticipated and initiate end of life care is appropriate (DoH, 2008). This is covered elsewhere in the handbook (Chapter 16.4).

For residents in whom death is not anticipated, and where no decision has been made not to resuscitate that person, the presumption should be towards attempting basic life support.

If it is not known whether a decision has been made about resuscitation, it is important that some staff members attempt to find out urgently. However, this should not delay attempts at resuscitation being made.

Collapse and cardiac arrest may, of course, occur in anyone, including visitors and staff, so it is important to be familiar with basic life support techniques.

Please refer to the *Basic Life Support Algorithm* (Figure 9.7.1) while following the instructions below.

Upon discovering someone collapsed/unconscious

1. Ensure your own, and others' safety before approaching the resident.
2. Check for a response – ask if they are alright, while shaking the individual gently.
3. If there is no response – call for help.
4. Turn the resident on to their back.

Assess the: **Airway, Breathing, Circulation**.

- *Open the airway* using the *head tilt/chin lift* technique (Figure 9.7.2).
  a. Place one hand on their forehead and tilt the head back.
  b. Place two fingers of your other hand under the hard part of their chin, and gently lift.

The Care Home Handbook, First Edition. Edited by Graham Mulley, Clive Bowman, Michal Boyd and Sarah Stowe.
© 2015 John Wiley & Sons, Ltd. Published 2015 by John Wiley & Sons, Ltd.

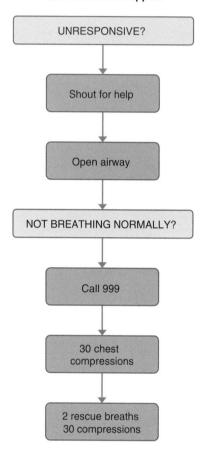

Adult Basic Life Support

UNRESPONSIVE?

↓

Shout for help

↓

Open airway

↓

NOT BREATHING NORMALLY?

↓

Call 999

↓

30 chest compressions

↓

2 rescue breaths 30 compressions

Figure 9.7.1 Basic life support algorithm. Reproduced with kind permission of the Resuscitation Council (UK).

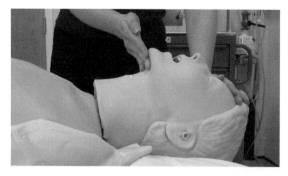

Figure 9.7.2 Head tilt/chin lift technique of opening airway.

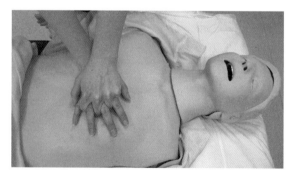

Figure 9.7.3 Correct placement of hands for chest compressions.

c. If there is any visible obstruction within easy reach, try and remove with a finger, or with suction.

- What is the *breathing* like? Taking no more than 10 seconds and while keeping the airway open
  a. *Look* for the chest moving.
  b. *Listen* for breathing.
  c. *Feel* for exhaled air on your cheek.

↓

NORMAL BREATHING	NOT BREATHING or OCCASIONAL GASPS
Place them in the recovery position.	Ask someone to call an ambulance.
Ask someone to call an ambulance.	**The person is in cardiac arrest**.
Stay with the person until help arrives.	**Start cardiopulmonary resuscitation (CPR)**.

How to perform CPR

1. If you have not already done so, turn the resident on to their back.
2. Start performing *chest compressions*:
   - Place hands in the centre of the chest (Figure 9.7.3).
   - Depress chest 5–6 cm.
   - Perform at a rate of 100–120 per minute.
3. If you have not been trained, or are unhappy to give rescue breaths, perform continuous chest compressions.
   If rescue breaths are to be given, after 30 compressions open the airway and give two breaths:

- Pinch the soft part of the resident's nose closed and form a seal over their mouth. Breathe for 1 second and watch for the chest to rise. Allow them to exhale for 1 second.
- Repeat.
- If using a pocket mouth, place over their nose and mouth to form a seal. Again give two breaths, this time through the mouth piece.
4. If possible, switch staff every 2 minutes so that the person performing compressions doesn't tire.
5. Continue until you are relieved by the ambulance crew, or until the resident appears to be regaining consciousness, that is:
   They seem to be breathing normally AND one of
   - opening their eyes
   - coughing
   - purposefully moving
   - speaking.

Finally: make sure that you know the local procedures for summoning paramedics or the ambulance and make sure that you are familiar with the equipment (such as masks) within the home.

References

DoH. 2008. End of life care strategy. Department of Health, July 2008. Available at www.cpa.org.uk/ [Accessed October 2013]

ONS. 2010. Regional Trends, No. 42 Edition - Ageing across the UK. Available at www.ons.gov.uk/ons/index [Accessed October 2013]

Resuscitation Council (UK). 2011. *Advanced Life Support* (6th Edn). Resuscitation Council (UK), Jan 2011. Available at: www.resus.org.uk [Accessed October 2013]

9.8 Tachycardia and bradycardia

Josie Clare[1] and Mary Burke[2]

[1]*Cork University Hospital, Ireland*
[2]*Killure Bridge Nursing Home, Waterford, Ireland*

> **Key points**
> * Always take the pulse in an ill resident.
> * Palpate the pulse at the wrist for a minute.
> * The pulse rate can be fast (tachycardia), slow (bradycardia) or normal.
> * A fast or slow pulse might be the cause or consequence of an underlying condition – the reason should always be determined.
> * The checklist of associated symptoms, signs and action required should help the front-line nurse in knowing what to do and when to get urgent medical help.

A normal heart rate for an old person is usually 60–85 beats per minute (bpm).

* A tachycardia (fast heart rate) is over 85 beats per minute.
* A bradycardia (slow heart rate) is less than 55 beats per minute.

It is important to monitor pulse rates for a resident in order to detect trends. A pulse rate of 49 bpm would be more concerning for a resident who normally has a pulse rate of 85 bpm than a resident who normally has a pulse rate of 55 bpm.

Pulse measurement

* If possible, measure the pulse under the same conditions each time.
* Ideally, the resident should refrain from physical activity for 20 minutes before the pulse is measured as exertion can cause tachycardia. Ensure that the resident is comfortable and relaxed.
* Place the first and second finger along the radial artery at the wrist and apply light pressure until the pulse is felt.
* The pulse should be counted for 60 seconds. If the pulse is regular and of good volume subsequent readings may be taken for 30 seconds and then doubled to give beats per minute.

For a resident who is unwell or not their usual self, it is important to check:

* Pulse rate (radial pulse at the wrist).
* Blood pressure.
* The ABCDE assessment (Airway, Breathing, Circulation, Disability, Exposure) to identify residents who are critically ill.

Presenting symptoms and/signs

Indications of *critical illness* include:

* Low blood pressure.
* Increased breathing rate (tachypnoea).
* Altered consciousness level.

A resident may present less acutely. Other signs or symptoms may include:

* Near fainting (pre-syncope) or fainting (syncope).
* Weakness.
* Tiredness.
* Shortness of breath.
* Chest pains.
* Confusion.

Tachycardia or bradycardia may be either:

* a consequence of a person being unwell for other reasons, for example severe infection, OR
* the reason for the person being unwell, for example heart block or ventricular tachycardia.

Please refer to Tables 9.8.1, 9.8.2 and 9.8.3 for more detail.

The Care Home Handbook, First Edition. Edited by Graham Mulley, Clive Bowman, Michal Boyd and Sarah Stowe.
© 2015 John Wiley & Sons, Ltd. Published 2015 by John Wiley & Sons, Ltd.

Table 9.8.1 Some conditions which can cause bradycardia or tachycardia.

	Possible symptoms and signs with which the older person may present	Action required
Shock (usually causes tachycardia but can cause bradycardia)	Evidence of fluid loss or blood loss Evidence of infection e.g. chest or urinary Shortness of breath Low blood pressure Symptoms are likely to have developed over minutes or hours	Urgent medical review
Myocardial infarction	Chest pain – but older people do not necessarily present with pain Nausea and vomiting Sweating Blood pressure may be low Generally unwell	Urgent medical review
Pain (Chapter 8.6)		Analgesia Explore the cause of pain and manage as appropriate

Table 9.8.2 Other causes of tachycardia.

	Possible symptoms and signs with which the older person may present	Action required
Medications Inhalers Nebulisers	Tremor may occur	Review of medications Urgency of medical review will depend on the clinical condition of the resident. It may be reasonable to make a telephone call and agree to hold medications pending medical review
Congestive cardiac failure	Shortness of breath Ankle swelling If the person is very unwell, they may have a low blood pressure and be clammy	Medical review. Urgency will depend on how suddenly the symptoms have developed
Pulmonary embolism	Shortness of breath Coughing blood Chest pain – often worse on breathing in	Urgent medical review
Hyperthyroidism	Weight loss Heat intolerance	Blood test to check thyroid function
Arrhythmia e.g. Supraventricular tachycardia Fast atrial fibrillation Ventricular tachycardia	The tachycardia may be persistent or intermittent Presentation will vary from being asymptomatic to in a state of collapse with a very low blood pressure	Urgency of medical review will depend on the clinical condition of the resident An ECG assists in making the diagnosis

Table 9.8.3 Other causes of bradycardia.

	Possible symptoms and signs with which the older person may present	Action required
Medications		
Digoxin	Nausea Confusion	Review of medications
Beta blockers e.g. bisoprolol, atenolol	Tiredness Collapse	Urgency of medical review will depend on the clinical condition of the resident
Calcium channel blockers e.g. diltiazem	Confusion Blood pressure may be low	It may be reasonable to make a telephone call and agree to hold medications pending medical review Checking Digoxin levels and electrolytes advised
Hypothyroidism (underactive thyroid)	Tiredness Cold intolerance Symptoms may present over weeks or months	Blood test to check thyroid function
Hypothermia	Cold. Temperature at or below 35 °C Unwell Fall or collapse Intercurrent infection	Warm the resident Seek medical advice
Increased intracranial pressure	Very unwell with decreased conscious level Neurological signs may be present Blood pressure is likely to be very high	Urgent medical review
Myocardial infarction	Chest pain – although older people do not necessarily present with pain Nausea and vomiting Sweating Blood pressure may be low Generally unwell	Urgent medical review
Atrio–ventricular block	The bradycardia may be persistent or intermittent Presentation will vary from the resident being asymptomatic to being in a state of collapse with very low blood pressure	Medical advice – urgency will depend on the clinical condition of the resident

Useful web site

www.resus.org.uk [Accessed October 2013]
Medical Emergencies and Resuscitation – standards for clinical practice and training, 2006.

9.9 Hypothermia

Aidan Dunphy and Simon Conroy

University Hospitals of Leicester NHS Trust, Leicester, UK

Key points

- Hypothermia is when the core temperature is 35 °C or less.
- Coolness of the abdomen should raise the possibility of hypothermia.
- A low reading thermometer is needed to confirm the presence of hypothermia.
- If the hypothermic resident is unconscious, get emergency medical help.
- There are many predisposing and precipitating causes of hypothermia.
- In every case, consider the possibility of underlying infection.
- Avoid active rewarming.
- Do not diagnose death in someone who is unconscious and hypothermic.

What is hypothermia?

Hypothermia is when the core body temperature is below 35 °C. This is a very serious condition that should not routinely occur in a care home. However, an instance such as a resident absenting themselves from the home in adverse weather may lead to hypothermia.

An unconscious, hypothermic patient is a clinical emergency. You need to seek immediate medical support and begin appropriate resuscitation techniques.

Hypothermia can result from environmental exposure (primary) and/or a medical illness (secondary).

- Signs and symptoms.
  1. A core temperature that is below 35 °C / 95 °F. The most accurate measure is obtained this using a low grade rectal thermometer (see Chapter 15.4). Oral and tympanic thermometers are not always accurate.

     We recommend all care homes have a low grade rectal thermometer.

     It is common for old people to have cold peripheries. However, if an old person is in a normal temperature environment, dressed or well covered in bed, and the abdomen feels cold, then hypothermia should be considered and a low reading thermometer used. Freshly passed urine will also reflect core temperature.
  2. Shivering – this stops at lower temperatures as the body tries to conserve core temperature (as shivering may encourage peripheral dilation and therefore increase heat loss).
  3. The heart may slow and/or become irregular and the pulse become less palpable.
  4. Breathing may slow and become shallow.
  5. Skin may be cold to touch and pale, especially in areas that would normally be warm (such as the armpits and the groin).
  6. Sleepiness, reduced conscious level, possibly confusion/irritation and poor coordination brought about by a lower blood volume circulating and reduced O2 and nutrients reaching the brain. This may lead to lethargy and the desire to sleep.
  7. On initial assessment, a hypothermic resident may appear to be dead.
- Causes:
  1. Extended exposure to a cold atmosphere or via contact (commonly prolonged contact with the floor following a fall).
  2. Wet clothing: this increases heat loss by 5–10 times – even during the summer. However, clothing should only be changed when the resident is in a sheltered environment with dry clothing to change them into.

The Care Home Handbook, First Edition. Edited by Graham Mulley, Clive Bowman, Michal Boyd and Sarah Stowe.
© 2015 John Wiley & Sons, Ltd. Published 2015 by John Wiley & Sons, Ltd.

3. Poor heating in a home can cause a gradual reduction in core temperature.
4. Some drugs can have an effect on body temperature (such as beta-blockers).
5. Exhaustion.
6. Poor diet.
7. Alcohol.
8. Medical conditions that make the older person more susceptible include hypothyroidism and diabetes.
9. Underlying infection, such as chest or urinary infection. While many frail old people become pyrexial with infections, others become hypothermic – especially with septicaemia.

   The possibility of infection should always be considered in a case of hypothermia.

Remember authorities have the power to close care homes which fail to provide adequate heating or nutrition that may result in hypothermia.

- Immediate treatment:
  1. In general, it is best to avoid active rewarming an old person with hypothermia.

     It might be reasonable to place warmed blankets over the torso.

     If the opportunity allows, get a colleague to put a few in the tumble dryer in your linen room.
  2. The resident should receive very close care, ideally one to one, and always have a means to summon support.
  3. Remove the resident from a cold, moist environment and change them into dry clothing.
  4. Check the blood glucose level.
  5. If conscious and able to swallow, the resident should be given warm liquids. Don't give liquids to residents you think may have

had a stroke (Chapters 8.1 and 8.2); *never give alcohol.*

6. *If the resident is not conscious, immediate medical care should be sought, resuscitation should be undertaken under close supervision because of the risk of cardiac arrhythmias.*

   Remember always to ensure a full medical and drug history is passed to the resuscitation team.

7. *Do not* rub the skin as this may cause further peripheral dilation and contribute to heat loss.

8. *Keep interventions to a minimum – the less the resident is disturbed, the better the outcome.*

Alert: severely hypothermic patients may mimic death due to slow shallow breathing and altered/slow heart rate. Remember your **ABCDE** (**A**irway **B**reathing **C**irculation **D**isability **E**xposure).

Take great care not to certify death in someone who is hypothermic (see Chapter 16.5).

Remember people with dementia may not express feeling cold and are at the highest risk.

Further reading

Campbell, D, Travis DD. 1997. Chronic subclinical hypothermia: home care alert. *Home Healthcare Nursing* 15: 727.

Irvine RE. 1974. Hypothermia in old age. *Practitioner* 213: 795.

Useful web site

http://www.resus.org.uk/pages/GL2010.pdf   [Accessed October 2013]

9.10 Hot painful joints

Sadia Ismail

Leeds Teaching Hospitals NHS Trust, Leeds, UK

Key points

- A hot, red, painful joint is often a medical emergency which may have several causes, including infection and gout.
- It is very important to get medical help with diagnosis and treatment: the doctor will insert a needle into the joint in order to obtain fluid for analysis.

Causes

There are several causes of hot painful joints, most of which will need urgent medical attention. Be aware of symptoms and signs which may indicate a more serious cause as these can help you decide whether to ask for urgent help.

If in doubt, call the doctor right away.

Most hot joints that are inflamed are also swollen and red to some degree and this can give a clue as to the cause of the hot joint.

History

It is important to document the history of the joint, as well as some of the symptoms reported by the resident, as this can be very useful for the assessing doctor.

The doctor will wish to ascertain:

- For how long has the joint been swollen/hot/red/tender?
- How quickly did it come on?
- Is it improving or getting worse?
- Is the pain, heat or redness actually in the joint or in the skin around it?
- Do the symptoms appear to be moving from one joint to another?
- Are the symptoms spreading while continuing in the original joint?
- Has the resident been unwell with a fever or any obvious signs of infection?
- Any previous similar episodes?

- Any history of joint problems?
- Any surgery on that joint in the past?
- Any recent injury to that joint?

Investigations and treatment

These will often depend on the cause of the hot joints but will often include x-rays of the inflamed joint, blood tests and (most importantly) removing some fluid from the joint with a needle, to check for infection or gout.

Problems and pitfalls

- Sometimes cellulitis can be mistaken for septic arthritis or gout.
- Some people with gout may also have a high temperature which can make clinical assessment especially difficult.
- Septic arthritis is most likely to affect joints which are already damaged
- *If an area of redness or heat is very tender and is rapidly and visibly spreading call for medical assistance urgently as this may indicate a very serious infection needing immediate treatment.*

Acknowledgement

I wish to thank Debra Sager for her helpful advice on this chapter.

The Care Home Handbook, First Edition. Edited by Graham Mulley, Clive Bowman, Michal Boyd and Sarah Stowe.
© 2015 John Wiley & Sons, Ltd. Published 2015 by John Wiley & Sons, Ltd.

Further reading

Acute monoarthritis. Article available from patient.co.uk: http://www.patient.co.uk/showdoc/40001605/ [Accessed October 2013]

Hot swollen joints. Article available from patient.co.uk: http://www.patient.co.uk/doctor/Hot-Swollen-Joints.htm [Accessed October 2013]

The approach to the painful joint. Article available from: http://emedicine.medscape.com/article/336054-overview [Accessed October 2013]

9.11 Acute lower limb ischaemia

Simon Conroy and Aidan Dunphy

University Hospitals of Leicester NHS Trust, Leicester, UK

Key points

- Acute limb ischaemia is a medical emergency: treatment must begin within six hours or the leg may need to be amputated.
- Sudden vascular blockage of the leg can be recognised by the 6 P's: Pain, Paraesthesia, Pallor, Pulselessness, Paralysis and Perishing cold.

Acute limb ischaemia is the *sudden* occlusion of blood flow to a limb (usually a leg). This is not the same as critical limb ischaemia (CLI), which may develop over a couple of weeks in a limb already demonstrating signs of ischaemia (such as resting leg pain, ulceration or gangrene).

Alert: Acute limb ischaemia is a *clinical emergency*. You need to seek immediate medical support to begin appropriate treatment.

Common causes of acute limb ischaemia (in the absence of trauma)

1. Dislodged blood thrombus or clot (embolic) travelling to the affected limb. There is usually an underlying cardiac cause.
2. Blood clot (thrombotic) formation in a narrowed (atherosclerotic) artery. This is similar to the blockage of an artery that occurs in a heart attack, but affects the limbs, not the heart.

Risk factors

- Cardiac arrhythmia, recent myocardial infarction and valvular heart disease.
- High cholesterol.
- Diabetes.
- Smoking.

- Hypertension.
- Peripheral vascular disease.

Symptoms of acute ischaemia are known as the 'The 6 P's':

1. Pain.
2. Paraesthesia (tingling or numbness of the leg).
3. Pallor (whiteness).
4. Pulselessness (unable to feel the pulse in the affected limb).
5. Paralysis (unable to move the affected limb).
6. 'Perishing' cold.

Two of the most important distinguishing *signs* are related to pallor:

- when the limb turns quickly white (sometimes a mottled blue/grey) and is perishing cold,
- when touched, the limb might feel like 'refrigerated meat'.

Both can indicate an irreversible outcome.

Actions

- *Remember*: If treatment is not sought *within six hours* the tissue will start to die, leading to amputation and/or death.
- Emergency hospital admission is a priority.
- *Important*: Ensure that the resident's clinical history is passed on to the surgical team, as it will help

The Care Home Handbook, First Edition. Edited by Graham Mulley, Clive Bowman, Michal Boyd and Sarah Stowe.
© 2015 John Wiley & Sons, Ltd. Published 2015 by John Wiley & Sons, Ltd.

determine the cause of the ischaemia (embolic/thrombotic) and therefore guide treatment.

Treatment during hospital admission may include surgical intervention.

- Heparinisation (blood thinning medication given as a drip or injection) – this helps stabilise the clot.
- Pain relief, for patient comfort and to relieve anxiety.
- Emergency surgery to remove the clot ('embolectomy').
- Injection of a 'clot-busting' drug into the artery ('intra-arterial thrombolysis').

Long-term care needs.

An assessment of underlying causes will inform on-going care around individual risk factors such as:

1. Further medical treatment for:
   - cardiovascular disease
   - diabetes
   - hypertension.

2. Education support for:
   - smoking cessation
   - nutrition.

In older subjects, it may mean an extended hospital stay, and residents may need ongoing physiotherapy and occupational therapy to regain their former levels of activities of daily living.

Further reading

Hansa CP, Holtveg HM, Rasch L, Holsten P. 1992. Thrombo-embolectomy in geriatric patients from long-stay wards. *Danish Medical Bulletin* 39: 570–572.

Useful web sites

http://www.patient.co.uk/doctor/Limb-Embolism-and-Ischaemia.htm [Accessed October 2013]

http://www.surgical-tutor.org.uk/default-home.htm?system/vascular/acute_ischaemia.htm~right [Accessed October 2013]

The debate over surgical intervention versus thrombolytic therapy is summarised here: http://onlinelibrary.wiley.com/doi/10.1002/14651858.CD002784/abstract [Accessed October 2013]

9.12 Nausea and vomiting

Sean Ninan[1] and Lisa Wickens[2]

[1]*Yorkshire and the Humber Deanery, UK*
[2]*Hull and East Yorkshire Hospitals NHS Trust, Hull, UK*

Key points

- Nausea and vomiting have many causes and diagnosing them early is very important.
- A flow chart and list of Red Flags (Box 9.12.1) will help you in assessing the resident with these symptoms.
- Nauseated residents may be come dehydrated.
- Vomiting with fever and diarrhoea suggests gastroenteritis.
- Vomiting with pain and tenderness suggests pancreatitis or cholecystitis.
- Vomiting with no passage of stools suggests bowel obstruction.
- Vomiting with headache suggests meningitis or raised intra-cranial pressure.

Introduction

- Nausea is the sensation of needing to vomit, the act of forceful expulsion of stomach contents through the mouth.
- Nausea and vomiting are common in elderly care home residents
- These symptoms may be acute or chronic (lasting more than a month).

Vomiting

If there is acute vomiting associated with diarrhoea, fever, cramping abdominal pain, headache and feeling generally unwell, than the diagnosis of gastroenteritis is most likely.

- However, many conditions may present with acute vomiting.

All of the below warrant urgent medical review:

- If there is acute vomiting with abdominal pain, then the possibilities of *pancreatitis* and *cholecystitis* should be considered, which usually present with pain and tenderness in the upper abdomen.
- Vomiting, abdominal pain and tenderness with a failure to pass stools per rectum should prompt the possibility of *bowel obstruction*.

Box 9.12.1 Red Flags: When to get help

Vomiting associated with new headache, especially if new photophobia (unable to tolerate the light), neck stiffness, confusion or rash.

- Recent head injury.
- Severe abdominal pain associated with absence of bowel movement.
- Vomiting fresh blood or altered blood ('coffee ground' vomiting).
- Resident unable to maintain adequate oral intake.
- Resident hypotensive, tachycardic or oliguric (reduced urine output).

- A history of sudden onset headache with vomiting may suggest *infection*, for example meningitis *or increased intra-cranial pressure*, for example subarachnoid haemorrhage.

Causes of vomiting are outlined in Figure 9.12.1.

Nausea

Nausea has many causes. We should ask:

- Have there been any changes in medication or are there medications that may cause nausea? (See Box 9.12.2.)

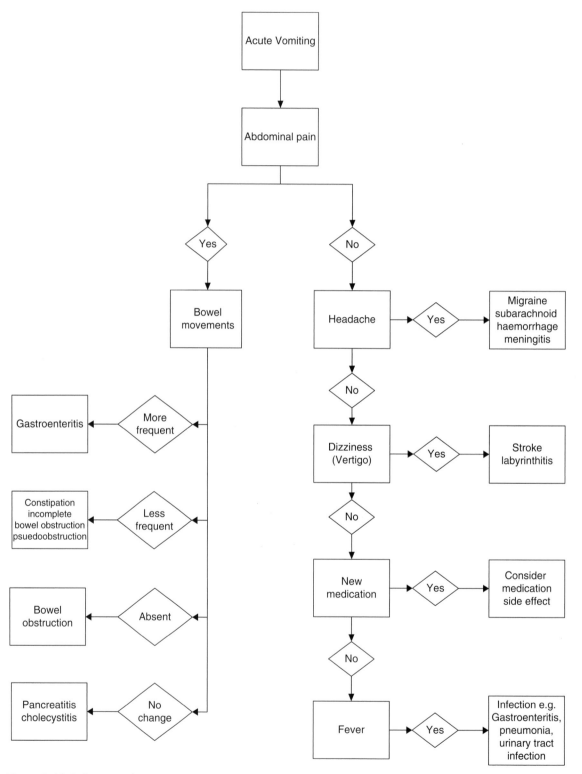

Figure 9.12.1 Causes of acute vomiting.

Box 9.12.2 Medications that may cause nausea

- Anti-arrhythmics, for example amiodarone, digoxin.
- Anti-hypertensives.
- Antibiotics, for example erythromycin.
- Chemotherapy.
- Diuretics.
- Oral hypoglycaemics.
- Opiate analgesia, for example codeine, tramadol, morphine.
- Theophyllines, for example uniphyllin.

Box 9.12.3 Management of nausea

- Drink little and often
- Avoid carbonated drinks
- Give oral rehydration salts
- Try diluted fruit juice
- Eat small meals of plain food
- Avoid fatty or spicy foods
- A blended or liquid diet may sometimes be helpful
- These measures should be considered only if there are no Red Flags.
- *If in doubt, do not give anything by mouth and ask the doctor to come as soon as possible*

- Is there any indication of infection, for example fever, urinary symptoms, chest symptoms, earache?
- Are there any symptoms of gastro-oesophageal reflux disease, for example heartburn or indigestion?
- Are there any symptoms of vertigo ('room spinning')? This may suggest a disorder such as labyrinthitis or Meniere's disease
- Is there a history of headache, for example migraine?

Management

Management of nausea and vomiting should address the identification and management of the underlying cause, treatment of the symptoms and the prevention of associated complications, such as dehydration, renal failure, electrolyte imbalance (Box 9.12.3).

The resident should be examined for signs of hypovolaemia. The heart rate and blood pressure should be checked and mucous membranes examined (dry lips or dryness under the tongue) (see Chapter 5.3).

Nauseated residents may maintain an adequate fluid and electrolyte intake by taking simple measures.

Once the cause has been identified, anti-emetics may be prescribed to ease the symptoms of nausea and vomiting. These are summarised in Table 9.12.1.

Table 9.12.1 Anti-emetics.

Drug	Use	Caution
Anti-histamines, e.g. cyclizine	Effective in wide range of conditions	• May cause dry mouth, blurred vision, constipation, urinary retention. • Avoid if constipated or history of glaucoma or prostate enlargement. • Avoid with other anti-muscarinics, e.g. Amitriptyline, oxybutynin, Buscopan etc.
Dopamine antagonists, e.g. domperidone, metoclopramide	Act directly on gastrointestinal tract. Useful in gastroduodenal, hepatic and biliary disease.	Metoclopramide should be avoided in elderly people because of dystonic reactions and Parkinsonian side-effects.
5HT3 receptor antagonists, e.g. ondansetron	Work on GI tract and central nervous system. Good for symptoms related to chemotherapy	May cause constipation
Antipsychotics, e.g. haloperidol, levomprazine	Terminal care	May cause Parkinsonian and dystonic side-effects

Other points

- It is vital to maintain good hygiene in cases of suspected infectious gastroenteritis to prevent infection spreading to staff and other residents.
- Hands should be washed before and after contact and protective aprons should be worn while carrying out nursing procedures (see Chapters 12.1 and 12.2).

- The resident should avoid using shared toilets, flannels or towels and surfaces and handles should be disinfected.

Further reading

Quigley EMM, Hasler WL, Parkman HP. 2001. AGA technical review on nausea and vomiting. *Gastroenterology* 120: 263–286.

Section E

Mental Health Problems

Chapter 10
Dementia, Delirium and Depression

10.1 Dementia

Ben Shaw[1], Sean Page[2] and Alistair Burns[3]

[1]*Royal Bolton Hospital, Bolton, UK*
[2]*University of Bangor, Glan Clywd General Hospital, Rhyl, UK*
[3]*University of Manchester, Manchester, UK*

Key points

- Dementias are a range of conditions that interfere with everyday living.
- They are characterised by loss of memory, altered mood, problems with communication, recognition, reasoning and orientation.
- Alzheimer's disease is the commonest type: it has a gradual onset and gradually progresses. The resident often lacks insight into their loss of memory.
- A full knowledge of the individual is important in planning person-centred care.
- We offer tips on how to manage behavioural problems that may occur in dementia.

Introduction

About two-thirds of people living in care homes have a form of dementia, and being involved in their care can be rewarding, but also challenging. Many people working in care homes lack confidence in providing dementia care, and some feel they lack knowledge.

Dementia can be a distressing condition, both for the person affected and those around them. This condition gives the opportunity to strive for excellence in care, and you can make a huge difference in the quality of life of residents with dementia.

Dementia: what is it and who does it affect?

Worldwide, about 30,000,000 people have a dementia. Dementia is an umbrella term that describes a range of symptoms, including: memory loss; mood changes; problems with communication; difficulties with dressing and personal care; problems with recognition, calculation and reasoning; and disorientation to time and place. When such problems interfere with daily life, then they are termed a dementia.

There are a number of different types of dementia, with *Alzheimer's dementia* being the most common, making up around 62% of cases.

- Alzheimer's is a progressive illness, with a gradual onset.
- A person who has Alzheimer's may not be aware they have problems with their memory, and may find it very difficult when others point this out.
- They may start to experience mood changes and anxiety.
- They may struggle to recognise places and people.
- Initially, their short-term memory is more affected than their memory of long ago, and sometimes they will talk more about past experiences.
- Word finding difficulties are common, and can be very frustrating.

Alzheimer's dementia is caused by a build up of protein *plaques* and *tangles* in the brain. These lead to brain cell death, and abnormal levels of certain chemicals (principally acetylcholine) in the brain. It is the levels of these chemicals that the dementia drugs (donepezil, rivastigmine, galantamine and memantine) work on.

Vascular dementia is the second most common dementia, and accounts for about a fifth of cases.

- It occurs when the blood vessels to the brain become narrowed and the blood supply is reduced or stopped.
- The onset may be sudden, for example after a stroke, and there may be a stepwise progression.

- People with vascular dementia may vary from day to day in how much their dementia affects them.
- Similarly, there may be times of the day, particularly early evening or at night, when they appear to become more confused.

Around 10% of people with dementia will have a *mixed dementia*, with features of both Alzheimer's and vascular dementia.

Rarer, but important, causes of dementia are fronto-temporal dementia, and Lewy body dementia.

In *fronto-temporal dementia* the first symptoms may be ones of behavioural or personality change, rather than memory difficulties. Sometimes the individual's behaviour may become socially inappropriate, or out of character. It is an important cause of dementia in people under 65.

In *Lewy body dementia* a person may show marked variation in their symptoms.

They may be troubled by complex *visual hallucinations*, often of creatures or animals.

As their dementia progresses, they may develop symptoms of Parkinsonism, such as shuffling when walking; a tremor; rigidity to their limbs; and reduced facial expressions. As with Alzheimer's dementia, it is caused by protein deposits in the brain, so called 'Lewy bodies', and can also be treated with the memory drug rivastigmine.

Guiding principles for dementia care

One of the criticisms of the biomedical model approach to dementia, illustrated above, is that it characterises 'sufferers' by their 'deficits', rather than considering what is still possible. Moreover, this approach does not consider what life may be like for the person with dementia, or the effect it has on those around them.

An alternative view is to highlight the importance of the person with dementia, and the reality that someone with a dementia is no less a person than one without. In this way the importance of 'personhood' can be highlighted. Personhood has been defined as 'the status and standing bestowed upon one human being by others … it implies recognition, respect and trust'.

Ideas of personhood form the foundation of person-centred care in dementia, whereby the focus is on empowerment, enablement and independence (see Chapter 3.4).

Inherent within person-centred care is valuing the person with dementia. The aim is to create care for that person that has incorporated what is known about their views and choices. If it is to succeed, it also requires a broader environment that seeks to ensure and maintain the resident's well-being.

Person-centred care

The idea of person-centred care, as well as society's role in providing that care, form the basis of the recommendations of the National Institute of Clinical Excellence (NICE) in the UK, and worldwide work is being done to establish a consensus for standards in dementia care. The NICE guidance considers a *social model of care*, whereby a person's impairments become disabilities due to social processes. By emphasising this dynamic relationship, they highlight the following principles that can be used to guide dementia care:

- The condition is not the 'fault' of the individual.
- The focus is on the skills and capabilities the person retains, rather than those lost.
- The individual can be fully understood (his or her history, likes/dislikes, and so on).
- An enabling or supportive environment can exert a positive influence.
- Appropriate communication is an integral part of care.
- Opportunities should be taken for rehabilitation or re-enablement.
- The responsibility to reach out to people with dementia lies with people who do not (yet) have dementia.

Unusual or troubling behaviours

Though not all people with dementia will display unusual behaviours, there are certain behaviours that are more common.

These may be frustrating and challenging to manage, and can cause distress in both the resident and their carers. Often, this distress can be eased by trying to understand where these behaviours arise from, what their purpose may be, and how they can be overcome. The use of medication for challenging behaviours should only be considered when there is 'severe distress or an immediate risk of harm to the person with dementia or others'. The use of restraint would not be recommended unless in situations of immediate risk of harm to the resident or others, and should only be carried out by staff who have been appropriately trained (see Chapter 4.2).

Below we detail some of the behaviours that can commonly occur. This is by no means an exhaustive list, and the Alzheimer's Society web site is recommended for a more detailed explanation.

Restlessness

- People with dementia can often appear restless. They may fidget, or pace and wander.
- Restlessness can be a sign of physical discomfort, pain or need to use the toilet.
- It can be a side-effect of medication.
- It may reflect boredom or physical inactivity in a previously active person.
- *It is important to establish what is causing the restlessness, and address the cause.* If it relates to a lack of stimulus, it may help to engage the person in an activity, or to give reassurance where needed.
- If they regularly pace, checking their shoes are comfortable, and their feet have not become sore, is imperative. Due to their high level of activity, these people may require extra nutritional support to ensure they do not lose weight.

Shouting out

- Shouting out or screaming can be extremely disturbing to staff and other residents, particularly if it is persistent or loud.
- Try to establish why the person is shouting out, as it may reflect a number of physical needs that the person is unable to verbalise appropriately.
- Sometimes shouting out comes from the distress when a person forgets there is someone nearby to help. It may be that the person is troubled by anxiety. *More rarely they may be frightened by hallucinations, and if this is suspected they should be reviewed by the GP or a member of the mental health team.*

Exposing/dressing problems

- These difficulties can vary from problems dressing oneself, through to undressing and exposing oneself inappropriately.
- At times the person may touch or handle their genitals, or fiddle with their clothing (consider delirium, see Chapter 10.2). Such behaviours may cause offence. Try to approach the situation calmly, and in a way that preserves the person's dignity.

- Dementia can cause people to not recognise what is appropriate social behaviour, or not inhibit their sexual impulses. People may continue to have physical needs and desires, and it may be possible to help them to attend to these privately in a way that does not offend (see Chapter 2.6).

Sleep disturbance

Sleep disturbance can be a common feature of dementia, and can lead to a complete reversal of the sleep–wake cycle. It is first important to ask the question: who is this a problem to? A person may sleep with adequate duration and quality, but at an anti-social time. If this is in a setting where it can be managed, then it could be argued that it is not in itself a problem.

When considering sleep disturbance, there is a number of physical causes that must be excluded: needing to empty one's bladder; pain; depression; or side-effects of medication. Having addressed these, one should consider techniques to improve sleep hygiene.

- Keeping a person stimulated during the day will minimise daytime sleeping.
- Avoid caffeine, excessive fluids or diuretics in the evening.
- Make sure the bedroom environment is warm, quiet and free from disturbance.
- Try to establish calming routines, such as a bath or a milky drink.

The use of medication for sleep disturbance should only be considered after the above techniques have been tried. Hypnotic medication carries a risk of cognitive decline and behavioural disturbance. If it is to be used, it should be as a short-term measure, with a clear plan of review.

Repetition

- People with dementia often repeat questions, phrases or actions. This may reflect the deterioration in their short-term memory so they do not recall what they have asked or been told.
- It may be that they repeat actions relating to their past employment of hobbies. If this is apparent, ask them about their life.
- Often repetitive behaviours reflect underlying anxiety and the need for reassurance. Again this can be irritating and difficult for carers to manage, but a calm and consistent approach can provide the reassurance needed.

Suspicious behaviour

- Sometimes people with dementia may become suspicious, or feel threatened and paranoid. This may result from confusion, or not being able to interpret others' actions.
- They may not recognise previously known people.
- They may misplace things and believe they have been stolen.
- They may react to these experiences with anger, or become distressed.
- Do try to keep calm, and remain consistent. If accusations have been made, a balance must be struck between allowing the person to feel listened to, while also evaluating the evidence for the accusations. At its most extreme, such suspicions may become fixed and a person may ruminate upon them repeatedly. *If so, consider involving the GP or mental health team.*

The role of the GP and the mental health team

Prolonged periods of disturbed or agitated behaviour can signify an underlying physical or mental health problem that requires review by the GP or mental health team.

People with dementia are more at risk of anxiety and depression, as well as unusual experiences such as hallucinations.

The person may struggle to explain what is happening and how they are feeling.

However, with the right approach, much can be done to alleviate this distress. It may be that the person is already known to the community mental health team, and has a community nurse who will review them and work with a psychiatrist. If this is not the case, the GP may be able to make an initial assessment, and refer on as needed.

Training and support for carers

NICE have made recommendations for training for all those involved in the care of people with dementia, which includes training in communication skills and person-centred care. They have recommended that there are links between local mental health services and care homes for communication and consultation.

It is imperative that all those who care for people with dementia have clearly defined sources of support and supervision.

References

NHS Choices. 2011. Alzheimer's in the News. Fear and Fascination. www.nhs.uk/news [Accessed 5 February 2014].

Department of Health. 2009. Living Well with Dementia: A National Dementia Strategy. www.dh.gov.uk/dementia [Accessed 5 February 2014].

NICE Guidelines. Alzheimer's in the News. Fear and Fascination. http://www.nice.org.uk/nicemedia/live/10998/30318/30318.pdf [Accessed 5 February 2014].

10.2 Delirium

Alison Cracknell

Leeds Teaching Hospitals NHS Trust, Leeds, UK

Key points

- Delirium is common in care home residents, developing in over 30% of residents.
- Delirium is commonly referred to as an 'Acute Confusional State'.
- It is often under-recognised, delayed or misdiagnosed by healthcare professionals.
- Its prevention or early detection and management can result in fewer hospitalisations, a reduction in the development of short- and long-term morbidity and mortality, and bring benefits to the resident experience.
- All healthcare providers should feel empowered to help with early detection and prompt management of this unpleasant, frequently avoidable condition.

Delirium is a clinical syndrome characterised by the following features:

1. *Disturbed consciousness* (reduced ability to focus, sustain or shift attention).
2. *Change in cognition* (such as memory deficit, disorientation, language or perceptual disturbance).
3. *Develops over a short period* (usually hours to days) and tends to have a *fluctuating course*.
4. *Organic illness is evident* (from history, examination and investigations).

Up to one-third of cases of delirium are preventable. Avoiding possible precipitants and promptly managing those at increased risk of delirium and those who develop it improves outcomes.

Any older resident can develop delirium. To identify the risk of delirium developing it can be helpful to consider both:

- the vulnerability or pre-disposition of the individual; and
- the precipitating factors or stressor events that may trigger delirium in that individual.

A person with high vulnerability may only need a minor insult/precipitant (e.g. dehydration) to develop delirium (Boxes 10.2.1 and 10.2.2).

Box 10.2.1 Pre-disposing risk factors (or vulnerability) for developing delirium

- Old age
- Dementia or previous episode of delirium
- Frailty
- Visual and or hearing impairment
- Severe illness
- Recent surgery
- Polypharmacy
- Alcohol excess
- Renal impairment

Box 10.2.2 Precipitating factors (or stressors) for delirium

- Immobility
- Use of bladder catheter
- Dehydration
- Intercurrent illness
- Malnutrition
- Use of physical restraint
- Change of environment

The Care Home Handbook, First Edition. Edited by Graham Mulley, Clive Bowman, Michal Boyd and Sarah Stowe.
© 2015 John Wiley & Sons, Ltd. Published 2015 by John Wiley & Sons, Ltd.

Types of delirium

- 'Hyperactive':
  - characterised by increased motor activity with agitation, restlessness, hallucinations and inappropriate behaviour. These residents may be aggressive.
- 'Hypoactive' or 'quiet' delirium:
  - is more common, and characterised by reduced motor activity and lethargy. Residents may be withdrawn and drowsy.
- 'Mixed':
  - the commonest type, with features of both hyperactive and hypoactive delirium.

Hypoactive and mixed delirium types are often more difficult to recognise.

It is important to differentiate delirium, which can be the sole manifestation of serious underlying illness in older people, from other causes of confusion, which include: dementia, depression, schizophrenia and mania (see Chapters 10.1, 10.3 and 10.4). The main differences between dementia and delirium are highlighted in Table 10.2.1.

Cognitive assessment

- It is helpful to have *a baseline assessment* of cognitive function on residents admitted to care homes. *Repeat measurements* can then detect the development of delirium and its resolution.
- Cognitive screening tools such as the Abbreviated Mental Test Score (AMTS) and Mini-Mental State Examination (MMSE) are frequently used, but do not distinguish between delirium and other causes of cognitive impairment (see Appendix 1, 1.7).
- Inexperienced healthcare professionals may use the terms 'vague', 'difficult historian' or 'uncooperative'. These cues should alert those responsible for care to consider delirium as a potential diagnosis.
- A history from a relative or carer of the onset and course of confusion is essential to make the diagnosis of delirium, alongside the use of the Confusion Assessment Method (CAM) by healthcare professionals.

Confusion Assessment Method

To have a positive CAM result the resident must display:

1. Presence of acute onset confusion and fluctuating course
   and
2. inattention (e.g. counting down 20–1 with reduced ability to maintain attention or shift attention)
   and either
3. disorganised thinking (disorganised or incoherent speech)
   or
4. altered level of consciousness (usually lethargic or stuporose).

Physical assessment

Figure 10.2.1 shows the steps that should be taken by the multi-professional staff managing each resident with delirium, including care support workers, nurses and the responsible physician.

Causes of delirium

The underlying cause of delirium is often multi-factorial, see Box 10.2.3.

Management of delirium

1. Detection and treatment of underlying cause.
   - The most important step in management of delirium is identification and treatment of the

Table 10.2.1 Main differences between dementia and delirium.

	Dementia	Delirium
Onset	Gradual (months to years)	Acute (hours to days)
Progression	Progressive	Non-progressive
Duration	Usually irreversible	Days to weeks
Impaired inattention	Mild except in severe dementia	Prominent feature
Level of consciousness	Mild except in severe dementia	Fluctuating (often impaired)
Organic cause	Usually NOT found	Usually found

Step 1: Comprehensive Physical Assessment

Vital signs: temperature, pulse, blood pressure, respiratory rate, oxygen saturations, capillary blood glucose

Assess: hydration and nutritional status, for signs of constipation and urinary retention, look for evidence of infection

Perform: urine analysis

Step 2: Neurological and Cognitive Assessment

Record: Glasgow Coma Scale

Perform: Confusion Assessment Method (CAM) and a cognitive screen using Abbreviated Mental Test Score (AMTS) or Mini-Mental State Examination (MMSE)

Step 3: Review Medication Chart

In particular review anti-cholinergics, sedatives and opiates

---

Step 4: Investigations

The following are usually indicated in residents with delirium in order to identify the underlying cause:

Bloods: full blood count, urea and electrolytes, calcium, liver function test, C-reactive protein, glucose.

In addition consider: urine culture, blood culture, thyroid function tests, B12 and folate, chest x-ray, electrocardiogram.

CT head is unhelpful if used routinely, but consider if an intracranial lesion is suspected.

Figure 10.2.1 Assessment steps.

underlying cause. *Residents who appear to be developing delirium require a prompt medical assessment, examination and investigation.*

○ Care staff should undertake observations and ensure medication charts are readily available.

○ Delirium may require admission to hospital for investigation and treatment. However delirium can be exacerbated by admitting the resident to hospital away from their 'normal' environment. Therefore, each case should be assessed accordingly as to whether hospital admission is appropriate.

○ Carers with good knowledge of the resident and relatives play an important role: in corroborating the history, reporting symptoms suggestive of underlying cause, functional deficits, nutritional status, comorbid function and sensory deficit. The benefit of a collateral history surrounding events and background cannot be understated as this will often lead to identifying the underlying

Box 10.2.3 Common causes of delirium

- Infection (e.g. pneumonia, urinary tract infection, biliary infection)
- Electrolyte abnormality (e.g. dehydration, hyponatraemia, hypoglycaemia, renal failure)
- Cardiac illness (e.g. acute coronary syndrome)
- Respiratory illness (e.g. pulmonary embolism, hypoxia)
- Neurological illness (e.g. stroke, epilepsy, subdural, encephalitits)
- Drugs (especially opiates, steroids, anti-Parkinsonian drugs, anti-cholinergics)
- Drug withdrawal (e.g. benzodiazepines or alcohol)
- Urinary retention
- Faecal impaction
- Uncontrolled pain

Box 10.2.4 Ensuring an appropriate sensory environment

- Appropriate lighting for time of day
- Use of clocks and calendars to improve orientation
- Hearing and visual aids available and working
- Regular and repeated cues to improve personal orientation
- Continuity of care from staff
- Gentle approach (including verbal and when physically handling)
- Reduce background noise
- Regular visits from friends and family, encourage them to bring in familiar objects and photographs
- Encouragement of mobility and engagement in activities
- Good diet and fluid intake
- Good sleep pattern
- Consider regular analgesia (e.g. paracetemol)

cause, prompt treatment of which may avoid hospitalisation.

2. *Increase supervision* and increase frequency of monitoring, including measuring of vital signs.
3. Environmental measures.
   In addition to treating the underlying cause, there are many steps that can be taken to relieve the symptoms of delirium. The same approach can reduce the occurrence of delirium in those at high risk. Residents should be managed in a positive sensory environment with a reality-orientated approach (Box 10.2.4). Inform and involve family members as soon as possible.
   Avoid physical restraint, constipation, catheters and keep drug treatment to a minimum.
4. Pharmacological measures.
   Most cases of delirium do *not* require sedation: their use should be kept to a minimum, titrated cautiously and only considered in the following circumstances:
   ○ To allow essential investigations or treatment to be carried out.
   ○ To prevent residents endangering themselves or others.
   ○ To relieve distress in a highly agitated or hallucinating resident.
   The preferred drug option is usually haloperidol, starting at the lowest possible dose and taken orally if possible. Lorazepam is an alternative, especially in those with Parkinson's disease.
5. Prevention of complications.
   Box 10.2.6 lists some complications of delirium.
   It is often preferable to nurse the resident on a low bed, or place the mattress directly on floor.

Box 10.2.5 Special consideration: wandering behaviour

Residents who wander require close observation.

- First, attempts should be made to address the cause of agitation, for example pain, thirst, need to toilet.
- If the cause is not clear or cannot be remedied, the next step is distraction. Relatives and carers who know the resident well are best placed to offer this.
- Restraint and use of sedation are last resorts (see Chapter 4.2). One-to-one supervision may be necessary.

Box 10.2.6 Complications of delirium

- Falls
- Functional impairment
- Over-sedation
- Malnutrition
- Functional impairment
- Continence problems
- Infections

Regular toileting, optimising nutrition and taking into account the resident's preferences (hyperactive delirium leads to increased metabolic needs) and maintaining functional ability are important.

Box 10.2.7 Special consideration: the use of restraints

Restraints (including cot sides and special 'geriatric seating') have not been shown to reduce falls and may increase the risk of injury (see Chapter 6.6).

Post-delirium management

Patients who have suffered delirium often recall some or all of the events related to the episode. These can be unpleasant. Consideration should be given to provide support for those who have been through the experience. Remember that these residents are potentially at risk of further delirium or developing dementia and thus should be followed up, ideally by clinicians with a specialist interest in delirium through the community mental health team (see Chapter 17.2), but all members of the care team can ensure the appropriate environmental steps are taken to reduce recurrence.

A stepwise approach to the prevention, diagnosis and management of delirium

Step 1: Identify residents with cognitive impairment on admission.

Step 2: Consider delirium in all patients with confusion and known risk factors. Use the CAM screening instrument.

Step 3: Identify and treat the cause of delirium.

Step 4: In residents with delirium and those at high risk, maintain an optimal sensory environment with personal orientation.

Step 5: Use sedation only if essential and at the lowest possible dose.

Step 6: Take steps to prevent recurrence and ensure all members of the multi-professional team caring for older residents have training in delirium.

Further reading

British Geriatrics Society and Royal College of Physicians. 2006. Guidelines for the prevention, diagnosis and management of delirium in older people. London, Royal College of Physicians.

National Institute for Health and Clinical Excellence. 2010. Delirium: diagnosis, prevention and management. NICE clinical guideline 103. London, National Institute for Health and Clinical Excellence.http://www.nice.org.uk/nicemedia/live/13060/49909/49909.pdf [Accessed October 2013].

10.3 Anxiety and depression

Rachel Thompson[1] and David Jolley[2]

[1]*Royal College of Nursing, London, UK*
[2]*Personal Social Services Research Unit, The University of Manchester, Manchester, UK*

Key points

- Anxiety and depression are experienced as normal variants but may become dominant and pathological.
- Admission to a care home can be a major stressful event.
- Recognition of anxiety and depression requires vigilance and sensitivity.
- Unrecognised or poorly treated depression can be extremely debilitating. Nursing has a significant role in identifying and supporting residents experiencing anxiety and depression.
- With time, sensitive listening and careful, tailored therapy people can be helped to find a new healthy adjustment of mood.

A care home is a closed community made up of individuals who have come together, usually as a result of increasing frailty and dependency on others.

While social relationships with others have a significant impact on our well-being, it is unlikely that those individuals will have chosen their co-residents for their qualities of personality, behaviour or sociability.

Yet these are factors which are likely to influence the peace of mind, confidence and happiness of residents singularly and in their interactions day by day.

Moving into a care home

A number of questions and concerns will be raised by those considering a move into a care home:

- Who will I be with?
- Who will provide the intimate care I may need?
- Will they be kind and gentle or brisk and rough?
- Will I feel I can trust them with my body or my thoughts of fun, fear, regrets and lingering desires?
- Who will come to spend time with me?
- Can I look forward to pleasure, time out, laughter and music?
- Will pain be relieved?

Some residents may find it difficult to remember daily events due to cognitive changes and some will have difficulty understanding their environment and relating to others. Many will have limitations of sight or hearing or both; balance can no longer be assured and falls may occur even when residents remember to use walking aids.

This is a time of understandable anxiety and stress with possible fears of a hostile world, fuelled by pervasive images in the media and negative perceptions of residential care.

The surprise and reassurance is that most residents, most of the time are *not* consumed by feelings of fear, suspicion or anxiety. Most residents, most of the time are *not* prisoners of fear, despair and depression. In fact most residents with the right support will adapt and adjust to their new surroundings remarkably well and can have a good quality of life.

We bring into every situation our former selves and something of our inheritance from previous generations. Some are easy-going and flexible in new situations, relishing challenges and opportunities. Others will be, by nature, more reserved, private and need to have control of what is to be done, with whom and at what pace.

The Care Home Handbook, First Edition. Edited by Graham Mulley, Clive Bowman, Michal Boyd and Sarah Stowe.
© 2015 John Wiley & Sons, Ltd. Published 2015 by John Wiley & Sons, Ltd.

Anxiety

Faced with the prospect of personal control shared or transferred to others, feelings of apprehension and persistent anxiety are more likely in those who are more reliant on personal or family routines

Anxieties are likely to peak in anticipation of moving into care, to continue within the first days and weeks, but hopefully to be resolved with time, sensitivity of staff and familiarity. They may re-emerge when there are additional changes: of staff, other residents or families; or changes in the general health, dependency, of the individual, or other residents within their circle.

Anxiety includes subjective feelings of doubt and fear and biological changes:

- tremor
- tachycardia
- raised blood pressure
- tachypnoea (a rapid respiratory rate)
- weakness
- sleep may be difficult, disturbed or unsatisfactory.

Symptoms of anxiety may be misinterpreted as 'difficult' or 'confused behaviour' – especially in those with a dementia or delirium – and it is essential that possible causes are investigated.

Depression

Depression is a darker, more debilitating disorder and *is the most common psychological disorder of later life*.

- Symptoms of anxiety and depression usually co-exist.
- Predisposition to depression, as for anxiety, may rest in personal history, individual make-up and experiences past and current.
- Some individuals carry a history of relapsing mood disorder over many years: uni-polar of bi-polar. Life events, particularly those which carry stress or represent loss, can precipitate depression at any age.
- For some, the losses of health, independence, freedom, wealth and status associated with late life and the particulars of life in care, are sufficient to produce depression – even when they had previously shown robust resilience.
- Pain may be pervasive.
- Medications, notably hypotensive agents and anti-Parkinsonian medicines, may drain the brain of the chemicals which maintain good moods.

Depression, like anxiety, is most likely at times of stress and change. Its subjective feelings of hopelessness, loss of confidence and self-worth, loss of interest, and impaired concentration may develop to psychotic intensity with a conviction that death is nigh.

Common depression signs and symptoms

- subjective feelings of hopelessness
- loss of confidence and self-worth
- loss of interest in usual activities and in others
- impaired concentration
- reduced appetite
- weight loss
- diminished muscle strength
- sleep may be significantly disturbed.

Although suicide is rare among the residents of care homes, perhaps in part due to limitations on independence, it remains a notable feature of late life in general.

Suicidal ideation is not uncommon (though perhaps unspoken) and should be explored carefully.

Recognising anxiety and depression

Depression and anxiety are serious conditions. They dangerously span the range of 'normal', 'understandable' to pathological and debilitating. Their recognition and interpretation requires awareness based on knowledge of the individual and open, non-threatening availability, skill and sensitivity on the part of the nurse and others. Sometimes clues come through other people who are trusted more or who are able to give time and a listening ear at the right time. This may be a visiting friend or a domestic cleaner. It often includes night staff.

Whatever the route, these are important symptoms and demand careful attention and sensitive responses. Appreciation of the altered mood should be shared within the caring team. Particular initiatives may become the responsibility of one or more individuals. Awareness and more listening will be the first steps in therapy. An assessment of the individual, their current mood as well as their personal history, life experiences and individual make-up will facilitate understanding.

Help in coming to terms with the new situation takes time and the development of supportive relationships will help the person adjust and assimilate losses. Social relationships and inclusion have a significant influence on mental health and well-being, and efforts to help the person maintain or develop relationships both inside and outside the care home are vital.

When symptoms are fierce or persistent, a medical review of physical and mental health, symptoms and medication is essential. Further advice or the involvement of a mental health nurse, psychiatrist or clinical psychologist should be considered early rather than late.

Additional therapy, including counselling, psychotherapy, cognitive behavioural therapy an antidepressant or other medicine may be life-changing and should not be ruled out for those with dementia.

A number of scales are available which are designed to identify or monitor the presence and severity of anxiety or depression (see Appendix 1, 1.8). They have virtue but should be used with respect for their limitations.

Anxiety and depression are conditions which are commonly missed or misunderstood in residents of care homes and it is imperative that we identify these as significant conditions and offer the right support

Further reading

Bell M, Goss A. 2001. Recognition, assessment and treatment of depression in geriatric nursing home residents. *Clinical Excellence for Nurse Practitioners* 5(1): 26.

Burns A, Lawlor B, Craig S. 1999. *Assessment Scales in Old Age Psychiatry*. London, Martin Dunitz.

Cahill S, Diaz-Ponce A. 2011. I hate having nobody here. I'd like to know where they all are. *Aging and Mental Health* 15(5): 562–572.

Dohrenwend BS, Dohrenwend BP. 1974. *Stressful Life Events: Their Nature and Effects*. New York, John Wiley and Sons.

National Institute for Health and Clinical Excellence Guidance. 2007. (CG22) (2007) Anxiety. Available at: http://www.nice.org.uk/nicemedia/pdf/CG022NICEguideline amended.pdf [Accessed October 2013]

National Institute for Health and Clinical Excellence. 2009. Guidance: (CG90) Depression in adults. Available at: http://www.nice.org.uk/nicemedia/live/12329/45896/45896.pdf [Accessed October 2013]

Weyerer S, Hafner H, Mann A, Graham N. 1995. Prevalence and course of depression among elderly residential home admissions in Mannheim and Camden, London. *International Psychogeriatrics* 7(4): 479–495.

10.4 Psychosis

John Holmes[1] and Ceri Edwards[2]

[1]*University of Leeds, Leeds, UK*
[2]*Leeds and York Partnership NHS Foundation Trust, York, UK*

Key points

- Psychotic symptoms can occur in a range of conditions, including dementia, delirium, depression and schizophrenia.
- Delusions and hallucinations are real to those experiencing them, and challenging individuals about them may provoke an adverse reaction.
- Anti-psychotics are not without problems and should be reserved for when symptoms are severe or distressing.

There is a common misconception that schizophrenia causes a split personality. The reality is that people with schizophrenia experience psychotic symptoms, which are some of the most difficult symptoms of mental disorder to understand. We have all been low in mood or anxious at some stage, but few of us hear voices or have ideas that our neighbours are plotting against us. Although closely linked with schizophrenia, these symptoms occur in a wide range of conditions, including dementia, delirium, severe depression and mania. Here, we will concentrate on schizophrenia, a relatively rare condition in old age that affects about 0.3% of the older population in the UK.

This is not an exhaustive guide, but a pointer towards better care, and those who want to know more can refer to the additional material at the end of the chapter.

Most older people with schizophrenia will have had it for much of their adult lives, although it is possible to develop schizophrenia in old age. Most people with schizophrenia in care homes are there for reasons of physical dependency, and staff should have the skills to deal with both their physical and mental health problems. Unfortunately, general nursing training in the UK includes very little training on mental health issues, meaning that staff may lack the knowledge and skills to nurse residents with schizophrenia and other mental health problems successfully. Initiatives such as the development of this handbook, and the existence and expansion of care homes liaison mental health teams, aim to improve knowledge and skills so that residents with schizophrenia may receive better care.

Before we go further, we need to understand some definitions:

- Hallucinations. A hallucination is a sensory experience that does not have a stimulus, for example the experience of hearing people speaking where there is no noise. Hallucinations are possible in any sensory modality, and the commonest are auditory (voices or other noises) and visual (seeing lights, figures or other complex images). Hallucinations are real to the person at the time, although some people can recognise them as unreal after the event.
- Illusions. An illusion is a sensory experience that does have a stimulus, but the stimulus is processed incorrectly so that what the person experiences is not what they would normally do. An example is the experience of seeing snakes arising from a floral-patterned carpet, seeing a coat hung on the back of a door and perceiving a person, or hearing a noise and thinking a name has been called out. Illusions are more common in people with poor sight or hearing.
- Delusions. A delusion is a false and unshakeable belief; an idea that is not true and is outside the person's usual cultural and religious beliefs. Delusions come in different types. They may be

persecutory, with ideas of state surveillance, poisoning of the water or air, or the plotting of physical or other harm. People with grandiose delusions have ideas 'above their station'; they may believe that they are royalty or have exceptional powers, such as the ability to predict the future. Severely depressed people may believe that they have caused a natural disaster such as an earthquake or, in extreme cases, may believe themselves to actually be dead. Because the delusion is unshakeable, no amount of discussion or argument will persuade the person that they are wrong

People with schizophrenia have other symptoms that are outside our usual experience. They may feel that other people are putting thoughts into their heads, stopping their thoughts from happening or taking their thoughts away. They may feel their thoughts being sent or broadcast to other people. Some experience external control of movement or emotions. All of these experiences have the potential to be very distressing, and may bring risks to care staff if the person believes that staff are implicated in some kind of conspiracy.

Negative symptoms

The psychotic symptoms already mentioned fit the general public's perception of mental disorder. However, people with schizophrenia also get a range of symptoms – often called negative symptoms – that may hamper their day-to-day living. Apathy and social withdrawal are common, low or flattened mood may exist, problems remembering facts may exist and a general lack of care about self or others may develop. These symptoms can be very disabling, especially in the presence of physical rehabilitation needs where the person needs to engage with rehabilitation staff and work hard to meet rehabilitation goals.

Treatment

Treatment of schizophrenia encompasses a range of approaches across biological, psychological and social areas. Psychological approaches can help some of the disordered thinking that people with schizophrenia experience and people can be encouraged to think about recovery rather than permanent disability, with a strong emphasis on self-determination. Social isolation can be addressed in care homes by encouraging mixing with others, although this may be difficult. At the heart of the treatment of schizophrenia is anti-psychotic medication, drugs which are sometimes called neuroleptics. These are usually taken orally but sometimes are given in the form on long-lasting injections, or depot medication, where there are concerns over adherence. Older drugs, such as chlorpromazine and haloperidol, have mainly been superseded by newer drugs, such as risperidone, olanzapine, quetiapine and amisulpride. These are all similarly effective, differing mainly in price and in the different side-effects. When commenced, medication will not be effective straight away, taking a few weeks to begin to have an effect, although side-effects will be experienced during this period.

Immediate-side effects include:

- tremor (much like the tremor seen in Parkinson's disease),
- drowsiness,
- low blood pressure,
- falls and
- hypothermia.

Longer term side-effects include:

- Weight gain, hyperglycaemia and diabetes.
- Cardiac arrhythmias, rarely causing sudden death
- An increased risk of stroke.
- People with epilepsy may be more prone to having fits if taking anti-psychotics.
- A rare, but potentially fatal, side-effect is called Neuroleptic Malignant Syndrome, which brings pyrexia, muscle rigidity, fluctuating consciousness and autonomic dysfunction. *These symptoms in someone on anti-psychotics indicate the need for urgent medical attention.*

As with all medication, there are risks and benefits to taking anti-psychotics. They do not work in all people, and are not very effective against the negative symptoms of schizophrenia.

In older people, anti-psychotics should not be used for mild and moderate psychotic symptoms, particularly where they are not causing distress. Where they are used in this population, the initial dose should be half of that used in adults of working age and should be titrated carefully and reviewed regularly.

There is particular concern over the use of anti-psychotics in dementia, and treatment in these cases should be initiated by a specialist.

Assessment and care planning

Residents with schizophrenia will have their own individual care needs and likes and dislikes; for example, preferences for particular kinds of food or for being addressed in a certain way. In this way they are no different from any resident. Nursing care for people with schizophrenia involves a holistic assessment of needs. This should draw upon information from a range of sources that might include relatives, primary care and mental health services. Some residents with schizophrenia may already have a mental health care coordinator, who will be a useful source of information on personalised care planning; where there is a care coordinator, they should ideally be involved in ongoing care planning. The care plan may need to involve items in the 'do's and don't's of care' listed below.

Therapeutic activities

These should be in place and available for all residents, including those with schizophrenia. Puzzles and problem solving are examples of techniques that may help, and exercise enhances physical fitness as well as mental well-being. Where present, activity coordinators should be aware of the personalised needs of all residents to deliver tailored therapeutic programmes for all.

Environmental aspects

The ideal care home environment is calm and not over-stimulating. Individual rooms will be preferred by those who want little social contact, whereas others may want more company. Many of the features associated with good environments for dementia will also apply here.

Do's and don't's of care

The nursing assessment of residents with psychosis does not differ from that of other residents. Different care homes will adopt various nursing models but all should ensure that there is an individualised assessment and inclusion of the resident (and their significant others, where appropriate) in the development of their care plan.

Any plan should include the resident's goals and responsibilities, as well as those of the care establishment. An assessment of risks should take place on initial assessment and at agreed appropriate intervals and if the resident's presentation changes.

There is no single care plan that will meet the needs of every resident with psychotic symptoms as each resident is different. The following tips may help staff caring for someone with psychotic symptoms, whatever their cause.

- Nurse people with psychotic symptoms in a safe environment which is not overly stimulating. Avoid complex patterns, lighting effects and keep noise levels, including radio and television, to minimal levels.
- Adopt a non-threatening and open body posture, ensuring your arms are not folded, eye contact is maintained but not too focused and your facial expression indicates you are actively listening to the person.
- Avoid touching residents without warning.
- Ensure your language is non-confrontational and non-ambiguous. Check that the resident has clearly understood you. Maintain a calm tone of voice throughout and try not to raise it.
- Adopt a consistent approach when undertaking any physical care; if possible, do this in short repeated contact until trust is established.
- Ensure that you explain to the person what you are about to do and the reason why, wherever possible encouraging them to maintain their independence in meeting their self-care needs.
- Avoid arguing with the person about any hallucinations or delusions they may be experiencing as these belief(s) are very real to them and may be causing them to feel distressed and frightened.
- Staff may in some cases need to avoid the use of humour, as this may be open to misinterpretation.
- Do not reinforce any abnormal beliefs; acknowledge that the hallucination/delusion is real to the person but that you are unable to share their experience. Do not discourage the resident from sharing their hallucinations/delusions, as these can give clues to their level of distress and the risks they pose to themselves and others.
- Ensure that throughout your interaction with the resident that you reinforce and focus on reality without escalating the situation and causing them to feel more distressed.
- Be honest when making promises, do not say you will return in 5 minutes when this is unrealistic because of commitments you may have to other residents.
- Cautiously use PRN medication aimed at reducing distress/anxiety caused by the hallucinations/delusions. Be aware of side-effects, such as increased risk of falls and Parkinsonism.

Further reading

Shah SM Carey IM, Harris T, et al. 2011. Antipsychotic prescribing in older people living in care homes and in the community in England and Wales. *International Journal of Geriatric Psychiatry* 26: 423–434.

Useful web site

Further information about schizophrenia from the Royal College of Psychiatrists can be found at: http://www.rcpsych.ac.uk/expertadvice/problems/schizophrenia/schizophrenia.aspx [Accessed October 2013]

Medicines Management

Chapter 11

The Management of Medications

11.1 Reviewing prescriptions

Adam Gordon[1], Sandra Jackson[2] and Sandra Horton[2]

[1]Nottingham University Hospitals NHS Trust, Nottingham, UK
[2]Provectus (UK) Limited, Mansfield Woodhouse, Nottinghamshire, UK

Key points

- In advanced long-term medical conditions, drug treatments are often less effective and frequently may produce more side-effects than benefits.
- Starting treatments is easy when new diagnoses are made.
- Removing treatments that have outlived their usefulness – or are producing more side effects than benefit – requires a combination of observation, experience and expertise. The benefits to the individual can be astonishing.

Residents are frequently prescribed more medications than they require (sometimes called polypharmacy, literally meaning 'many drugs').

This can lead to:

- an accumulation of side-effects,
- unintended interactions between prescribed drugs,
- difficulties with compliance, as residents struggle to take all of their medicines.

One consequence of moving into a care home is that a resident who was previously poorly compliant becomes much more reliable in taking their medicines because of the support of care home staff. This can increase the likelihood of adverse drug reaction during the time immediately following admission.

A rarer, but equally important, problem is residents who are not prescribed medicines from which they might benefit. Important examples are the anti-cholinesterase medications (donepezil, galantamine, rivastigmine) and memantine, which are used to treat dementia (see Chapter 10.1).

An important consideration in elderly care is *the principle of minimal medication*:

- *The lowest effective dose.*
- *The shortest effective duration of drug administration.*
- *The fewest number of drugs.*
- *The use of non-drug alternatives.*

In order to review medications, regular input from a resident's GP, or a representative of the GP, is required.

Care home residents should have a medication review at least every 6 months and more frequently if their condition is changing and/or they are on a large number of medications (six or more).

Prescription reviews should be accompanied by a review of the residents' diagnoses and current clinical status. Reviews will therefore work best if undertaken in the care home.

Prescription reviews are more effective if the GP has the support of a pharmacist with expertise in prescribing for older people.

In reviewing medications, the following steps are advised:

- The resident should be reviewed, face-to-face, in order to identify new medical conditions, chronic conditions which have become more or less severe, or previous diagnoses which have resolved.
- The GP and/or an advanced nurse practitioner should be present. Often these will be part of the primary care team, but sometimes the doctor and nurse practitioner will be care home staff. Their role is to lead decision making. Care home staff should be there to advise on observed side-effects and issues of administration. If the resident has capacity to participate in discussions about medications, they should be fully involved, providing further information on effects, side-effects

The Care Home Handbook, First Edition. Edited by Graham Mulley, Clive Bowman, Michal Boyd and Sarah Stowe.
© 2015 John Wiley & Sons, Ltd. Published 2015 by John Wiley & Sons, Ltd.

and opinions on the risk–benefit ratio of medications. If run as a multi-disciplinary case conference (MDT), several residents can be reviewed during a single afternoon.

- The medication review should use an up-to-date list of diagnoses and medications, which should be viewed side-by-side with the medication administration record (MAR).

The MAR is the care home's record of which medications are prescribed and given and is similar to a hospital drug card. It contains a list of medications, usually printed by the pharmacy, with instructions on dose, route and timing of administration. There are gaps for care home staff to document whether a medication was taken. It is important, where a medication is not taken, that this is also recorded in the MAR along with a reason for non-compliance. These reasons, where documented, are an important consideration at medication review.

- Each medication should be matched to a diagnosis. If no diagnosis is apparent to support a prescription, the resident's medical history should be reviewed. If no indication for the drug is found, it should be stopped.
- Those medications remaining should be reviewed, one by one, considering compliance, interactions and witnessed side-effects. If the adverse effects outweigh the benefits of the medication, it should be stopped.
- In reconciling multiple prescriptions, it is useful to weigh which medications are 'absolutely essential' – that is the resident will definitely come to harm if they are discontinued – against those which are 'indicated but not essential'.
- Finally, the list of diagnoses should be reviewed to ensure that the resident is receiving the best-evidenced treatment for each diagnosis. Both addition and substitution of medications should be carefully considered, remembering the potential harm of polypharmacy.

Medication reviews are a good opportunity for care home staff to have their questions about drugs answered. It is essential that nurses and carers administering drugs, treatments and medications understand the reasons for prescription, what side-effects might be expected and the correct dosage (refer to the Nursing and Midwifery Council Standards for Medicines Management).

Medication review also represents an excellent opportunity to consider non-pharmacological alternatives to commonly prescribed medications. Examples include non-pharmacological behavioural strategies for agitation in dementia (see Chapter 10.1), sleep-hygiene programmes for insomnia, bladder training or regular toileting for urinary incontinence and dietary treatments for chronic constipation. Such treatments are safer and better tolerated than the drugs they replace and, when used appropriately, can be as effective.)

Explicit criteria to avoid inappropriate prescribing have been developed and can be used to guide medication reviews. In Europe, the Screening Tool for Older People Prescriptions (STOPP) and Screening Tool to Alert Doctors to Right Treatment (START) criteria are commonly used, whilst in the USA, the Beer's Criteria are commonly applied. These tools can be long and practically challenging to use, but they can be a good focus for educational sessions on inappropriate prescribing, or used to train teams who are new to care home medication reviews.

Further reading

Barber ND, Alldred DP, Raynor DK, et al. 2009. Care homes' use of medicines study: prevalence, causes and potential harm of medication errors in care homes for older people. *Quality and Safety in Health Care* 18: 341–346.

Hamilton H, Gallagher P, O'Mahony D. 2009. Inappropriate prescribing and adverse drug events in older people. *BMC Geriatrics* 9: 5. Available online at http://www.biomedcentral.com/1471-2318/9/5 [Accessed October 2013]

11.2 Self-medication

Adam Gordon[1], Sandra Jackson[2] and Sandra Horton[2]

[1]Nottingham University Hospitals NHS Trust, Nottingham, UK
[2]Provectus (UK) Limited, Mansfield Woodhouse, Nottinghamshire, UK

Key points

- Self-medication may be desirable for residents to maintain autonomy and control over an important aspect of their health. This is particularly true for residents who may be returning to independent living in the community.
- Residents need to demonstrate competence in taking their medication at the right time, at the correct dose and in the correct manner, before they can be regarded as having capacity to self-medicate.
- Care homes staff must ensure that medications are stored and managed safely when residents self-medicate.

In order to ensure the safety of self-medication, it is essential to consider whether the resident has the mental capacity to manage their own prescriptions. The test of mental capacity (see Chapter 4.6) and capability has four components:

1. Can the resident *understand* their medications?. They should be able to describe the indication for each medication and, ideally, they should also have some insight into the important side-effects of each.
2. Can the resident *retain information* about their medications? They need to remember when to take their medicines and how to take them.
3. Can the resident *take responsibility* for their medications? They should be able to describe the importance of following their prescription and what will happen if they do not.
4. Is the resident able *to communicate information* about their medications to care home staff? This does not mean that the resident needs to communicate verbally.

If a resident has capacity to make their own decisions, but the home wishes to administer the medicines for the resident, consent is required and this should be recorded in the care plan.

It is essential to consider safe storage when residents are self-administering. It may be necessary for the resident to have a locker in their room, for which they hold the key, to protect their medications from other residents.

Reference

Gloucestershire NHS Primary Care Trust. Self Medication Assessment Tool. Available online at: http://www.glospct.nhs.uk/chst/documents/medicines/Sample%20Self%20medication%20assessment%20checklist%20-%20finalised%2002-06-10.pdf [Accessed October 2012]

Further reading

Hughes CM, Goldie R. 2009. "I just take what I am given": adherence and resident involvement in decision-making on medications in nursing homes for older people: a qualitative survey. *Drugs Aging* 26: 505–517.

11.3 Inhalers

Adam Gordon[1], Sandra Jackson[2] and Sandra Horton[2]

[1]*Nottingham University Hospitals NHS Trust, Nottingham, UK*
[2]*Provectus (UK) Limited, Mansfield Woodhouse, Nottinghamshire, UK*

Key points

- Inhaled drugs are the mainstay of the treatment of asthma: they can be delivered by inhalers or nebulisers.
- There are two main categories of drugs: relievers and preventers.
- Inhaled drugs may be in the form of soft mist or dry powder.
- The technique of using inhalers is important: some older residents have difficulty in using them.
- There are modified inhalers which can be useful in residents with arthritis and those who have problems timing the administration of the medication.

There are several types of inhaler. It is useful to understand how each of these works.

Types of inhaler

- *The Metered Dose Inhaler* (MDI – see Figure 11.3.1) – this has been the most commonly used type of inhaler. It is still used frequently because it is cheaper than other forms of inhaler and just as effective when the resident can use it correctly. In order to use it, the resident must shake it, exhale fully, and then inhale fully, while depressing the inhaler canister and ensuring that their lips are sealed tightly around the mouthpiece.
  Some residents with arthritis find this type of inhaler difficult to use and a number of lever devices such as the Haleraid™ have been developed to enable such residents to use MDIs. For residents who struggle with timing, a spacer device can be used (Figure 11.3.2). This means that the resident does not need to synchronise inhalation with depressing the canister.
- *The dry-powder inhaler* – these come in a number of shapes and sizes. Commonly used ones are the accuhaler™ (Figure 11.3.3), the turbohaler™ (Figure 11.3.4) and the handihaler™ (Figure 11.3.5). The accuhaler™ is activated by pressing on a trigger, the turbohaler™ by twisting the inhaler top, and the handihaler™ by introducing a capsule which contains the medication.
  There is no need to synchronise breathing with administration of the drug as the dosage is released only when the resident inhales. In order to use these, a resident must exhale fully, seal their lips tightly around the mouthpiece, and then inhale deeply.
- *The soft mist inhaler (respimat™)* – in the UK, this is currently only available for the medication tiotropium (Figure 11.3.6). It was introduced for this medication in particular because residents with arthritis struggled to use the handihaler device. It is activated by twisting the headpiece of the inhaler. Like dry powder inhalers, it is activated by the resident's breath.

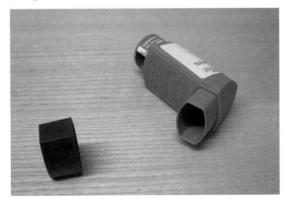

Figure 11.3.1 A metered dose inhaler.

The Care Home Handbook, First Edition. Edited by Graham Mulley, Clive Bowman, Michal Boyd and Sarah Stowe.
© 2015 John Wiley & Sons, Ltd. Published 2015 by John Wiley & Sons, Ltd.

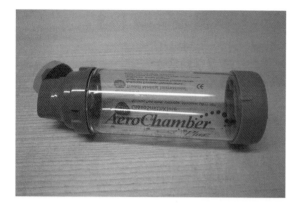

Figure 11.3.2 A spacer device.

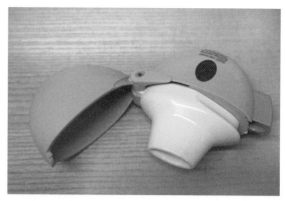

Figure 11.3.5 A handihaler™.

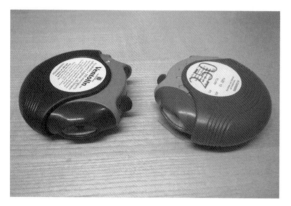

Figure 11.3.3 An accuhaler™.

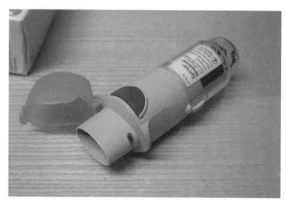

Figure 11.3.6 A soft mist inhaler (respimat™).

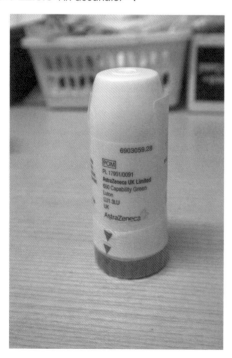

Figure 11.3.4 A turbohaler™.

Nebulisers are no more effective than normal inhalers, but they are useful in residents with very advanced airways disease, who struggle to activate dry powder or soft mist inhalers, and in residents with dementia, who sometimes cannot understand how to manipulate their inhaler.

- They are administered using a face mask and reservoir.
- Usually in a care home they will be *air driven* and the resident will have a compressor (Figure 11.3.7) which is used to drive the nebulizer.
- Rarely, they will be *oxygen driven* and, for these, residents will have either an oxygen cylinder or oxygen concentrator. Prescribing doctors should specify whether a nebulizer is to be air- or oxygen-driven and ensure appropriate equipment to deliver the medicine. Where oxygen therapy is being used, it is important that all concerned understand the dangers of oxygen and naked flames (see Chapter 11.9).

Devices should be used according to the manufacturer's instructions to ensure accurate delivery of the inhaled medication. It is important that the devices are checked

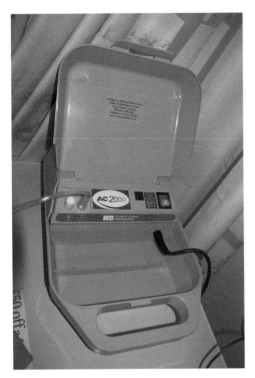

Figure 11.3.7 A compressor.

frequently, serviced in accordance with manufacturer's instructions and a record should be kept of dates when the service has been done.

Drugs delivered via inhaler or nebulizer can be split into two main categories: relievers and preventers.

- *Relievers* – these are drugs that open up the airways and provide immediate relief from distressing breathlessness. The main drugs in this category are salbutamol and terbutaline. They do not need to be taken except when the resident is breathless.
- *Preventers* – these include drugs that help to keep the airways open longer term (salmetarol, formetarol, ipratropium and tiotropium) and also steroid drugs, which act to reduce inflammation in the airways (beclomethasone, fluticasone, budesonide, ciclesonide). In practice, they are often given as compound preparations, such as seretide™, symbicort™ and fostair™, which are a combination of steroids with medications to open the airways. They should be taken regularly, *even when the resident is not breathless.* Often there will be a requirement for the resident to gargle with water after using a steroid preparation in order to prevent oral thrush, which is a side-effect of inhaled steroids.

For further details on asthma, see Chapter 9.2.

Useful web site

Asthma UK. "Using your inhalers", available online at http://www.asthma.org.uk/about-asthma/medicines-treatments/using-your-inhalers [Accessed October 2013].

11.4 Suppositories and enemas

Adam Gordon[1], Sandra Jackson[2] and Sandra Horton[2]

[1]*Nottingham University Hospitals NHS Trust, Nottingham, UK*
[2]*Provectus (UK) Limited, Mansfield Woodhouse, Nottinghamshire, UK*

Key points

- Suppositories and enemas are administered rectally for the treatment of constipation and faecal incontinence.
- There are three main types: softeners, stimulants and osmotic laxatives.
- This approach is also used for some non-laxative medications, including analgesics, drugs for epilepsy and certain antibiotics.

A suppository is a solid medication and an enema a liquid. Both are administered rectally. Medications are most commonly delivered via these routes for treatment, or prevention of constipation and faecal incontinence. In this regard, the most commonly used medications are:

- *Faecal softeners* (glycerol suppositories and arachis oil enemas): these are used to loosen hardened stool which can block the rectum resulting in constipation or 'overflow' incontinence, where liquid faeces trickles down from above.
- *Stimulant laxatives* (bisacodyl enemas): these are used to stimulate rectal contraction and promote emptying of the rectum. As they can result in painful rectal contractions when used with very hard faeces, they are more commonly prescribed where there is softer, 'clay' consistency faeces in the rectum. They are sometimes used after a few days' treatment with a softener.
- *Osmotic laxatives* (phosphate enemas): these are used to clear the rectum before residents attend for investigative procedures such as sigmoidoscopy or colonoscopy. They represent a large volume and as such can be both uncomfortable and difficult to retain. They can result in painful and explosive faecal incontinence. They should not usually be used as a first-line treatment for constipation or faecal loading, although they can sometimes be used as a second-line therapy.

Documentation of stool type using the Bristol stool chart can be useful guide as to which of these agents should be used (see Chapter 5.5).

Suppositories and enemas can also be a useful way to deliver medications that are absorbed through the lining of the rectum and are used for their effects elsewhere in the body. This can be helpful where a resident is not able, or refuses, to take a medication by mouth (although it is important that when prescribing and dispensing medications by rectum for this reason that an assessment of capacity and best interests is undertaken).

Non-laxative medications that are commonly prescribed in this way include:

- paracetamol (for control of pain and to treat a high temperature);
- diazepam (usually in the context of an epileptic seizure, when it is difficult to give the medication by mouth); and
- a variety of antibiotics (which can be given rectally when the resident is delirious (see Chapter 10.2) and therefore unable to take medications by mouth).

Rectal administration of medication should only be undertaken by appropriately trained staff. If the patient has inflammatory bowel disease, rectal or anal pain, obvious rectal bleeding, or there is any evidence of local tissue trauma, it may be reasonable to seek assurance from the resident's GP that rectal administration is safe.

The Care Home Handbook, First Edition. Edited by Graham Mulley, Clive Bowman, Michal Boyd and Sarah Stowe.
© 2015 John Wiley & Sons, Ltd. Published 2015 by John Wiley & Sons, Ltd.

In giving a suppository or enema, the following steps should be undertaken:

- Privacy should be assured: the resident should be taken to their room or, if they share a room, to a bathroom or other private area. Curtains on exterior windows should be drawn. A 'do not disturb' sign should be placed on the door until the procedure is completed. Toilet facilities, or a commode or bedpan (depending on the resident's mobility), should be close to hand, in case they feel the urge to defecate either during, or immediately after, the procedure.
- Staff should work in teams: because of the intimate nature of rectal administration, it is important that more than one staff member is present to ensure that care is managed delicately and to minimise the possibility of accusation of abuse (see Chapter 4.3). It can be useful for one member of staff to remain in front of the resident, holding a hand and making eye contact, to minimise the distress associated with the procedure. At least one member of staff, if possible, should be the same gender as the resident.
- Staff should wear appropriate protective clothing: latex gloves and an apron. A number of alternative gloves are available for staff or patients who are allergic to latex. When handling body fluids, nitrile gloves should be used and not those made from vinyl. Continence sheets should be placed on the bed under the resident in case of leakage.
- The resident should be positioned appropriately: if possible on their left side, with knees drawn up to abdomen. If possible, a bed or couch which is height-adjustable should be used. This should be raised to a level that will allow the procedure to be completed with minimal strain for the staff involved.
- Before inserting the medication, a digital rectal examination should be performed to find out whether the rectum is faecally loaded. If there is gross faecal loading, it might not be possible to introduce large volume enemas, such as phosphate. Rectal examination should be done using the index finger of the right hand, which should be lubricated with an aqueous gel.
- The tip of the suppository, or introducer for an enema, should be lubricated with aqueous gel. For bullet-shaped suppositories, there is no particular consensus as to whether they should be introduced blunt or sharp tip first, either will do. For enemas, remember to keep the bottle squeezed until withdrawn from the rectum, or else it may fill with liquid faeces – unpleasant and difficult to dispose of.
- Finally, the resident should be cleaned around the anus and perineum. Gloves and aprons should be disposed of in a clinical waste bag (see Chapter 12.8). The resident should be encouraged to retain the enema for as long as possible. They should give sufficient warning if they need to go to the toilet, to avoid an episode of incontinence.

Further reading

Higgins D. 2007. Bowel care Part 6 – Administration of a suppository. *Nursing Times* 103(47): 26–27.

Kyle G. 2007. Bowel care Part 4 – Administering an enema. *Nursing Times* 103(45): 26–27.

11.5 Vaccinations

Adam Gordon[1], Sandra Jackson[2] and Sandra Horton[2]

[1]Nottingham University Hospitals NHS Trust, Nottingham, UK
[2]Provectus (UK) Limited, Mansfield Woodhouse, Nottinghamshire, UK

Key points

- A pneumococcal vaccine should be considered for all new care home residents.
- An influenza vaccine should be considered every year for all residents and staff.

Vaccination is generally the responsibility of primary care or public health.

Two are particularly relevant to care home residents: pneumonia and influenza.

The World Health Organization recommends that all adults over the age of 65 are vaccinated against pneumonia with 23-valent Pneumococcal vaccine (PPV23). Although there is some evidence that the vaccine is less effective in care home residents due to changes in immunity in advanced old age, the recommendation still stands for this group. Residents under the age of 65 may also be recommended to have the vaccine where they suffer from chronic heart, lung, kidney or liver disease, or diabetes. Once vaccination is given, revaccination is not routinely recommended. *It is therefore reasonable to consider pneumococcal vaccination as part of the admission assessment to the care home.*

Influenza vaccination does not seem to affect the rate of influenza infection in care home residents, but there is good evidence that it prevents life-threatening complications, such as pneumonia. It is most effective when *all* residents and staff are vaccinated. Because the influenza viruses undergo changes annually, *it is important that flu vaccination is repeated once per year – usually in the autumn or early winter, since infection rates are highest over the winter months.*

Nobody can be made to take the vaccination against their will, but both staff and residents should be strongly encouraged to take it.

Inactive trivalent influenza vaccine is safe in those with asthma. It is probably safe to give influenza vaccines to residents with egg allergy. However, there is a small risk of anaphylaxis and therefore standard precautions should be taken (see Chapter 9.1)

Further reading

Gordon AL, Ewan V. 2010. Pneumonia and influenza – specific considerations in care homes. *Reviews in Clinical Gerontology* 20(1): 69–80.

Kelso LM. 2012. Safety of influenza vaccines. *Current Opinion in Allergy and Clinical Immunology* 12: 383–388.

11.6 Intra-muscular and intra-venous drugs and syringe drivers

Adam Gordon[1], Sandra Jackson[2] and Sandra Horton[2]

[1]*Nottingham University Hospitals NHS Trust, Nottingham, UK*
[2]*Provectus (UK) Limited, Mansfield Woodhouse, Nottinghamshire, UK*

Key points

- Practitioners should not attempt to administer medications sub-cutaneously, intra-muscularly or intra-venously unless they have received specific training and have been signed off as competent.
- If a resident with an intra-venous access device shows signs of infection (temperature, fast heart rate, low blood pressure), this is a medical emergency and a GP should see the patient within a matter of hours. If the resident looks critically unwell at any point, the safest place to manage them will be in acute hospital and an ambulance should be called.
- Regular refresher courses are required to ensure that practitioners maintain the basic competencies in these routes of administration.

Sub-cutaneous (SC), intra-muscular (IM) or intra-venous (IV) therapy is increasingly used in care homes. This approach is usually restricted to nursing homes, although care assistants can sometimes play a role (such as in residential homes where care staff might assist a resident to administer sub-cutaneous insulin or pain relief with the primary care team).

Sub-cutaneous (SC) medications have a particular role in the management of *diabetes* (insulin is given via this route) and in the *palliative care* of patients in the last few weeks or days of life. Treatment can be delivered either as an injection or as an infusion, using a special giving set and infusion driver. Fluids can also be administered via this route to prevent residents becoming dehydrated.

SC fluids can be used to either supplement inadequate fluid intake (see Chapter 5.3) by other routes or as a short-term 'bridging' measure until definitive measures for hydration can be established. Other forms of hydration will need to be established (oral, nasogastric or PEG). Relying on subcutaneous fluids to support life beyond a bridging period is more likely to prolong a patient's death, rather than maintain their life.

The *IM route* is used for injections only; infusions cannot be administered via this route. They are most commonly administered into the vastus lateralus (thigh), dorso-gluteus (buttock) or deltoid (shoulder) muscles. Each of these has specific surface landmarks which are taught as part of the training in how to deliver an IM injection.

Intra-venous therapies can be administered in care homes. Medications can be given by the approved practitioners within a home with nursing, or by visiting nurses within a residential home. These therapies will usually be commenced in a hospital, before a resident is discharged to their care home. The most common indication is for an infection that requires a prolonged course of antibiotics. It is important before accepting a patient for such care that the care home team establishes the following:

- A definitive vascular access device is in place – an intra-venous cannula (venflon™) will not suffice for long-term community management. Acceptable alternatives are a peripherally inserted central cannula (PICC) line; or a tunneled central catheter (either a Hickman line or portacath device).
- That the resident's GP is happy to accept medical responsibility for management of the vascular access device and course of medication and that there is a named hospital service that can respond rapidly to problems with the device. A clear

The Care Home Handbook, First Edition. Edited by Graham Mulley, Clive Bowman, Michal Boyd and Sarah Stowe.
© 2015 John Wiley & Sons, Ltd. Published 2015 by John Wiley & Sons, Ltd.

specialist care plan should be available pre transfer/admission for safety.

- That the visiting nursing service, or nursing home staff, who are to look after the device have adequate training to support the full course of therapy – if this is to run for several weeks or months, then staff will have to be available to support the therapy throughout.

- That plans are in place for regular review of the vascular access device by an appropriately trained member of nursing or medical staff and for its removal after the course of treatment is completed.

Syringe drivers are used only in a minority of care home residents, usually with advice from the palliative care team.

Further reading

Kinley J, Hockley J. 2010. A baseline review of medication provided to older people in nursing care homes in the last month of life. *International Journal of Palliative Nursing* 10: 216–223.

11.7 Controlled drugs

Adam Gordon[1], Sandra Jackson[2] and Sandra Horton[2]

[1]*Nottingham University Hospitals NHS Trust, Nottingham, UK*
[2]*Provectus (UK) Limited, Mansfield Woodhouse, Nottinghamshire, UK*

Key points

- Controlled drugs are subject to strict regulations regarding storage, prescribing, dispensing and disposal.
- These drugs should only be given to named individuals.
- Controlled drugs must be kept in a locked cupboard. Whenever drugs are taken out of the cupboard, two members of staff must be present.

Drugs that are 'controlled' are commonly abused and, as such, have a 'street value'. Controlled drugs which are commonly used in care homes include morphine, buprenorphine and fentanyl (used for pain); and temazepam and zolpidem (used for sleep).

Most regulatory authorities expect care homes to treat these drugs in the way that hospitals and clinics would, as the drugs are both dangerous and a focus for regulatory scrutiny.

The guidelines on prescribing, dispensing and administration vary depending upon the drug. For example, in the UK:

- Morphine and fentanyl (which in the UK are called schedule 2 drugs) are subject to the strictest regulations.
- Buprenorphine and temazepam are schedule 3 drugs.
- Zolpidem is a schedule 4 drug.
- Each schedule requires less strict regulations than the one before it. Each care home will have to make a decision about how to manage these medications but it can, in practice, be easier to treat all medications as if they are schedule 2 medications – this will depend on the number of residents prescribed controlled drugs and staff availability to support the strict administration criteria for schedule 2 medications.

The guidelines generally mean that:

- Prescriptions have to follow very specific requirements – it is therefore important that care home staff give GPs adequate notice when a repeat prescription is required.
- Drugs should only be prescribed for fixed time intervals. This is often a month at a time. Frequent requests for repeat prescriptions are therefore required.
- Medications are usually prescribed for a named resident and cannot be transferred between residents (although some homes will have arrangements in place that allow them to hold a stock of more commonly prescribed medications, such as morphine, this is not normal practice).
- Medications must be held in a special locked 'controlled drugs' (CD) cupboard – to which a restricted number of staff have access.

Whenever a drug is removed from the cupboard and administered, two members of staff should be involved.

Administration should be documented in a controlled drug register, as well as the residents' MAR (Medical Administration Record) (see Chapter 11.1). This should be a bound book, with individually numbered pages.

There should be a separate page for each resident receiving a CD and for each CD that they receive. It should record the date, the amount of drug removed from stock, the amount of stock remaining in the CD cupboard, the amount of drug actually administered to the resident, the name of the staff member administering the drug and the name of the staff member who witnessed the administration.

The Care Home Handbook, First Edition. Edited by Graham Mulley, Clive Bowman, Michal Boyd and Sarah Stowe.
© 2015 John Wiley & Sons, Ltd. Published 2015 by John Wiley & Sons, Ltd.

It will, from time to time, be necessary to dispose of controlled drugs. Nursing home staff are required to obtain a CD denaturing kit from their supplying pharmacy before disposing of them via their normal licensed waste company. These usually consist of a jar or bottle containing a denaturing agent, into which medicines are placed before disposal. Residential homes should return the CD to their supplying pharmacy. When drugs are disposed of, or returned to pharmacy, this should be witnessed and documented in the CD register.

Further reading

British National Formulary No. 63 (March 2012). London, Pharmaceutical Press.

Pharmaceutical Press. 2012. *Guidance on Prescribing – Controlled Drugs and Drug Dependance*.

The Royal Pharmaceutical Society of Great Britain. 2009. The handling of medications in social care, available online at http://www.rpharms.com/ [Accessed October 2013]. London, Royal Pharmaceutical Society.

11.8 Disposal of drugs

Adam Gordon[1], Sandra Jackson[2] and Sandra Horton[2]

[1] Nottingham University Hospitals NHS Trust, Nottingham, UK
[2] Provectus (UK) Limited, Mansfield Woodhouse, Nottinghamshire, UK

Key points

It may be necessary to dispose of drugs when:

- A resident's treatment is changed or discontinued.
- A resident moves to another care service (though ideally, their medication should be transferred with them).
- A resident dies. In this instance, their drugs should be kept for seven days before disposal, in case the Coroner's Office (or, in Scotland, the Procurator Fiscal) asks for them.
- A medicine reaches its expiry date.

Your care home will have a written policy for the safe disposal of surplus, unwanted or expired medicines – *if you are unsure where this is kept, ask your manager.*

When medications are disposed of, the following information should be recorded and held on record:

- Date of disposal/return to pharmacy.
- Name and strength of medicine.
- Quantity removed.
- Name of the resident for whom the drug was prescribed.
- Signature of the member of staff who arranged disposal of the medicines.

There are specific arrangements for disposal of controlled drugs (see Chapter 11.7).

Some community pharmacists organise the disposal of medications.

Further reading

Denham MJ, Barrett NL. 1998. Drug therapy and the older person: role of the pharmacist *Drug Safety* 19: 243–250.

The Royal Pharmaceutical Society of Great Britain. 2009. The handling of medications in social care, available online at http://www.rpharms.com/ [Accessed October 2013]. London, Royal Pharmaceutical Society.

The Care Home Handbook, First Edition. Edited by Graham Mulley, Clive Bowman, Michal Boyd and Sarah Stowe.
© 2015 John Wiley & Sons, Ltd. Published 2015 by John Wiley & Sons, Ltd.

11.9 Oxygen therapy

Adam Gordon[1], Sandra Jackson[2] and Sandra Horton[2]

[1]*Nottingham University Hospitals NHS Trust, Nottingham, UK*
[2]*Provectus (UK) Limited, Mansfield Woodhouse, Nottinghamshire, UK*

Key points

- Oxygen is administered in care homes for one of two indications:
  - In end-stage Chronic Obstructive Pulmonary Disease (COPD), where it is usually prescribed for 16–18 hours per day, to prevent the long-term cardiac complications of that condition.
  - For symptomatic relief of breathlessness, usually in palliative care. There is no minimum requirement for the number of hours of therapy in this instance.
- Oxygen can be dangerous in those with COPD and in those who smoke.
- It should be carefully prescribed by the GP.

In either end stage COPD or in palliative care, it is unlikely that the resident will come to harm if their oxygen is taken off for a few minutes to complete a particular activity of daily living. Where a resident struggles to undertake activities of daily living because of breathlessness, staff must ensure that they give them adequate time to do these at their own pace.

Oxygen, where it is administered, should be prescribed. This can either be on the MAR (see Chapter 11.1), on a separate oxygen prescribing sheet, or both. *It is important that the prescription is adhered to and not deviated from, except in consultation with the resident's GP. Some people with COPD can become critically unwell if their oxygen levels are allowed to climb too high.*

Oxygen saturations should not be routinely measured unless specified by the prescribing doctor. *It is important if a doctor asks for saturations to be measured using a pulse oximeter that they specify, in writing, how they want care home staff to respond to these measurements.* It may be that they simply want a diary to be kept, or it may be that they want oxygen therapy to be adjusted to maintain saturations within a specific range. In this case, the desired saturation range should be written on the oxygen prescription. Once oxygen flow rate has been changed, oxygen saturations, as measured by pulse oximetry, will reach their new steady-state value within 2–3 minutes.

All residents on oxygen should, in addition, have a care plan for management of their airways and mouth care (see Chapters 5.7 and 5.8).

Oxygen will either be supplied as a cylinder, where therapy is expected to be short term (or the duration of therapy is uncertain), or an oxygen concentrator, where residents are expected to be on therapy for the majority of the day for the forseeable future. These will usually supplied with either nasal cannulae (Figure 11.9.1) or a Venturi mask (Figure 11.9.2).

Nasal cannulae can be used for any flow rate of oxygen up to 4 litres.

The Venturi mask comes with a specified flow rate and oxygen concentration on the nozzle. When a particular nozzle is attached, the Venturi mask can only reliably deliver the specified concentration of oxygen at the specified flow rate. To change this, a different nozzle is required to be fitted. In particular, *turning the oxygen flow rate up on a Venturi mask will not deliver a higher rate of oxygen.* Other types of oxygen mask are not usually used within care homes.

Oxygen is highly combustible and, where it used within a care home, staff, relatives and the resident must be advised not to smoke. Open flames for cooking or heating should not be used in the same room as an oxygen cylinder or concentrator.

Increasingly, care home residents are being put on Non-Invasive Positive Pressure Ventilation (NIPPV) therapy for the treatment of sleep apnoea, obesity

The Care Home Handbook, First Edition. Edited by Graham Mulley, Clive Bowman, Michal Boyd and Sarah Stowe.
© 2015 John Wiley & Sons, Ltd. Published 2015 by John Wiley & Sons, Ltd.

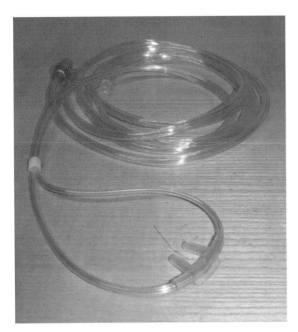

Figure 11.9.1 Nasal cannula.

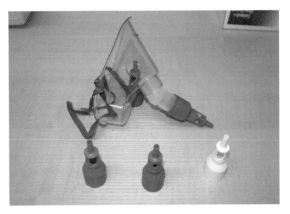

Figure 11.9.2 Venturi mask.

hypoventilation syndrome or musculoskeletal respiratory failure.

Care home staff should only assume responsibility for using these machines when they have undergone appropriate instruction in how to fit the mask, how to switch the machine on and off, and how to respond to alarms. This can be organised with the hospital that has prescribed the therapy and may involve staff attending the hospital for specific instruction.

It would usually not be appropriate for care home staff to be instructed in how to modify settings on an NIPPV ventilator.

Ventilator settings should usually be locked by hospital staff at the point of discharge to the care home.

The home must ensure that there is adequate battery back-up for the NIPPV machine as well as a spare in case of failure.

Further reading

Kelly C, Lynes D. 2008. The use of domiciliary oxygen therapy. *Nursing Times* 104(23): 46–48.

11.10 Crushing tablets for people with swallowing difficulties

Adam Gordon[1], Sandra Jackson[2] and Sandra Horton[2]

[1]*Nottingham University Hospitals NHS Trust, Nottingham, UK*
[2]*Provectus (UK) Limited, Mansfield Woodhouse, Nottinghamshire, UK*

Key points

- Do not crush enteric coated or modified-release tablets.
- If in doubt about opening or crushing tablets, ask the pharmacist for advice.

Swallowing difficulties (dysphagia) are common in care home residents, particularly those with stroke or dementia. It is also increasingly common for residents to be fed via percutaneous entero-gastrostomy (PEG) tube. Tablets and capsules can be difficult for patients with swallowing difficulties to manage and it is impossible to administer them via PEG tube.

The alternatives are to:

- Use dispersible medications, suspensions or syrups.
- Crush tablets or open capsules and administer them as a powder, or by mixing with food or drink (see Chapter 11.11).

Many tablets remain effective when crushed. There are two main types of medication that should *not* be crushed or opened:

- Enteric coated medications – these are designed with a special coating so that they are not broken down by the acid in the stomach. This is either because they damage the stomach, are damaged by stomach acid, or are absorbed more effectively further down the intestine.
- Modified release preparations (sometimes called slow- or controlled-release preparations) – these are designed to be released over a long period of time and they can be toxic, less effective or ineffective if crushed or opened.

Medications should therefore only be crushed or capsules opened when:

- A pharmacist has advised it is safe to crush or open the medication.
- The medication label and the MAR (see Chapter 11.1) has been altered to indicate that the medication should be crushed or opened.

It may be necessary to administer multiple drugs or medications via the PEG tube at the same time. It is usually advised that the medications are injected into the PEG one at a time, with a flush of water between each drug – this is to stop the PEG tube becoming blocked.

Further reading

Cornish P. 2005. "Avoid the crush": hazards of medication administration in patients with dysphagia or a feeding tube. *Canadian Medical Association Journal* 172: 871–872.

Williams NT. 2008. Medication administration through enteral feeding tubes. *American Journal of Health-System Pharmacy* 65: 2347–2357.

11.11 Disguising medication

Adam Gordon[1], Sandra Jackson[2] and Sandra Horton[2]

[1]*Nottingham University Hospitals NHS Trust, Nottingham, UK*
[2]*Provectus (UK) Limited, Mansfield Woodhouse, Nottinghamshire, UK*

Key points

- Disguising medications without the resident being aware of this must only be done after expert input from a consultant.
- Whenever possible, the resident and their family must be informed.

Regulatory authorities often have very clear guidance on disguising medication and covert administration. Care home staff should be familiar with this.

Mixing medications with food or drink can take place where the resident has capacity and wishes their medicines to be given with food such as yogurt (some residents with swallowing difficulties may find this easier).

Occasionally, disguising medication in food or drink is deemed to be in the best interests of a resident who lacks capacity – perhaps because of advanced dementia. Because of the potential harm from this practice and the complexity of best-interest assessments in this context, *it should only take place after expert input, usually from a geriatrician or old age psychiatrist.* Doctors undertaking these decisions need expertise in both the Mental Capacity and Mental Health Act.

In all instances, where possible, the resident, as well as their next of kin, should be informed of the plan to administer medication in food or drink and this should be documented in the care plan.

Medications should only be given in food or drink when it is specified on either the medication label, or the MAR (see Chapter 11.1), that it is safe to do so. A pharmacist therefore needs to be consulted. The pharmacist can also give advice on which foods or drinks can be mixed with medications. This is both in order to avoid unpleasant tastes and textures and to ensure that the food does not in any way deactivate or alter the medication. The pharmacist can also advise on which combinations of medications can safely be given within a single food or drink.

It is good practice to inform the resident that they are receiving their medication in food or drink at each administration. This does not have to be unduly formal and can be achieved simply by pointing out, for example, that the residents' morning medications are mixed in with their porridge (just make sure this is in the resident's room and bowls don't get mixed).

Further reading

UK Nursing And Midwifery Council. Covert Administration of Medication in Food and Drink, available online at http://www.nmc-uk.org/Nurses-and-midwives/Advice-by-topic/A/Advice/Covert-administration-of-medicines/ [Accessed October 2013].

Waite J, Harwood R, Morton I, Connoly D. 2008. Chapter 4. Treatment. In: *Dementia Care: A Practical Manual*. Oxford, Oxford University Press.

11.12 Eye drops

Adam Gordon[1], Sandra Jackson[2] and Sandra Horton[2]

[1]*Nottingham University Hospitals NHS Trust, Nottingham, UK*
[2]*Provectus (UK) Limited, Mansfield Woodhouse, Nottinghamshire, UK*

Key points

- Always inform the resident before you apply eye drops or ointment.
- Carefully wash and dry your hands before giving these medications.
- Eye drop dispensers are available for cases where residents have problems inserting eye medications.

Some medications commonly used in care home residents are administered as eye drops or eye ointments (see Chapter 7.1).

Eye drops are usually a clear, water-like liquid and usually come in a bottle with a drop dispenser attached.

Eye ointments look much more like creams, and often come in a tube. In order to administer them, the following steps should be followed:

- Staff members should wash, thoroughly rinse and dry their hands before administration (see Chapter 12.1).
- The resident should be informed of what is about to take place and that it might be uncomfortable.
- Gently shake the bottle of eye drops.
- The resident should be asked to tilt their head backwards slightly and look up.
- The lower eyelid should be gently pulled back to form a 'pocket' to receive the drop.
- The bottle should be turned upside down and one drop administered into the pocket.
- Unless instructed otherwise, only one drop should be administered per eye. Additional drops may result in side-effects from the medication.
- The patient's eye will automatically close by

reflex after administration. You should encourage them to keep it closed for a minute or so, until it feels comfortable to re-open the eye.

- Excess medication, or tears, escaping from the closed eye can be gently blotted with a clean tissue.
- If more than one medication is required to be administered, 5 minutes should be left between each medication. Drops should be applied before ointments.

Eye drop dispenser devices are available for residents who struggle to comply with the standard mode of administration, perhaps as a consequence of dementia. A pharmacist or occupational therapist can advise on which will best suit your resident.

Further reading

National Institutes of Health Clinical Center. How to put in your eye drops. Available online at http://www.cc.nih.gov/ccc/patient_education/pepubs/eyedrops.pdf [Accessed October 2013]

Pharmaceutical Press. 2012. 11.1 Administration of Medications to the Eye. British National Formulary No. 63 (March 2012). London, Pharmaceutical Press.

The Care Home Handbook, First Edition. Edited by Graham Mulley, Clive Bowman, Michal Boyd and Sarah Stowe.
© 2015 John Wiley & Sons, Ltd. Published 2015 by John Wiley & Sons, Ltd.

11.13 Mistakes with medication: what to do

Adam Gordon[1], Sandra Jackson[2] and Sandra Horton[2]

[1] Nottingham University Hospitals NHS Trust, Nottingham, UK
[2] Provectus (UK) Limited, Mansfield Woodhouse, Nottinghamshire, UK

Key points

- All errors in administering medications must be reported and logged.
- If there is any chance that the error could result in harm, medical advice must be sought at once.
- All care homes should have a review process for the audit of medication errors.

Errors in the administration of medications are an unfortunate fact of life. It is important that when they do occur that they are reported, first to avoid any harm to the resident and second to understand why the error occurred so that it will hopefully not be repeated.

Not all drug errors result in harm but, depending on the drug and resident involved, there can be significant adverse effects.

It may be necessary for the resident to be admitted to hospital.

When care staff realise that an error has occurred, they must report it to their shift manager immediately. The shift manager must consider the likelihood that the error will have caused any harm to the resident. *If there is any uncertainty, the advice of a doctor should be sought immediately.*

If out-of-hours, then in England and Wales it would be appropriate to contact NHS direct (NHS24 in Scotland), who would be able to provide advice on any potential harm and whether any further action is required.

If the incident has occurred out-of-hours and there is possible or actual harm to the resident, the GP responsible for the resident should be notified on the next working day.

The resident should be made aware that an error has occurred at the time of the error. If they lack capacity to participate in discussions about their medication then their next-of-kin should be notified – if out-of-hours, this notification should take place the following day.

Each home should have in place processes for the review of untoward incidents, including medication errors. This should include the keeping of an incident log. In the case of a medication error, it would be normal for the home manager to undertake a root cause analysis (RCA) to understand why the error occurred and to attempt to learn lessons so that the error is not repeated. It is important that staff, residents and next-of-kin understand that this process is not about attributing blame and that staff, in particular, feel they can contribute openly without their reputation or job being endangered.

If a resident has suffered harm as a consequence of a medication error, the home has an obligation under the UK Health and Social Care Act 2008 to report this as an injury to the Care Quality Commission. This should be done on the next working day. Advice on how to make these notifications can be found on the CQC web site at: http://www.cqc.org.uk/organisa tions-we-regulate/registered-services/notifications/ notifications-non-nhs-providers.

Useful web site

Care Quality Commission
Notifications for non-NHS providers, available online at http://www.cqc.org.uk/organisations-we-regulate/regis tered-services/notifications/notifications-non-nhs-providers [Accessed October 2013]

The Care Home Handbook, First Edition. Edited by Graham Mulley, Clive Bowman, Michal Boyd and Sarah Stowe.
© 2015 John Wiley & Sons, Ltd. Published 2015 by John Wiley & Sons, Ltd.

Section G

Infection Prevention and Control

Chapter 12

Infection Prevention

12.1 Hand hygiene

Jean Lawrence

Retired Infection Prevention and Control Nurse, (IPS) Yorkshire, UK

Key points

- Hand hygiene remains a most important measure in the prevention and control of infection and can save lives.
- Hands must always be washed at the start of the working day as well as before and after many nursing tasks.
- Washing your hands is about protecting the person being cared for, staff and families of staff.

Always ask

- What have I just done?
- What am I about to do?
- What are the risks?
- Do I need to wash my hands?

When

- Before and after contact with a person in your care and any procedures in their immediate environment.
- Before clean/aseptic procedures.
- After handling laundry, waste or potentially contaminated equipment.
- After using or cleaning the toilet and after assisting someone with toileting.
- After exposure to blood and body fluids.
- Before preparing and giving medication/treatments.
- After handling or cleaning up after pets (see Chapter 2.7).
- After blowing/touching nose or covering a sneeze or cough.

(This is not an exhaustive list as you must always assess each task and action.)

How

- Remove wrist watches, bracelets and stoned rings. Plain wedding bands only.
- Keep fingernails short, clean and free of varnish and false nails.
- Use elbow/wrist taps where available.
- Wet hands first before soap application (Figure 12.1.1).
- Apply liquid soap/cleanser to produce a good lather.
- Cover all areas of the hands and wrists remembering tips of fingers, thumbs and in between fingers and the palm of the hand using the defined technique shown.
- Rinse hands and wrists well under running water.
- Dry using disposable paper hand towel.
- Turn of taps using 'hands free' technique, for example elbows or wrists. Paper towels can be used to turn off taps if no hand free taps are in place.
- Dispose of used paper towels into the domestic waste system.

Technique

Please see Figure 12.1.1.

- Wet your hands with warm running water using a mixer tap if possible.
- Apply liquid soap from a dispenser and cover all your hands to create a lather.
- Rub your hands palm to palm.
- Rub the back of each hand with the palm of the other hand and interlace your fingers.
- Rub palm to palm with fingers interlaced.

The Care Home Handbook, First Edition. Edited by Graham Mulley, Clive Bowman, Michal Boyd and Sarah Stowe.
© 2015 John Wiley & Sons, Ltd. Published 2015 by John Wiley & Sons, Ltd.

Hand hygiene technique with soap and water

🕐 **Duration of the entire procedure:** 40–60 seconds

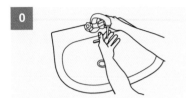

0 Wet hands with water;

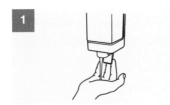

1 Apply enough soap to cover all hand surfaces;

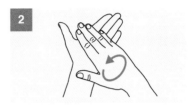

2 Rub hands palm to palm;

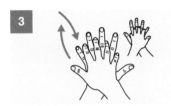

3 Right palm over left dorsum with interlaced fingers and vice versa;

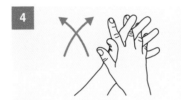

4 Palm to palm with fingers interlaced;

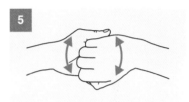

5 Backs of fingers to opposing palms with fingers interlocked;

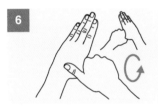

6 Rotational rubbing of left thumb clasped in right palm and vice versa;

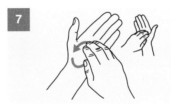

7 Rotational rubbing, backwards and forwards with clasped fingers of right hand in left palm and vice versa;

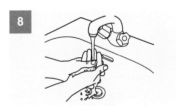

8 Rinse hands with water;

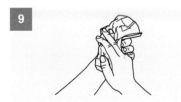

9 Dry hands thoroughly with a single use towel;

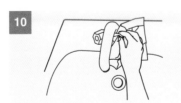

10 Use towel to turn off faucet;

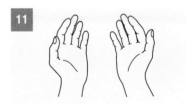

11 Your hands are now safe.

Figure 12.1.1 Hand hygiene (WHO 2009).

- Rub the back of your fingers to the opposing palm with fingers interlocked.
- Rub each thumb in turn, holding it in the opposite hand using a rotational movement.
- Rub the tips of your fingers in the opposite palm in a circular motion.
- Rub each wrist with the opposite hand.
- Rinse your hands with running water.

- Turn off taps – if you have long- handled taps, use your elbow, if not use a paper towel.
- Dry your hands thoroughly with a single-use paper towel.
- Dispose of the paper towel in the bin.

Points to note

- Any cuts, nicks or abrasions should be covered with a waterproof plaster.
- Liquid soap contained within a dispenser is the recommended standard. Bar soap must not be used as it can become contaminated. Bottles of liquid soap should not be replaced, topped up or re-used.
- Disposable paper hand towels are recommended for drying hands. Never use cotton towels that are shared.

Alcohol hand rubs

- They can only be used when no hand wash sinks are readily available with soap.
- They must not be used on hands that are physically dirty and not free of dirt and organic material.
- They must not be used during outbreaks of infection such as Norovirus or *Clostridium difficile* as they are not effective (see Chapters 13.2 and 13.4).
- Alcohol hand rub should not be used more than five consecutive occasions. Hands must be washed using soap and water after using the alcohol rub five times.
- Cleaning hands properly with an alcohol hand rub should take 15–30 seconds and the technique used is the same as for handwashing.

Hand hygiene and residents

- Encourage and assist residents to wash their hands before eating and drinking and after visiting the toilet or when hands are physically dirty.

Hand care

- Avoid perfumed soap and solutions that can cause skin problems. Aim for uncoloured and unperfumed soap. Any staff who consider there is a problem must report to their manager and seek advice on which solutions to use.
- Hand creams can be used but ensure they are not in a communal tub or jar.
- Do not use residents' bar soaps.

Hand hygiene and visitors

- Ensure visitors are made aware of hand hygiene techniques when using soap and alcohol-based hand rubs.
- Make information available on hand hygiene, such as a leaflet, or within information for visitors.

Further reading

Department of Health. 2006. Infection Control Guidance for Care Homes. Available at: www.dh.gov.uk [Accessed October 2013]

Department of Health. 2010. December 2010 The Health and Social Care Act 2008 Code of Practice for health and social care on the prevention and control of infctions and related guidance. Available at: www.dh.gov.uk [Accessed October 2013]

Health Protection Scotland. 2012. National Infection Prevention and Control Manual. January 2012. Available at: www.hps.scot.nhs.uk/haiic/index.aspx [Accessed October 2013].

Lawrence J, May D. 2003. *Infection Control in the Community*. London, Churchill, Livingstone.

Useful web site

www.who.int/search?q=hand [Accessed October 2013]

The World Health Organization had numerous guidelines and information. For example 'Five moments for Hand Hygiene'.

12.2 Personal protective equipment (PPE)

Jean Lawrence

Retired Infection Prevention and Control Nurse, (IPS) Yorkshire, UK

Key points

- PPE is an essential health and safety measure used to protect residents and staff and is a requirement of health and safety legislation.
- PPE is used when there is a risk that contamination will occur following handling and contact with blood and body fluids and contaminated equipment.

What is PPE?

- Disposable gloves.
- Disposable plastic aprons.
- Facial protection such as mask/eye protection.

When and how to use it

- Always ask yourself if gloves are appropriate for the individual care activity.
- Disposable plastic aprons and gloves are used once only then discarded. They must never be re-used for another activity.
- Contaminated gloves and aprons must be disposed of safely into the correct colour-coded waste bin.
- Glove selection must be in accordance with local policy.
- Gloves must be fit for purpose and well fitting to allow for dexterity.
- Do not wear jewellery under gloves.
- Ensure the correct colour-coded PPE is worn for the task.
- Never wash disposable gloves or use alcohol hand rub on them.
- Always wash hands after removal of disposable gloves.
- Facial protection should be available for use in any situation where a procedure or task will create splashing or aerosol into the face and eyes (such as coughing, sputum induction, chest physiotherapy, tracheotomy care). This protection can be a combined mask with visor, or a mask and goggles for the eyes. Goggles should cover all areas around the eyes including side protection.

Remove PPE in the following order

- Gloves.
- Apron.
- Facial protection.

Remember

- All staff must be trained in the use of PPE. See Table 12.2.1.
- Adequate supplies of PPE must always be available.

Table 12.2.1 Example of risk assessment for PPE.

Question	Answer	PPE Requirement
Will there be contact with blood or body fluid?	No	No protective clothing required
Will there be contact with blood and body fluids and a risk of splashing or aerosol of low volume?	Yes	Disposable plastic apron and gloves
Will there be contact with blood and body fluids and a risk of splashing and aerosol of high volume?	Yes	Disposable plastic apron, gloves and facial protection

The Care Home Handbook, First Edition. Edited by Graham Mulley, Clive Bowman, Michal Boyd and Sarah Stowe.
© 2015 John Wiley & Sons, Ltd. Published 2015 by John Wiley & Sons, Ltd.

Further reading

Department of Health. 2006. Infection Control Guidance for Care Homes. Available at: www.dh.gov.uk [Accessed October 2013]

Department of Health. 2007. Uniforms and Workwear: an Evidence Base for Developing Local Policy (January 2007). Available at: www.dh.gov.uk [Accessed October 2013]

Department of Health. 2010. December 2010. The Health and Social Care Act 2008 Code of Practice for health and social care on the prevention and control of infections and related guidance. Available at: www.dh.gov.uk [Accessed October 2013]

Pratt RJ, Pellowe CM, Wilson JA, et al. 2007. *epic2* National Evidence Based Guidelines for Preventing Healthcare-Associated Infections in NHS Hospitals in England. *Journal of Hospital Infection* 65, Supp 1: 1–64.

12.3 Management of blood and body fluid spillage

Jean Lawrence

Retired Infection Prevention and Control Nurse, (IPS) Yorkshire, UK

Key points

- All blood and body fluids may be a source of infection.
- Spillages must be handled safely and effectively to prevent transmission of infection and comply with health and safety legislation.

Blood and body fluid spills include:

- blood and blood-stained fluid
- wound drainage fluid
- vaginal secretions
- faeces
- urine
- vomit
- semen
- pleural fluid
- saliva
- pus from wounds
- sputum.

Procedure for cleaning blood spillage

- The use of a Spill Kit (which contains disposable gloves, apron, cleaning cloths, disinfectant, scoop for spill and a waste bag) is commonly used for blood spillage.
  - Note: these kits are in wide use – not only in acute care.
  - The recent DVD for care homes (NES Scotland) and infection control demonstrates their use.
  - The alternative is to make up the kit from supplies in the care home.
  - Spill kits are easier to purchase and easier and safer to use.
- Any chlorine agents (such as bleach derivatives) and hypochlorite cannot be used on carpets and soft furnishings.
- Blood spillage on carpet should be dealt with by mopping up the spillage immediately using water and detergent to clean.
- Shampooing the area with an industrial cleaner is recommended. Always refer to local policy.

For spillage on other floors and surfaces the following procedure is advised

- Follow instructions as given by the manufacturer of the spill kit.
- Put on gloves and apron.
- Cover the spill completely with the granules or solution.
- Follow manufacturers' instructions for the time to be left on the spill.
- Remove granules/solution along with soaked up spillage using a paper towel and scoop if provided and dispose of into the correct colour code waste bag.

The Care Home Handbook, First Edition. Edited by Graham Mulley, Clive Bowman, Michal Boyd and Sarah Stowe.
© 2015 John Wiley & Sons, Ltd. Published 2015 by John Wiley & Sons, Ltd.

- Wash the area using detergent and water.
- Remove protective clothing and dispose of it.
- Wash hands thoroughly.

Procedure for cleaning other body fluid spills

- Put on gloves and apron.
- Cover the spill with disposable paper towels to blot/soak up the spill.
- Gather the towels with the soaked spill and place in a yellow waste bag and place in the clinical waste bin.
- Wash the area using detergent and water followed by a solution of disinfectant. This will be available in a kit if used.
- Remove protective clothing and dispose of in the yellow waste bin.
- Wash your hands thoroughly.

General points

- Do not use chlorine solutions for urine spills as this can cause the release of chlorine gas.
- Spills on communal equipment should be treated in the same manner as floors and surfaces.
- Follow all advice regarding Control of Substances Hazardous to Health (COSHH) regulations when handling chemicals.

- When using the spillage kit for blood and body fluids, always ensure that the manufacturer's instructions for use are followed.
- Do not use alcohol solutions to clean spillage of blood and body fluids.

Further reading

Department of Health. 2006. Infection Control Guidance for Care Homes. Available at: www.dh.gov.uk [Accessed October 2013]

Department of Health. 2010. December 2010. The Health and Social Care Act 2008 Code of Practice for health and social care on the prevention and control of infections and related guidance. Available at: www.dh.gov.uk [Accessed October 2013]

HSE Books. 2002. Control of substances hazardous to health. The Control of Substances Hazardous to Health Regulations.

National Clinical Guideline Centre. 2012. Partial update of NICE Clinical Guideline 2. Infection: prevention and control of healthcare-associated infection in primary and community care. Clinical Guideline: Methods, evidence and recommendations. (New and updated evidence reviews and recommendations are shaded pink with 'Update 2012' in the right hand margin.)

NHS. 2012. HPS Model Infection Control Policies. Available at: http://www.hps.scot.nhs.uk/haiic/ic/modelinfection controlpolicies.aspx [Accessed October 2013]

12.4 Management of occupational exposure (including sharps)

Jean Lawrence

Retired Infection Prevention and Control Nurse, (IPS) Yorkshire, UK

Key points

You must be aware of good practice in relation to occupational exposure. This includes:

- Correct handling of all sharp items.
- Correct and safe sharps containers.
- Safe disposal of all sharp items.
- Correct procedure following any injury with a sharp item.

Accidental exposure to blood and body fluids can occur through:

- Incorrect handling and disposal of sharps.
- Splashes of blood and body fluid on broken skin.
- Splashes of blood and body fluids into eyes and mouth.
- Bites that cause the skin to break.

Sharps items

These include:

- needles
- stitch cutters
- disposable razors
- lancet devices for blood testing
- cannulae
- broken glass.

Sharps containers

- Sharps containers must conform to national standards.
- Assemble sharps containers following the manufacturer's instructions.
- Label them with the date brought into use, your signature and name.
- Place in a safe area out of reach; never place them on the floor or anywhere with unauthorised access.

Sharps use

- Never leave any sharp item lying around.
- Do not walk with sharps unguarded in your hands.
- Do not place needles or syringes in your pockets.
- Always request assistance when dealing with un-cooperative residents.
- Always take the sharps container to where you will be carrying out the procedure.
- *Never re-sheath, bend or break a needle.*

Sharps disposal

- Always supply a sharps container for a visiting health professional to use if required.
- Dispose of syringe and needle as a complete unit.
- Dispose of sharp item immediately following use and at the point of use.
- Dispose of only in the sharps container; *not in clinical waste bags.*

The Care Home Handbook, First Edition. Edited by Graham Mulley, Clive Bowman, Michal Boyd and Sarah Stowe.
© 2015 John Wiley & Sons, Ltd. Published 2015 by John Wiley & Sons, Ltd.

- The sharps container needs to be closed when it is three-quarters full and should not be overfilled. A line marking is indicated on the container.
- Do not press down sharps to 'make more room'.
- Never retrieve any item from a sharps container.

Sharps container closure and disposal

- Seal the container as directed in the manufacturer's instructions, before removal from the clinical area, when three-quarters full.
- Always carry sharps disposal containers with the handles provided and hold it away from you.
- Label it with the point of origin and date sealed, then follow local waste management policy.
- Place damaged used sharps containers into a larger secure container and properly label the outer container.
- Do not allow sharps containers to accumulate. Convey to a secure storage area while awaiting final disposal.
- Do not place used sharps containers into plastic waste bags.

Sharps container spillage/sharp items spill/stray sharps

- Seek help to guard the area while dealing with the spillage.
- Collect together a new correctly assembled sharps disposal container, personal protective equipment and items to disinfect the area after removal of the spillage.
- Wear disposable gloves, or preferably gauntlets if available, apron and eye protection or other personal protective equipment as appropriate.
- Employ a 'non-touch technique' using, for example, a pair of tongs or a plastic dustpan and brush (*which is used for this purpose alone*), and carefully collect spilled items and transfer to them to the new sharps container. Do not rush this procedure.
- Seal the sharps container.
- Clean the contaminated area as per the technique for spillage.
- Discard disposable protective clothing/equipment as clinical waste and wash hands thoroughly.
- Complete an incident/accident form report as directed in the local policy.

Accidental inoculation injuries

Exposure to blood and body fluids can occur from a sharps injury, bites, splashing onto skin abrasions and into the eyes or mouth.

It is important that all staff know that in the unlikely event that the resident who was involved during the needle stick or similar injury is HIV-positive, the member of staff should receive medical attention within one hour for consideration of post-exposure prophylaxis.

The immediate use of hepatitis B vaccine (with or without anti-hep B immune globulin) should also be considered because of the risk of this blood-borne viral infection.

Procedure following injury

Always follow local policy when an injury occurs. The issue that concerns most people who sustain inoculation injury is the danger of blood-borne infection. Injury may also lead to physical trauma (puncture wounds, lacerations etc.) and the risk of other infections (such as tetanus) from inoculation by dirty sharps.

- *Bleed t*he wound by encouraging it to bleed by gentle squeezing. DO NOT suck the area.
- *Wash* the area thoroughly with detergent and warm running water. Do not scrub the area.
- *Irrigate* eye or mouth splashes thoroughly with water. Treat mucosal surfaces, such as mouth or conjunctiva, by rinsing with warm water or saline. Water used for rinsing the mouth must not be swallowed.
- *Report* it to your manager and *seek medical advice immediately.*

Bites

If the skin has been broken by a bite, treat it as advised above (under inoculation).

Further reading

Department of Health. 2006. Infection Control Guidance for Care Homes. Available at: www.dh.gov.uk [Accessed October 2013]
Department of Health. 2007. Hepatitis B infected healthcare workers and antiviral therapy. Available from: www.dh.gov.uk [Accessed October 2013]

Department of Health. 2010. December 2010 The Health and Social Care Act 2008 Code of Practice for health and social care on the prevention and control of infections and related guidance. Available at www.dh.gov.uk [Accessed October 2013]

Health Protection Agency. 2008. Examples of good and bad practice to avoid sharps injuries. Available from: http://www.hpa.org.uk/Topics/InfectiousDiseases/ InfectionsAZ/BloodborneVirusesAndOccupational Exposure/ [Accessed October 2013]

Health and Safety Executive. 2001. Blood-borne viruses in the workplace: guidance for employers and employees – INDG342. London: HSE. Available from: www.hse.gov. uk/pubns/indg342.pdf [Accessed October 2013]

12.5 Management of care equipment

Jean Lawrence

Retired Infection Prevention and Control Nurse, (IPS) Yorkshire, UK

Key points

- Care of equipment is essential to ensure that the risks from infection are minimised.
- It is important that all staff are aware of the system that is in place and how the equipment is cleaned and by whom.
- The use of a policy that lists all the care equipment items in use is recommended.
- At all times ensure adherence to the Health and Safety regulations (in the UK this is through Care Of Substances Hazardous to Health (COSHH).
- Do not clean or re-use equipment that is termed a 'single-use item'. This is written on the outside of the pack and indicated by a 2 inside a circle with a diagonal line (Figure 12.5.1).

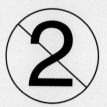

Figure 12.5.1 Single-use item symbol.

What is decontamination?

Decontamination is a term used to collectively describe the process of cleaning, disinfection and sterilisation (Table 12.5.1).

Disinfectant use

- This is a widely-used process to make items free from risk of infection and safe to handle.
- Where disinfectants are used, it is essential that the instructions for use from the manufacturer are followed correctly.
- Disinfectants *must not* be purchased from retail outlets by staff and brought in for use. (They may not be the correct type and dilution for recommended use.)
- Cleaning with detergent physically removes microorganisms and the organic material on which they survive. It is essential to clean with detergent before then using a disinfectant.

Example of equipment cleaning

1. Blood contamination.
   - Check manufacturers' instructions for suitability of cleaning products – especially when dealing with electronic equipment.
   - Decontaminate immediately, using disposable cloths and fresh detergent solution.
   - Wash, rinse and dry then follow with a solution of available chlorine (10,000 parts per million (ppm)) and rinse and dry again.
   - Some disinfectant solutions come ready prepared with 10,000 ppm combined with the detergent, and manufacturers' instructions must be followed for its use.

The Care Home Handbook, First Edition. Edited by Graham Mulley, Clive Bowman, Michal Boyd and Sarah Stowe.
© 2015 John Wiley & Sons, Ltd. Published 2015 by John Wiley & Sons, Ltd.

Table 12.5.1 Decontamination.

Cleaning	A process to physically remove microorganisms and the organic material on which they thrive. It is essential that this is carried out before any disinfection or sterilisation process. Cleaning can also remove any chemical residues, soil and dust, which can jeopardise the safe performance of the device.
Disinfection	A process which reduces the number of viable microorganisms but may not inactivate some bacterial spores. Disinfection is normally used for instruments, equipment and surfaces which are not intentionally invasive but are in contact with mucous membranes, blood, body fluids and other potentially infectious material.
Sterilisation	A process which removes or destroys all living micro-organisms, including bacterial spores. Recommended for items which penetrate intact skin, mucous membranes or enter body cavities.

Source: data from J. Babb in Lawrence & May (2003).

- Store equipment once dry in the correct storage area.
2. Urine, faeces or vomit contamination (also used on people with known or suspected infection).
    - Decontaminate equipment with disposable cloths/paper towel and a fresh solution of general purpose detergent and water or detergent-impregnated wipes.
    - Follow instructions from manufacturer for any dilutions and for contact time.
    - Using disposable cloths, clean using a fresh solution of detergent, rinse, dry then follow with a disinfectant solution of 1,000 ppm available chlorine, rinse and dry thoroughly.
    - Store cloths once dry in the correct storage area.

Reference

Lawrence J, May D. 2003. *Infection Control in the Community*. London, Churchill Livingstone.

Further reading

Department of Health. 2004. Standards for Better Health. Available at:http://www.dh.gov.uk [Accessed October 2013]

Department of Health. 2006. Infection Control Guidance for Care Homes. Available at: www.dh.gov.uk [Accessed October 2013]

Department of Health. 2010. The Health and Social Care Act 2008 Code of Practice for health and social care on the prevention and control of infections and related guidance. Available at: www.dh.gov.uk [Accessed October 2013]

HSE Books. 2002. Control of substances hazardous to health. The Control of Substances Hazardous to Health Regulations.

MHRA. Managing Medical Devices: Guidance for healthcare and social services organisations DB2006 (05) November 2006 and MDA DB2000 (04) Single Use Medical Devices. Available at: www.mhra.gov.uk [Accessed October 2013]

12.6 Management of the environment

Jean Lawrence

Retired Infection Prevention and Control Nurse, (IPS) Yorkshire, UK

Key points

- Cleaning of the environment is essential to ensure that the risks from infection are minimised.
- All staff must be aware of the system that is in place and how the schedules are carried out, and by whom, and follow local policy.
- Where residents clean their own rooms, this can be included in the care plan and advice given.
- During and after any outbreak of infection, or when a resident has had a particular infection, local policy must be followed.

Key points for cleaning

- Protective gloves should be worn for cleaning tasks. These should be sturdy, suitable for purpose and comply with the colour-coding system. Where the task involves the use of chemicals, the gloves should be certified as suitable for chemical resistance and in line with health and safety policy and/or local glove policy.
- Disposable, colour-coded plastic aprons should be worn.
- Sleeves on uniforms and personal clothing should either end above the elbow, or should be kept rolled up above the elbow when undertaking cleaning duties.
- Knowledge by all staff of cleaning procedures for the environment is important.
- Clear guidance must be available for the various cleaning tasks and areas and who is responsible for which tasks and areas concerned.

Colour coding

It is recommended that different areas have different equipment and that this is colour coded for ease of identification. This also prevents items being used in multiple areas, thus reducing the risk of infection.

Cleaning equipment

- All equipment in use should be fit for purpose, well maintained, clean and dry and stored correctly.
- Equipment cleanliness includes being visibly clean with no blood or body fluid substances, dust, dirt, debris or moisture present.
- Ideally a cleaning/storage area should be made available with a deep sink with hot and cold running water and storage shelving for equipment and chemicals. The store should be clean at all times.

Disinfectant use

- Cleaning with detergent physically removes microorganisms and the organic material on which they survive. It is therefore essential to clean with detergent before the use of a disinfectant.
- Instructions for use from the manufacturer must be followed.
- Disinfectants must not be purchased from retail outlets by staff and brought in for use.
- Refer to the local cleaning policy.

The Care Home Handbook, First Edition. Edited by Graham Mulley, Clive Bowman, Michal Boyd and Sarah Stowe.
© 2015 John Wiley & Sons, Ltd. Published 2015 by John Wiley & Sons, Ltd.

Control of Substances Hazardous to Health (COSHH)

All products in use for cleaning and disinfectants must be secure in a locked cupboard, store room or lockable cleaning trolley.

Cleaning frequencies

Follow local guidance and policy.

Cleaning with steam

This is a specialist cleaning method and can take place following gross spillage of blood and body fluids on a carpet or other area when extra cleaning is required. A risk assessment should be in place at the local level to determine its use.

- Deep cleaning involves the use of steam. It should be a planned system, for example carried out annually.
- Deep cleaning can help to emphasise the importance of cleanliness and reassure everyone of the care home's serious commitment to hygiene.

- It will require buying in a contractor to carry out the work.
- For further details see NPSA (2009).

Reference

National Patient Safety Agency (NPSA). 2009. *The Revised Healthcare Cleaning Manual*. National Reporting and Learning Service.

Further reading

Care Commission, Scotland. 2005. A Review of Cleanliness, Hygiene and Infection Control in Care Homes for Older People.

Department of Health. 2010. The Health and Social Care Act 2008 Code of Practice for health and social care on the prevention and control of infections and related guidance. Available at: www.dh.gov.uk [Accessed October 2013]

National Patient Safety Agency (NPSA) 2007. Safer Practice Notice: Colour coding hospital cleaning materials and equipment. January 2007 NPSA/2007/15.

National Patient Safety Agency (NPSA). 2010. The National Specifications for Cleanliness: Guidance on setting and measuring performance outcomes in care homes. August 2010.

12.7 Management of linen and laundry

Jean Lawrence

Retired Infection Prevention and Control Nurse, (IPS) Yorkshire, UK

Key points

- Used linen can harbour large numbers of microorganisms and these can be transferred through contact.
- Ideally the care home should establish designated 'clean' and 'dirty' areas in the laundry.
- Hand sluicing must not be carried out because of the high risk of spreading bacteria and viruses as aerosols and the subsequent risk of inhalation by both staff and residents, resulting in infection. Excess faecal matter should be removed using paper towels before putting clothing in a red laundry bag.
- Ensure that all laundry is washed effectively, that is never over-fill machines or contaminate clean linen.
- Staff must be trained in all aspects of laundering.
- Disposable aprons and gloves must be worn when dealing with used/fouled laundry.
- Skin lesions must be covered with a waterproof dressing.
- Hand-washing facilities should be available in the laundry room.
- Protective clothing should be removed and hands washed before returning to other duties.
- Eating and drinking must not to take place in the laundry room.

Handling and processing

- A colour-coded system is recommended for different types of soiled linen (see Table 12.7.1).
- Linen should be removed from a resident's bed with care, avoiding the creation of dust, and placed in the appropriate bag.
- Linen should never be sorted in the residential area.
- Aprons and gloves should be worn when removing linen from a bed for laundering.
- Hands should always be washed after handling linen.
- Red water-soluble bags should be used for all potentially contaminated linen.

Contracted laundry

If laundry is contracted out at the home, then colour-coded bagging should be undertaken in agreement with the contractor. This agreement must specify the colour coding for infected linen.

Storage of linen

Clean linen should be kept away from linen waiting processing. Once dried, linen should be kept in a dry area above the floor.

The Care Home Handbook, First Edition. Edited by Graham Mulley, Clive Bowman, Michal Boyd and Sarah Stowe.
© 2015 John Wiley & Sons, Ltd. Published 2015 by John Wiley & Sons, Ltd.

Table 12.7.1 Categories of linen (colour codes as directed by local policy).

Type of Linen	Colour Code	Suggested Recommended Practice
Used linen not fouled Fouled but not thought to be infectious/includes MRSA residents, unless visibly stained with body fluids		Follow all instructions for washing at 40°C. transfer to the laundry room in a secondary leak-proof bag place laundry in the machine using leak-proof gloves wash separately or with other non-infectious soiled laundry use a pre-wash first wash as directed in manufacturer's instructions wherever possible temperatures should reach thermal disinfection, i.e. 65°C for 10 minutes or 71°C for three minutes on removal from the machine, if still soiled, repeat process from beginning tumble dry the laundry as directed in manufacturer's instructions and then iron
Linen thought to be contaminated with gastro-intestinal pathogens, e.g. *Clostridium difficile* or blood borne viruses	Inner alginate plastic and outer linen/nylon bag	place in an alginate (water-soluble) membrane or bag place in an additional red bag unless thermal disinfection temperatures are attainable in the in-house machine, arrange for transfer to contracted agent for heat disinfecting the contractor must be informed of the possibility of infection
Personal and other heat labile laundry		Please refer to local policy
Heavily blood-soaked linen from residents with blood borne virus infection and/or CJD		Heavily blood-soaked linen from residents with Hepatitis B virus, HIV or Creutzfeldt Jacob Disease (CJD) should be placed in clinical waste bags for incineration

Further reading

Department of Health. 2010. The Health and Social Care Act 2008 Code of Practice for health and social care on the prevention and control of infections and related guidance. Available at: www.dh.gov.uk [Accessed October 2013]

NHS Executive. 1995. Hospital Laundry Arrangements for Used and Infected Linen HSG (95)18. London, HMSO.

12.8 Management of waste

Jean Lawrence

Retired Infection Prevention and Control Nurse, (IPS) Yorkshire, UK

Key points

- A waste system is essential to ensure that legislation and health and safety are being adhered to, and a local policy for the management of waste must be available to ensure that the collection, handling, disposal and transportation is safe and effective.
- A colour-coded system should be in operation in line with local and national policies.
- All waste bags must comply with the approved type.
- All staff should have been trained on the system in use and the regulations that apply.
- Clinical and hazardous waste is to be put in bins with foot pedals and lids.
- Dispose of waste should be as close as possible to the point of use.
- Waste bags should be no more than three-quarters full when ready for disposal.
- Use a ratchet type tie for closure.
- Use personal protective equipment (disposable gloves and disposable aprons).
- Hand hygiene after dealing with all waste is vital.

Categories and content

Check local and national policies and guidance that outlines the detail and legislative requirements.

- *Domestic* refers to black waste bags containing items such as newspapers and paper towels.
- *Clinical waste* refers to specifically coloured bags (usually orange) containing used dressings and personal protective equipment such as disposable gloves/aprons.
- *Hazardous waste* refers to often yellow (but may be a different colour in different locations) waste bags containing high risk/highly infectious material, such as infected human body parts.
- *Offensive hygiene* refers to waste items that were previously termed 'sanpro' and now are called Human Hygiene. In the UK, waste bags that are yellow with black stripes can be used. However, this may be different in other locations.

Collection and transportation

- Ensure a process is in place for the contractors to remove waste from the premises; this should include 'Consignment Notes' which require signatures.
- Provision of an area outside the premises to hold the waste awaiting collection securely.
- Collection times should be regular to ensure no waste accumulates or causes any hazard.

Further reading

Department of Health. 2010. The Health and Social Care Act 2008 Code of Practice for health and social care on the prevention and control of infections and related guidance. Available at: www.dh.gov.uk [Accessed October 2013]

The Care Home Handbook, First Edition. Edited by Graham Mulley, Clive Bowman, Michal Boyd and Sarah Stowe.
© 2015 John Wiley & Sons, Ltd. Published 2015 by John Wiley & Sons, Ltd.

12.9 Respiratory hygiene

Jean Lawrence

Retired Infection Prevention and Control Nurse, (IPS) Yorkshire, UK

Key points

- Colds and influenza can spread rapidly.
- Reducing the risk of respiratory infections is essential and the use of a coughing/sneezing etiquette must be followed.

General guidance

- Sneezing and coughing must be done into disposable tissues and they must be placed in the correct waste bin. Try to encourage sneezing and coughing into the lower arm area and not the hand. This is to try and reduce the number of microbes that are present on the hands after coughing into them.
- Hand washing must always be performed after coughing or sneezing into the arm or hand and after handling used tissues, as they contain secretions that can be transferred to others.
- Influenza immunisation is essential for all people of 65 years and over. Each year the Chief Medical Officers in each country informs on the requirements and any changes to the immunisation programme.
- *Staff are also recommended to have the influenza vaccine from their own GP for the protection of themselves, family and residents* (see Chapter 13.1).

Further reading

Health Protection Agency (HPA). 2008. Managing outbreaks of respiratory illness in care homes. Available at: http://www.hpa.org.uk/webc/HPAwebFile/HPAweb_C/1231490146703 [Accessed October 2013]

Health Protection Agency (HPA). 2010. Investigating acute respiratory infection in community settings: Principles for investigation of outbreak clusters in care homes. November 2010. Available at: http://www.hpa.org.uk/webc/HPAwebFile/HPAweb_C/1317136714703 [Accessed October 2013]

NHS Health protection Scotland (HPS). 2010. General information and infection control precautions to minimize transmission of Respiratory Tract Infection (RTI's) in the healthcare setting. December 2010 Version 2.0.

The Care Home Handbook, First Edition. Edited by Graham Mulley, Clive Bowman, Michal Boyd and Sarah Stowe.
© 2015 John Wiley & Sons, Ltd. Published 2015 by John Wiley & Sons, Ltd.

12.10 Providing care in the most appropriate place

Jean Lawrence

Retired Infection Prevention and Control Nurse, (IPS) Yorkshire, UK

Key points

- Sometimes it is necessary to segregate residents to prevent the spread of infection to others. This is part of breaking the chain of infection, by isolating the organism but not the resident.
- Standard infection prevention and control precautions are to be applied at all times.
- Staff should have instruction/education on the principles of resident place of care and standard precautions.
- Adequate resources must be in place to allow infection control measures to be implemented, for example personal protective equipment (see Chapter 12.2).
- Consult and obtain advice from infection control experts.
- Support staff in any corrective action or interventions if an incident occurs that may have resulted in cross-contamination.
- Staff with health concerns, or who become ill due to occupational exposure, are to be referred to the relevant agency, for example general practitioner or occupational health.
- Ensure effective communication at all times in the interest of resident safety and well-being.
- Ensure that evidence-based policies and procedures are in place.

Room

When a resident is isolated (see Table 12.10.1) in a room, the room must have its own toilet facilities and hand-washing sink. A nearby toilet can be allocated for the sole use of a resident if the room is not en-suite.

Table **12.10.1** Infections that might require isolating

Infection	Type	Virus/Bacteria
Influenza	Respiratory	Virus
Clostridium difficile	Diarrhoea/ gastrointestinal	Bacteria
Norovirus	Vomiting/ Diarrhoea/ Gastrointestinal	Virus
Shingles/ Chickenpox	Skin lesions	Virus

General information

When staff observe a resident with vomiting/diarrhoea or feeling unwell with a temperature, or signs and symptoms of delirium (see Chapter 10.2) that do not normally occur in that resident or residents, they must always report this to allow advice to be sought from the medical practitioner.

Reporting is essential as infections can spread rapidly.

Further advice on segregation and isolating residents should be sought from the health protection team and/or the infection prevention and control practitioner/nurse.

Placing a resident in a room and asking them to stay there may not always be easy. Being alone in a room can cause feelings of anxiety, depression and being 'shut in'. Frequent visits and explanations must continually take place to reassure the resident about the length of time needed in isolation. Careful

The Care Home Handbook, First Edition. Edited by Graham Mulley, Clive Bowman, Michal Boyd and Sarah Stowe.
© 2015 John Wiley & Sons, Ltd. Published 2015 by John Wiley & Sons, Ltd.

explanation and reassurance is also necessary to the residents' family, visitors and other carers on the reasons for the change in care.

Always advise on the need for good hand hygiene practices (see Chapter 12.1).

Further reading

Department of Health. 2006. Infection Control Guidance for Care Homes. Available at: www.dh.gov.uk [Accessed October 2013]

Department of Health. 2010. The Health and Social Care Act 2008 Code of Practice for health and social care on the prevention and control of infections and related guidance. Available at: www.dh.gov.uk [Accessed October 2013]

NHS Health Protection Scotland (HPS). 2009. Place of Care-Patient Placement Policy and Procedure. (Element of Standard Infection Control Precautions) February 2009. Updated Jan 2012. Available at: http://www.hps.scot.nhs.uk/haiic/ic/modelinfectioncontrolpolicies.aspx [Accessed October 2013]

NHS Health Protection Scotland (HPS). 2012. National Infection Prevention and Control Manual. January 2012. Available at: www.hps.scot.nhs.uk/haiic/index.aspx [Accessed October 2013]

12.11 Aseptic technique

Jean Lawrence

Retired Infection Prevention and Control Nurse, (IPS) Yorkshire, UK

Key points

- Aseptic technique is used to minimise the risk of introducing pathogenic organisms into a wound, or other susceptible sites, that could cause infection.
- It is used commonly for wound dressings, urinary catheterisation and related procedures, insertion of intra-venous cannulae, suturing and removal of sutures.
- It is important to follow local policy and procedure.
- Ensure that all equipment and fluids to be used are sterile.

Procedure principles

- All fluids and material must be sterile.
- Only sterile items should come into contact with the susceptible site.
- Use a clear surface/field from which to work.
- Ensure that no contaminated item is placed on the sterile field.
- Protect uniform or clothing with a disposable plastic apron.
- Use sterile gloves for manipulation of equipment and procedure.
- Single use equipment must not be re-used.
- Disposal of all waste must follow the local waste policy.
- Hand hygiene is necessary before the procedure and during the procedure, if the sterile field is broken and also on the removal of gloves.

Equipment

- A sterile dressing pack, containing items such as swabs, sterile field, disposable bag, gloves. Items may be supplied separately.
- Fluids for cleaning and/or irrigation.
- Other sterile items/equipment as required.
- Alcohol-based hand rub.
- A disposable plastic apron.
- A trolley/tray/surface in room for use as a working field.

Clean technique

This is a modified technique where the principles of asepsis are maintained. An example of this is the use of clean disposable gloves and a clean field from which to work. Examples of using clean technique can include chronic leg ulcers, minor wound grazes or vaginal examination. A non-touch technique is used and only the gloved hand or forceps are used when manipulating the procedure site. Hand hygiene must be carried out before and after the procedure is completed (see Chapter 12.1).

All waste is to be disposed of as directed in the local policy guidelines.

Further reading

Department of Health. 2006. Essential steps to safe, clean care. Available at: www.dh.gov.uk [Accessed October 2013]

Department of Health. 2010. The Health and Social Care Act 2008 Code of Practice for health and social care on the prevention and control of infections and related guidance. Appendix A Criterion 9b. Available at: www.dh.gov.uk [Accessed October 2013]

Pratt RJ, Pellowe CM, Wilson JA, et al. 2007. *epic2* national evidence based guidelines for preventing healthcare-associated infections in NHS hospitals in England. *Journal of Hospital Infection* 65, Supp 1: 1–64.

Preston RM. 2006. Aseptic technique: evidence-based approach for patient safety. *British Journal of Nursing* 14(10): 540–546.

The Care Home Handbook, First Edition. Edited by Graham Mulley, Clive Bowman, Michal Boyd and Sarah Stowe.
© 2015 John Wiley & Sons, Ltd. Published 2015 by John Wiley & Sons, Ltd.

Chapter 13

Managing Specific Infections

13.1 Influenza

Jean Lawrence

Retired Infection Prevention and Control Nurse, (IPS) Yorkshire, UK

Key points

- Always monitor residents with a temperature of 37.8 °C or above, or who experience a decline in physical ability.
- Report concerns of any flu-like symptoms as soon as possible to prevent rapid spread.
- Follow local guidance and policy for managing influenza.
- Protect yourself and others by having the influenza vaccine every year.

What is influenza?

Influenza is a respiratory illness that has a wide range of symptoms:

- A rapid onset of illness, fever, cough, headache, sore throat, and aching muscles and joints.
- It can spread rapidly from person to person when in close contact via the respiratory route or when talking, coughing and sneezing near someone who is infected.
- The acute symptoms can last up to a week but full recovery can take longer than this. If hands become contaminated, it can spread via the hand- to-face route.

Other facts of note include:

- It peaks between December and March in the northern hemisphere and June to August in the southern hemisphere.
- There are two main types that cause infection: influenza A and influenza B. Influenza A usually causes a more severe illness than influenza B.
- Common complications of influenza are bronchitis and secondary bacterial pneumonia.

These illnesses may require treatment in hospital and can be life threatening especially in elderly subjects, those with asthma and those in poor health.

Risk groups include:

- Those with immuno-suppression through disease (e.g. diabetes) or drug treatment (e.g. chemotherapy).
- People aged 65 years and older.

Clinical symptoms

- Fever of 37.8° C or above (oral temperature) (see Chapter 15.4).
- A sudden decline in physical or mental ability can be observed.

The following can be new or a worsening of existing symptoms:

- cough (with or without sputum)
- runny nose or congestion
- sore throat
- sneezing
- hoarseness
- shortness of breath
- wheezing
- chest pain.

Prevention and control

- Give careful consideration to the risks to admissions and transfers to individuals and the home during outbreaks of influenza.
- If admission to hospital is required in a clinical emergency, always advise the receiving ward/unit of the problem.
- Consider limiting the use of communal areas within the home to control infection.
- Avoid use of the communal areas by those affected.
- Plan staff to work in two teams to allow one team to care for those not affected and one for those who are ill.

The Care Home Handbook, First Edition. Edited by Graham Mulley, Clive Bowman, Michal Boyd and Sarah Stowe.
© 2015 John Wiley & Sons, Ltd. Published 2015 by John Wiley & Sons, Ltd.

- Staff especially agency staff should be advised not to work at other institutions during an outbreak.
- Advise elderly people and the very young not to visit the care home.
- Ensure supplies of tissues are available and pedal-operated bins for their disposal.
- Provide sputum containers with lids.
- Arrange for cleaning of the equipment and the environment, such as twice daily damp dusting of surfaces and frequently handled equipment.
- Use disposable aprons and disposable gloves for all procedures.
- Seek advice from health protection team regarding the use of facial protection (masks).
- Handwashing with soap and water after all contact with the affected person and after equipment handling, cleaning and removal of gloves (see Chapter 12.1).
- Alcohol hand rub can be used and placed in accessible areas for all.

Influenza vaccination

Residents

The aim of a vaccine is to produce a specific immune response against a particular microorganism without causing the actual disease.

Influenza vaccines are administered each year as new strains are evolving constantly. To allow time for vaccine manufacture, the decision about which strains to include is made about six months in advance of the start of the influenza season. This is done by the World Health Organization (WHO). The recommendations are based on the strains circulating at the time, as reported by countries across the globe.

Residents in long-stay care should receive a vaccine annually. The final decision as to who should be offered immunisation is a matter for the person's medical practitioner. This will be dependent on the general health and condition of the resident and the presence of any allergies (e.g. egg allergy – see Chapter 11.5). A programme for annual vaccination should be in place.

Immunisation and eligibility are regularly reviewed by the health departments for the countries involved and this is usually through annual information from the Chief Medical Officers.

Staff

Health and social care professionals have a duty and ethical responsibility to protect themselves by having the flu vaccine. Staff are caring for residents who are elderly and infirm: thus they are a vulnerable group who are at greater risk of acquiring influenza and its complications as a result of exposure to residents with the disease.

Vaccination for staff is highly recommended.

Delivery of the vaccine should be decided at the local level in collaboration with general practitioners and health protection staff.

Further reading

Department of Health. 2006. Immunisation against infectious disease. Available at: www.dh.gov.uk [Accessed October 2013]

Department of Health. 2012. The Flu Immunisation Programme 2012/13. Gateway reference number 17488. Available at: www.dh.gov.uk [Accessed October 2013]

The Scottish Government. 2012. Seasonal Influenza Vaccine Programme. SGHD/CMO (2012) 6. Available at: http://www.sehd.scot.nhs.uk/cmo/CMO(2012)06.pdf [Accessed October 2013]

The Scottish Government. 2012. Winter Flu: Vaccination of Healthcare Workers. Available at: http://www.sehd.scot.nhs.uk/mels/CEL2012_24.pdf [Accessed October 2013]

Wendelboe AM, Avery C, Andrade B, Baumbach J, Landen MG. 2011. Importance of employee vaccination against influenza preventing cases in long term care facilities. *Infection Control and Hospital Epidemiology*: DO1: 10.1086/661916.

13.2 Norovirus

Jean Lawrence

Retired Infection Prevention and Control Nurse, (IPS) Yorkshire, UK

Key points

- Norovirus is the most common cause of viral gastroenteritis.
- Typical symptoms are nausea, vomiting, diarrhoea, fever and aches and pains.
- Residents suspected of having this condition should be nursed in their room and stay there until they have been free from symptoms for 48 hours.
- Use soap and water for hand washing – alcohol rub is not effective in this condition.
- Standard infection prevention and control precautions apply at all times when dealing with norovirus.
- Inform the health protection team and the GP.
- Infected staff should stay away from work until they have been symptom-free for 48 hours.

What is it?

- Also known as 'Winter Vomiting Disease', norovirus is the most common cause of viral gastroenteritis. It used to be called 'Norwalk' virus, after the American town where it was first discovered.
- Outbreaks are common in semi-closed environments such as hospitals, care homes, schools and cruise ships.
- Spread occurs through contact with an infected person, consuming contaminated food or water and contact with contaminated surfaces or objects.
- It can survive on surfaces for at least a week.

Clinical symptoms

- Lasts from 12 to 60 hours
- Nausea
- Projectile vomiting (typically sudden onset)
- Watery diarrhoea
- Headaches
- Aching limbs, stomach cramps
- Raised temperature.

Prevention and control

- Inform the local health protection team and general practitioner of a suspected outbreak.
- Care for residents with symptoms in a room on their own where possible, where they should remain until they have been symptom free for 48 hours.
- Arrange for faecal specimens as soon as possible and send them to the laboratory.
- Closure of the care home to activities during the course of the outbreak is recommended – but always seek advice from the health protection team.
- Apply standard infection prevention and control precautions at all times and ensure hands are washed with soap and water. *Do not use alcohol hand rub as this is ineffective in this condition.*
- Cleaning to take place regularly and normal cleaning to be followed by the use of a chlorine-based disinfectant.

Staff illness

- Any members of staff with symptoms must be excluded from the care home and free of symptoms for 48 hours before returning to work.

The Care Home Handbook, First Edition. Edited by Graham Mulley, Clive Bowman, Michal Boyd and Sarah Stowe.
© 2015 John Wiley & Sons, Ltd. Published 2015 by John Wiley & Sons, Ltd.

Actions following the outbreak

- A thorough cleaning procedure is recommended throughout the care home. Seek advice from the health protection team or local public health authority/
- Continue to observe the residents for any symptoms as described, as re-infection can occur.

Further reading

Care Commission. 2005. Scottish commission for the regulation of care. Revised Health Guidance: The Use of the Infection Control in Adult Care Homes: Final Standards 2005. Revised 2008.

Department of Health. 2006. Infection Control Guidance for Care Homes. Available at: www.dh.gov.uk [Accessed October 2013]

Health Protection Agency. 2010. (South West London Health Protection Unit) Guidelines on Prevention and Management of Probable/Confirmed Viral Outbreaks of Diarrhoea and Vomiting in Care Homes, Schools, Nurseries and other Childcare Settings. Available at: http://www.hpa.org.uk/Topics/InfectiousDiseases/InfectionsAZ/Norovirus/GeneralInformation/ [Accessed October 2013]

NHS Scotland. Health Protection Scotland (HPS). 2009. Norovirus Outbreak: Control measures and practical considerations for optimal patient safety and service continuation in hospitals. December 2009

Norovirus Working Party. 2012. Guidelines for the management of norovirus outbreaks in acute and community health and social care settings. Available at: http://www.ips.uk.net [Accessed October 2013]

13.3 Scabies

Jean Lawrence

Retired Infection Prevention and Control Nurse, (IPS) Yorkshire, UK

Key points

- Scabies is a condition caused by mites.
- It causes intense itching and a rash.
- The ointment prescribed by the GP should be applied to cool dry, unbroken skin, preferably in the evening.
- If two or more residents are affected, then all those who are in contact with the residents must also be treated.
- A rare but severe form of the disease is called Norwegian (or hyperkeratotoic) scabies. This requires urgent medical attention and specific therapy.

Scabies is a clinical condition caused by infestation of the skin by mites. The main symptoms of the disease are caused by an allergic reaction to the presence of mites and their products under the skin. This subsequently causes an intense itching in particular areas of the body. Once the mites burrow, it takes up to 4 to 6 weeks before the itching starts.

Clinical symptoms of classical scabies

- Intense itching particularly at night.
- Rash: particularly the back, wrists, between the fingers, belt lines (Figure 13.3.1).

Transmission

- Prolonged skin to skin contact, for example sleeping together, holding hands, sexual contact.
- Through prolonged contact and general care, by nurses and carers.

Treatment for individuals

- Diagnosis and prescribing of treatment through the general practitioner.

- Follow manufacturer's instruction for application of the cream or lotion.
- Application of the cream or lotion is best applied in the evening before retiring to bed.
- Do not apply any cream or lotion to broken or infected areas of skin.
- Cream or lotion must be applied to cool dry skin to be most effective. *It is not recommended to have a hot shower or bath before any application.*
- All body areas from the neck down (the head, neck and ears are usually *treated in children) – including the palms of the hands and soles of the* feet – must have the cream/lotion applied.
- Cream/lotion must be re-applied to any parts of the body that have been washed (e.g. hands).
- Mites can be harboured under the nails, therefore ensure that nails are cut and groomed.
- After the treatment (8 to 12 hours) do not put the same clothes back on the resident. They may shower or bath as normal.
- Clothes and linen can be washed in the normal manner.
- All close family contacts to be treated whether a rash is present or not. It is important to have a medical assessment before others are given treatment.
- A second treatment may be required following assessment after seven days.
- The general practitioner can prescribe treatment for any itching.

The Care Home Handbook, First Edition. Edited by Graham Mulley, Clive Bowman, Michal Boyd and Sarah Stowe.
© 2015 John Wiley & Sons, Ltd. Published 2015 by John Wiley & Sons, Ltd.

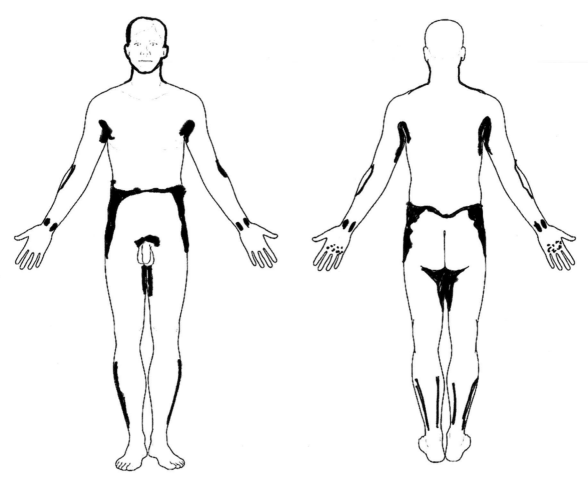

Figure 13.3.1 Scabies: distribution of the symmetrical rash. This does not correspond with the sites of predilection of the mites. Adapted from Lawrence & May (2003) with permission from Elsevier.

Hyperkeratotic scabies (Norwegian or crusted and atypical scabies)

- This is an unusual form of scabies that is highly infectious and is particularly seen in elderly people – especially those who are frail.
- Appears like a general dermatitis and is widely distributed, causing thickening of the skin with scales and crusting.
- Large numbers of mites are present and the scaling makes it highly contagious.

Treatment of hyperkeratotic scabies

- Two or three applications of treatment may be required daily to allow good penetration to kill the mites.
- If there is no response to treatment, an oral medication called Ivermectin can be prescribed (named person only) and used in combination with the topical treatments.

Treatment for outbreaks

When an outbreak is confirmed (two or more cases) arrangements must be made for treatment to take place at a specified time and date. It is advisable to delay treatment until plans have been properly made. Symptomatic relief can be given to residents if required and this must be prescribed by the general practitioner. It is important that the outbreak be managed by treatment of all residents, staff and close relatives *at the same time*. Seek advice from the health protection team.

- Treat individuals as described.
- Remove any pots of cream which are used daily from the residents' rooms and destroy them.
- Treat all close contacts of the infected residents. This includes family, staff and agency staff.
- After treatment, follow the same procedure as for individual cases.

Lotions and creams for treatment

- Permethrin 5% Dermal Cream (pyrethroid)
- Malathion 0.5% Liquid (organo-phosphate)
- The general practitioner will prescribe the appropriate lotion or cream.

Reference

Lawrence J, May D. 2003. *Infection Control in the Community*. London, Churchill Livingstone.

Further reading

Department of Health. 2006. Infection Control Guidance for Care Homes. Available at:www.dh.gov.uk [Accessed October 2013]
Health Protection Agency (HPA). 2010.The Management of Scabies Infection in the Community. August 2010. HPA North West. Available at:www.hpa.org.uk [Accessed October 2013]

13.4 *Clostridium difficile*

Jean Lawrence

Retired Infection Prevention and Control Nurse, (IPS) Yorkshire, UK

Key points

Clostridium difficile (*C. difficile*) infection (CDI) is an intestinal infection that can cause diarrhoea that is sometimes so severe that it can be life threatening.

- About 3% of healthy adults and 20% of hospitalized patients carry *C. difficile* in their gut without it causing them any harm. In older people, this may be between 20% and 50%.
- CDI occurs when the balance of the 'normal' bacteria in the large bowel is altered, allowing *C. difficile* to flourish.
- Complications can occur, such as psuedomembranous colitis (PMC), severe inflammation in the large intestine, which may lead to perforation and potentially be fatal.
- Sometimes people who have been treated and recovered from CDI will continue to carry *C. difficile* in their gut.

Risk factors

- Increased age (and increasingly in younger age groups).
- Current or recent use of antibiotics (anti-microbial agents).
- Recent or prolonged hospital stays (especially intensive care stays).
- Underlying diseases (comorbidity).
- Surgical bowel procedures.
- Immuno-compromising conditions (such as diabetes).
- Anti-ulcer medications, including proton pump inhibitors (e.g. Omeprazole).

Clinical symptoms

- Watery diarrhoea (smelly and green)
- Fever
- Loss of appetite
- Nausea
- Abdominal pain.

Prevention and control

See Figure 13.4.1.

Recommended actions

- *Inform the general practitioner and ask them to visit immediately when symptoms are suspected and illness present.*
- Seek advice early from the health protection team/infection prevention team.
- If severe diarrhoea, fever/other symptoms and any risk factors are present, admission to hospital should be considered as early as possible.
- Obtain a specimen of faeces as soon as possible and send to the laboratory. *Early diagnosis is essential.*
- Antibiotics are prescribed only if necessary, using the right antibiotic, correct dose and appropriate length of treatment. The antibiotic of choice is normally oral metronidazole 400–500 mg tds for 10 to 14 days for mild to moderate illness and vancomycin 125 mg qds for 10 to 14 days for

S	**Suspect that a case may be infective where there is no clear alternative cause for diarrhoea**
I	Isolate the resident and consult with the health protection team while determining the cause of the diarrhoea
G	Gloves and aprons must be used for all contacts with the resident and their environment
H	Hand washing with soap and water should be carried out before and after each contact with the resident and their immediate environment **Do not use alcohol-based hand rub**
T	Test the stool for toxin, by sending a specimen immediately

Figure 13.4.1 Sight. Source: *Clostridium difficile* infection: How to deal with the problem. Public Health England, January 2009.

severe illness (Department of Health and Health Protection Agency guidance 2008). (Guidance will be given by the general practitioner.)

- Meticulous hand hygiene with liquid soap and warm running water (staff, residents and visitors).
- *Alcohol-based hygienic hand rubs are not effective against C. difficile spores.*
- Use of disposable gloves and aprons.
- High standards of environmental cleaning, daily and after any spillage. Spores can spread rapidly in the environment.
- Cleaning and disinfection of contaminated equipment and environment with a chlorine-based agent is advised.

Staff

- Report any illness in residents promptly.
- Follow standard infection prevention and control precautions at all times.
- Ensure adequate handwashing facilities and resources and report when supplies are required.
- Ensure adequate supplies of equipment including personal protective equipment (PPE) and care equipment.
- Staff to assist residents/service users and relatives to undertake correct hand hygiene procedures.

Staff must be aware of in-house policies regarding infection prevention and control and follow all guidance as directed by the manager and the health protection/infection prevention team.

Staff must be aware of absence policies, including that they should not attend work if they have a sudden onset diarrhoeal illness (diarrhoea is defined as the passage of three or more loose or liquid stools per day, or more frequently than is normal for the individual). Seek advice from the general practitioner.

References

Department of Health and Health Protection Agency. 2009.*Clostridium difficile* infection: How to deal with the problem. (Gateway reference 9833) Available at: www.dh.gov.uk and www.hpa.org.uk [Accessed October 2013]

Further reading

Health Protection Agency. 2007. HPA Regional Microbiology Network January 2007. A Good Practice Guide to *C. Diff*. Available at: www.hpa.org.uk [Accessed October 2013]

NHS National Services Scotland. Health Protection Network. 2009. HPN 6 September 2009. Guidance on Prevention and Control of *Clostridium difficile* infection (CDI) in Healthcare Settings in Scotland (Section 2.2.12 CDI in the community). Available at: http://www.hps.scot.nhs.uk/haiic/sshaip/publicationsdetail.aspx?id=38848 [Accessed October 2013]

13.5 MRSA

Jean Lawrence

Retired Infection Prevention and Control Nurse, (IPS) Yorkshire, UK

Key points

- MRSA is a bacterium, not an illness itself. It can only be detected by a laboratory when a specimen is sent for testing, for example a wound swab.
- Thorough hand hygiene is the most important means of stopping the spread of MRSA.
- It is very important to follow all standard infection prevention and control precautions.

What is it?

MRSA stands for methicillin resistant *Staphylococcus aureus*. This bacterium can live harmlessly on the skin, but can sometimes cause infection. Around one in three people carry *Staphylococcus aureus* in the nose or on the skin. It is normally no risk to healthy people.

MRSA is a type of *Staphylococcus aureus* that has become resistant to commonly used antibiotics. MRSA can be treated and cured with certain antibiotics.

Clinical symptoms

MRSA is not an illness itself. It can only be detected by a laboratory when a specimen, such as a wound swab, is sent for testing. The terms 'colonized' and 'infected' are used to describe the spread of MRSA:

- *Colonization* means that the bacteria can grow and multiply in on or in the body but do not invade and cause damage.
- *Infection* is when the tissues are invaded (pathogenic microorganisms) and damage occurs, For example, MRSA can grow in the nose, groin or axilla and not cause any harm. The organisms can move to a susceptible site, such as a wound, and then infection can occur.

Prevention and control

- Thorough hand hygiene is the most important way to stop the spread of MRSA.
- Follow all standard infection prevention and control precautions.

- It is not always necessary to isolate someone with MRSA. Always check local policy to ensure that the correct procedures are being carried out.
- A person may require a specific washing regime and use of creams and lotions if they are about to have surgery and this will be recommended by the receiving hospital or unit.
- MRSA can survive in dust, therefore environmental cleaning regularly is important (see Chapter 12.6).
- Where antibiotic treatment is required (i.e. intravenous treatment), admission to hospital might be necessary.
- Visitors to the care home are not required to wear any protective clothing but should be advised on handwashing (see Chapter 12.1).

Other information

- MRSA should not be a contraindication to the transfer of a patient to a care home.
- Leaflets containing information about MRSA should be made available for residents and visitors.

Further reading

Association Medical Microbiologists and Health Protection Agency. 2007. MRSA Screening and Suppression. Quick Reference Guide for Primary Care. Available at: www.hpa.org.uk [Accessed October 2013]

Useful web site

www.hpa.org.uk Gives guidance and up to date information on MRSA.

13.6 Respiratory infections

Gurjit Chhokar[1] and Lisa Wickens[2]

[1] Yorkshire and Humber Deanery, Harrogate, UK
[2] Hull and East Yorkshire Hospitals NHS Trust, Hull, UK

Key points

- Infections can affect the upper or lower respiratory tract.
- Lower respiratory tract infections are the leading cause of infectious deaths.
- Monitor the respiratory rate, temperature and other vital signs.
- Contact the GP if symptoms are severe, if the resident has COPD or heart failure, if they become unrousable or if there are any other red flags.
- Optimum care includes fluids and nutrition, controlling the temperature, as well as early treatment with antibiotics and physiotherapy input.

A respiratory infection refers to any infectious disease involving the respiratory tract. These infections are classified as either *upper respiratory tract infections* (such as the common cold or influenza), or *lower respiratory tract infections* (pneumonia or bronchitis), which tend to be more serious.

Upper respiratory tract infections

The upper respiratory tract includes the nose, sinuses, pharynx and larynx (throat). Typical infections include tonsillitis, pharyngitis, laryngitis, sinusitis, otitis media (ear) as well as 'flu' and the common cold. These infections can easily be spread from staff and visitors via small drops coughed or sneezed into the air. Hand washing can reduce the transfer of infective organisms (see Chapter 12.1).

Symptoms

- Nasal discharge.
- Sore throat.
- Congestion.
- Fever.
- Cough.
- Wheeze.
- Muscle aches and pains.

Management and treatment

Most cases of upper respiratory infection are caused by viruses and therefore require no specific treatment (antibiotics do not improve viral infections).

- Antibiotics are sometimes used if a bacterial infection is suspected or diagnosed, such as 'strep throat' (caused by Streptococci, the commonest organism causing bacterial sore throats), bacterial sinusitis or infected tonsillitis.
- Rest, increased oral nutrition and fluids are advised.
- Symptoms can be treated with over the counter medications such as paracetamol, ibuprofen, cough medicines or anti-histamines.
- *If symptoms are severe or debilitating, a doctor should be consulted.*

Lower respiratory tract infections

- The lower respiratory tract consists of the trachea (wind pipe), bronchial tubes, the bronchioles and alveoli.
- Lower respiratory tract infections are generally more serious than upper respiratory infections.
- *They are the leading cause of death among all infectious diseases.*

The Care Home Handbook, First Edition. Edited by Graham Mulley, Clive Bowman, Michal Boyd and Sarah Stowe.
© 2015 John Wiley & Sons, Ltd. Published 2015 by John Wiley & Sons, Ltd.

- They include bronchitis, pneumonia and influenza (which can affect both the upper and lower respiratory tracts).

Symptoms and signs

- Productive cough or difficulty in expectorating.
- Pleurisy – chest pain on breathing.
- New or increase in purulent sputum.
- New crackles or wheeze on chest examination.
- Alterations in breathing especially rapid respiratory rate (over 30 respirations per minute; also Cheyne Stokes respirations).
- Rise or fall in temperature (including hypothermia).
- Flushed complexion.
- Shivering, sometimes violently.
- Increased heart rate.
- Decreased blood pressure.
- Confusion (see Chapter 10.2).
- Impaired consciousness.

Management and treatment

- Control increased temperature with paracetamol and damp cloths. If the resident feels cold, check for hypothermia and provide extra blankets.
- Encourage increased fluids, as much is lost with the extra breathing.
- Encourage nutrition, if possible soups and food which do not require much effort to eat.
- Collect sputum samples to observe and monitor and record colour consistency and volume of the sputum.
- Monitor vital signs (see Chapter 15.8).
- The resident may require antibiotics to be prescribed as early treatment of the infection will speed the recovery and reduce the work of extra breathing.
- Residents with chronic obstructive pulmonary disease (COPD) and congestive heart failure are at greater risk of complications and require consultation and assessment by the general practitioner earlier in the illness course.

> **How to reduce the spread of respiratory infections**
>
> - Aim to care for affected residents in single rooms away from others.
> - Avoid moving affected individuals from their rooms, if at all possible.
> - Reduce staff contact, if possible.
> - Use universal techniques at all times, face masks, and high standards of hand hygiene.

- Steroids may sometimes be used.
- Physiotherapists can perform or teach exercises that help with clearing the infected sputum.
- If the resident becomes unrousable and they are not receiving palliative care, consider getting urgent medical help – or call for an ambulance.

Aspiration

People with swallowing or speech difficulties may inhale food, leading to aspiration pneumonia. These people may cough and splutter when eating or drinking. If you suspect that this is the case, referral should be made for evaluation by the speech and language therapist (see Chapter 8.2). They may modify the consistency of a person's diet to avoid this.

TB

TB can infect any part of the body but is most commonly diagnosed in the chest. The disease is a particular concern in care homes as older people may have infections that "reignite" and staff from countries where the infection is more commonplace are at higher risk. For residents and staff who are persistently unwell without a good explanation the question, could this be TB? is worth asking.

It may have been caught in earlier life but as the person gets older and more frail, it can re-activate leading to coughing with or without sputum, fevers, night sweats, loss of appetite and weight loss. TB may collect in lymph nodes (lumps in the neck, armpits or groin).

If TB is suspected or diagnosed specialist advice and support must be sought for both the treatment and level of screening required.

COPD/asthma

Irritation to the lungs can lead to wheezing. This is caused by air passing through narrow airways. In asthma, this is caused by inflammation of normal airways and can develop fairly quickly (minutes to hours).

COPD is due to narrowing of damaged airways over time, by harmful agents, such as cigarette smoke or chemicals used in previous employment.

A chest infection in these residents can cause the airways to narrow suddenly, and will require rapid treatment.

Detecting and managing exacerbations early can prevent deterioration and hospital admission.

Make sure the resident is using their inhaler or nebuliser correctly. Contact a doctor to prescribe antibiotics and an increase in the frequency of bronchodilators.

NICE guidelines state that the initial management of COPD exacerbations should constitute:

- Increased frequency of bronchodilator use (see Chapter 9.2).
- Oral antibiotics if purulent sputum.
- Prednisolone 30 mg daily for 7–14 days for all patients with significant breathlessness (unless contraindicated).

Red flags: when to get help

- blue discolouration to lips and fingernails (cyanosis)
- respiratory rate over 20 breaths per minute (suggests a likely lung infection)
- becoming more breathless
- abdominal pain or diarrhoea
- confusion
- blood in sputum
- passing little or no urine
- general deterioration
- rapid deterioration with increased distress.

In each of these instances, you should contact the GP or emergency services.

Further reading

Beaglehole R, Irwin A, Prentice T et al. 2004. The World Health Report 2004 – Changing History. World Health Organization. pp 120–124.

Loeb M, Carusone SC, Goeree R, et al. 2006. Effect of a clinical pathway to reduce hospitalizations in nursing home residents with pneumonia: A randomized controlled trial. *Journal of the American Medical Association* 295: 2503–2509.

National Institute for Clinical Excellence. 2004. Clinical Guideline 12 Chronic Obstructive Pulmonary Disease.

13.7 Diarrhoea

Rhiannon Humphreys

Hull Royal Infirmary, Hull, UK

Key points

- Diarrhoea is common and can be fatal to elderly residents.
- Adequate hydration must be maintained and supplemented where necessary.
- Some residents may have non-specific signs and symptoms masking deeper infections.
- Be aware of red flags such as bloody diarrhoea.
- Avoid anti-diarrhoeal drugs until the cause has been found.
- Good hand hygiene is paramount in preventing the spread of infection.
- Relatives should be aware of the infection control policy if they have symptoms of diarrhoea.
- Always seek medical advice if there is any doubt or concern.

Diarrhoea is common in old age and has significant morbidity and mortality. In high-income countries, most deaths from gastroenteritis are in the over-70 age group. There is no increase in the incidence of infective diarrhoea in old age, but the impact is greater. Even a short period of diarrhoea can have serious consequences for an elderly resident with co-morbidities.

The aims of management are to:

- prevent complications, such as dehydration
- avoid delay in diagnosis
- avoid hospital admissions where possible.

If there is concern at any time, medical attention should be sought.

Definitions

- **Diarrhoea** – passing more than three loose or liquid stools in 24 hours, or an increased frequency than is normal for that individual.
- **Acute diarrhoea** – loose stools for less than 14 days (most likely to be infective).
- **Chronic diarrhoea** – loose stools for more than 30 days (unlikely to be infective).

Causes

The main causes of diarrhoea are listed below.

- Viral, for example norovirus (see Chapter 13.2)
- Medication side effects, for example lansoprazole, donepezil.
- Overflow diarrhoea due to constipation or faecal impaction
- Excess laxative use.
- Antibiotic use
  - side-effect
  - *C. difficile.*
- Bacterial, for example *Salmonella*, *Campylobacter*.
- Systemic illness for examples, sepsis
- Endocrine, for example hyperthyroidism.
- Cancer, for example colon cancer.
- Diverticular disease.
- Malabsorption.
- Enteral feeding, for example PEG or NG.
- Inflammatory bowel disease.
- Ischaemic bowel.

The most common cause is viral infection, such as norovirus. It is usually self limiting, lasting for up to five days.

Anti-diarrhoeals, such as loperamide, should be avoided until the cause is identified.

If food poisoning is suspected, then specific treatment may be needed, but the diarrhoea is usually self-limiting.

Food poisoning is a notifiable disease.

About 10% of care home residents have an episode of faecal incontinence (overflow diarrhoea or spurious diarrhoea) each week and 4% of residents have chronic diarrhoea.

The Care Home Handbook, First Edition. Edited by Graham Mulley, Clive Bowman, Michal Boyd and Sarah Stowe.
© 2015 John Wiley & Sons, Ltd. Published 2015 by John Wiley & Sons, Ltd.

Signs and symptoms of diarrhoea

Many residents will have non-specific symptoms that may mask an important problem. Figure 13.7.1 shows many of the symptoms or signs that may be present:

Red flag symptoms

Every resident with diarrhoea should be examined for red flag symptoms (Figure 13.7.2).

Medical attention should be sought for any resident who has red flag symptoms or about whom there is concern.

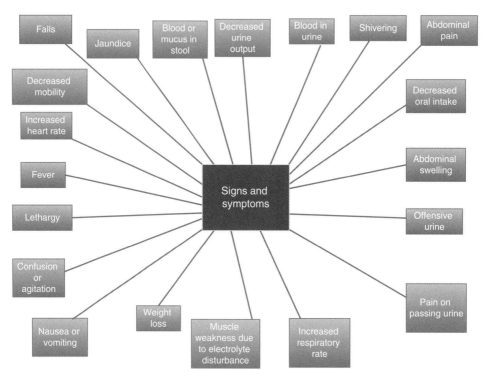

Figure 13.7.1 Signs and symptoms that may present in residents with diarrhoea.

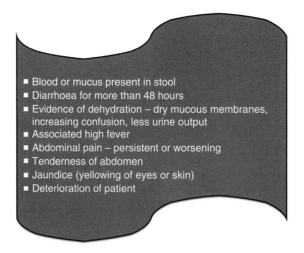

■ Blood or mucus present in stool
■ Diarrhoea for more than 48 hours
■ Evidence of dehydration – dry mucous membranes, increasing confusion, less urine output
■ Associated high fever
■ Abdominal pain – persistent or worsening
■ Tenderness of abdomen
■ Jaundice (yellowing of eyes or skin)
■ Deterioration of patient

Figure 13.7.2 Red flag symptoms.

Management of diarrhoea

Diarrhoea can be highly infectious and can spread rapidly in the care home.

It is imperative that a strict infection control protocol is followed for any resident with diarrhoea (see Chapters 12.1 and 13.4).

All staff should be trained in infection control protocols and proper hand hygiene. This training should be checked regularly.

It is also important that relatives adhere to the same protocol, as they can be both a source of infection and a cause for disseminating it. Relatives should be made aware of infection control policies, such as barrier nursing.

They should also be discouraged from visiting if they have symptoms of diarrhoea or vomiting themselves. They should not visit until they are more than 48 hours symptom free.

Case study

A 76 year old lady, Mrs. A, who is bed bound and has dysphagia following a stroke, is visited by her daughter and her grandson. Her grandson had vomiting and diarrhoea the day before but is now well. The next day, Mrs. A develops diarrhoea and vomiting. She quickly becomes dehydrated due to the diarrhoea and vomiting and her inability to feed herself. She requires hospital admission for fluid replace. Another 12 residents in the same nursing home are affected, two more requiring hospital admission. The hospital ward is closed as the infection has spread to other patients and is later identified as norovirus.

Management of resident with diarrhoea

- Isolate the resident.
- Barrier nurse – use gloves and aprons.
- Enforce rigorous hand hygiene *using soap and water*, before and after contact with the resident or their environment – *alcohol gel alone is not enough*.
- Send a stool sample for culture, viral studies and *C. difficile* screening as soon as possible.
- Document stool frequency and consistency using the Bristol Stool Chart (see Chapter 5.5).
- Document observations regularly.
- Ensure adequate hydration – supplemental fluids or oral rehydration salts, such as Dioralyte©, may

become necessary if there are copious amounts of diarrhoea.

- Ensure thorough cleaning of aids, such as commodes.
- Correct disposal of soiled linen is crucial to prevent the spread of infection.
- Ensure residents follow hand hygiene rules.
- Medications must be reviewed:
  - Stop laxatives.
  - Review need for antibiotics.
  - Other drugs may need to be discontinued (this should only be decided by a person who is competent to do so).
  - Some other drugs that cause diarrhoea are:
    - Diuretics – furosemide, bumetanide, spironolactone
    - Anti-hypertensives – bendroflumethiazide, amlodipine, ramipril, lisinopril.
- *If diarrhoea persists for more than 48 hours, concerns arise or there are red flag symptoms, then it is recommended that medical attention be sought.*

Figure 13.7.3 shows the management approach for acute diarrhoea.

Each resident should also have an infection checklist completed (Table 13.7.1).

Table **13.7.1** Infection checklist.

	Date achieved	Date result seen
Isolate patient		N/A
Stool sample for *C. diff* sent		
Stool sample sent for culture		
Relatives informed		N/A
Assessed for red flag symptoms		N/A
Fluid balance chart commenced		N/A
Stool chart commenced		N/A
Medication reviewed		N/A
Medical review		N/A

Summary

- There are many causes of diarrhoea.
- Diarrhoea may mask other pathology.
- Infection control protocols must be adhered to in order to prevent the spread of infection. Do be sure that relatives are aware of the protocol.
- All staff should be trained in infection control protocols and hand hygiene.

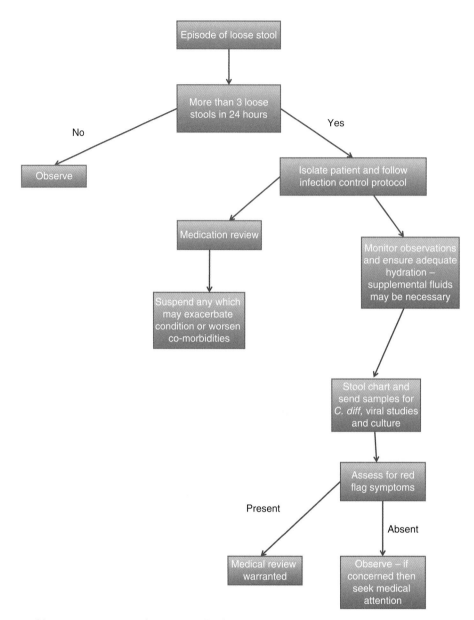

Figure 13.7.3 Management approach to acute diarrhoea.

- Infectious diarrhoea can spread rapidly in a care home.
- Ensure adequate hydration of residents.

  If in doubt, seek medical attention.

Further reading

World Health Organization. 2009. WHO Guidelines on Hand Hygiene in Health Care: a Summary. (Useful information on Health care associated infections as well as specific instructions on hand hygiene.)

Useful web site

Bristol stool chart – www.sthk.nhs.uk/library/documents/stoolchart.pdf

Health Protection Agency. Introduction to infection control in Care Homes www.hpa.org.uk/webw/HPAweb&Page&HPAwebAutoListName/Page/1229594195568?p=1229594195568 (contains videos on prevention of infection, management of equipment).

www.patient.co.uk – (has a good basic section on acute diarrhoea)

13.8 Intra-abdominal infections

Rhiannon Humphreys

Hull Royal Infirmary, Hull, UK

Key points

- Intra-abdominal infections can range from simple urine infections to life threatening infections.
- Most intra-abdominal infections will need medical review.
- More residents with severe intra-abdominal infections will require hospital admission.
- Elderly residents may have non-specific symptoms such as confusion or loss of appetite.
- If in doubt, seek medical attention

Intra-abdominal infections range from a simple urine infection with mild discomfort to severe life threatening sepsis.

Most intra-abdominal infections require medical review and many individuals will need admission to hospital for either investigation or management.

Some of the most common intra-abdominal infections and their symptoms are listed below. (Note that elderly residents may not present with typical features and non-specific symptoms may predominate.)

- **Urinary tract infections** – urinary frequency, offensive urine, pain on passing urine, lower abdominal pain (see Chapter 13.9).
- **Pyelonephritis** (kidney infection) – flank pain, fever, shivering, urinary symptoms.
- **Cholangitis** (infection of the biliary tree) – fever, abdominal pain, jaundice, shivers, nausea, vomiting.
- **Cholecystitis** (gallbladder inflammation) – nausea, vomiting, abdominal pain, jaundice.
- **Colitis** (infection or inflammation of the large bowel) – blood or mucus in stool, weight loss, fever, abdominal pain.
- **Pancreatitis** (inflammation of the pancreas) – central abdominal pain, nausea, vomiting, jaundice, fever.
- **Appendicitis** (inflammation or infection of the appendix) – lower right abdominal pain, fever, nausea, vomiting.

- **Diverticular abscess** (abscess formed in diverticular pouch) – fever, abdominal pain, diarrhoea, blood or mucus in stool.
- **Peritonitis** (infection or inflammation of the lining of the abdomen usually due to another cause) – abdominal pain, absent bowel sounds, abdominal tenderness.

The red flag symptoms are the same as those listed in the chapter on diarrhoea (see Chapter 13.7).

If there is concern about abdominal symptoms at any time, then you must call the GP or emergency services urgently.

Further reading

Sartelli M, Viale P, Koike K, et al. 2011. WSES consensus conference: Guidelines for first-line management of intra-abdominal infections. *World Journal of Emergency Surgery* 6: 2.

Useful web site

University of South Carolina School of Medicine. Microbiology and immunology on-line: Gastrointestinal and intra-abdominal infection. http://pathmicro.med.sc.edu/infectious%20disease/gastrointestinal%20infections.htm – (American on-line textbook, good explanations of different organisms and conditions, enables looking up of terms)[Accessed October 2013].

13.9 Urinary tract infections

Tanya Bish[1] and Michal Boyd[2]

[1] *Waitemata District Health Board, North Shore, New Zealand*
[2] *The University of Auckland, Auckland, New Zealand*

Key points

- Urinary tract infection is the most common bacterial infection in care homes.
- Older people commonly have asymptomatic bacteria in the urine.
- Only symptomatic urinary tract infections should be treated with antibiotics.

Definition of urinary tract infection (UTI)

Urinary tract infection is the most common bacterial infection in residents in care homes. Many older people chronically have bacteria in their urine (bacteriuria), but only *symptomatic* urinary tract infections should be treated.

The following criteria must be met for *symptomatic UTI*:

1. *The resident does not have an indwelling urinary catheter and has at least three of the following signs and symptoms:*
   - Fever (above 38 °C) or chills or increase of 1 °C above their normal temperature.
   - New or increased burning pain on passing urine, frequency or urgency.
   - New flank or supra-pubic pain or tenderness.
   - Change in character of urine (cloudy, milky or malodorous).
   - Worsening mental or functional status (may be also increased or new incontinence).
   - Urinalysis showing high level of nitrates.
2. *The resident has an indwelling catheter and has at least 2 of the following signs and symptoms:*
   - Fever (above 38 °C) or chills or increase of 1 °C degree above their normal temperature.
   - New flank or supra-pubic pain or tenderness.
   - Change in character of urine.
   - Worsening mental or functional status.

Care should be taken to rule out other causes of these symptoms.

Asymptomatic bacteriuria is not treated with antibiotics except in special circumstances, for example prior to surgery, where it may increase post-operative risk. There is no discernible benefit to the resident (when there are bacteria in the urine without symptoms) and there are risks of anti-microbial resistance and drug reactions.

Surveillance of asymptomatic bacteriuria is not recommended as this represents a baseline status for many residents.

If less than two of the above symptoms are presented, consider other causes such as dehydration (see Chapter 5.3).

Risk factors

- Factors that prohibit complete emptying of the bladder:
  - constipation
  - cystocele, uterine prolapse, urinary calculi, benign prostatic hypertrophy.
- Oestrogen deficiency.
- Oral anti-microbials.
- Immobility.
- Poor hygiene.
- Poor toileting habits.
- Faecal incontinence.
- Catheterisation.
- Diabetes mellitus.
- Dehydration.

The Care Home Handbook, First Edition. Edited by Graham Mulley, Clive Bowman, Michal Boyd and Sarah Stowe.
© 2015 John Wiley & Sons, Ltd. Published 2015 by John Wiley & Sons, Ltd.

Challenging assessment

- Some residents will *not* have an *elevated temperature.*
- Some may *not* have *chills* – their thermoregulation mechanism can be impaired.
- *Pain* – abdominal pain can be caused by GI problems, may be atypical or can be masked by medications.
- *New incontinence* – incontinence is chronic in 50% of the elderly population.
- *Altered mental health status* – helpful in diagnosing UTIs; manifested by acute confusion (see Chapter 10.2), lethargy or agitation.
- As a general rule, urine that is crystal clear to the naked eye is unlikely to be infected.

Collection of MSU

A urine specimen can take some time to collect. Alerting staff as soon as a UTI is suspected will assist in getting a specimen before any treatment is started. A urine specimen should always be obtained before treatment, because a negative urine culture is useful to exclude UTI.

A positive urine culture will show the microorganism's sensitivity to antibiotics, allowing for prudent prescribing (Figure 13.9.1). Anti-microbial resistance is becoming more problematic in residential care, increasing the importance of optimising anti-microbial therapy.

Treatment options

Treatment options need to be individualised for each resident. Deciding when to start antibiotics can be challenging and good assessment information can help the prescriber choose the best course of action.

Other treatments to consider:

- Adequate hydration to meet daily requirements.
- Attention to perineal hygiene and continence management.
- Cranberry capsules to reduce *E. coli* adherence to bladder wall (but there are no randomised controlled trials of cranberry juice in UTIs and no evidence of benefit in those who are catheterised).

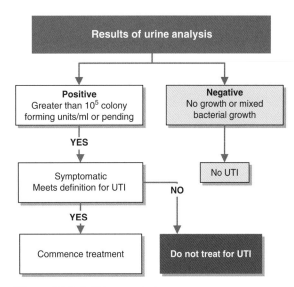

Figure 13.9.1 Urine analysis.

- Avoid catheterisation.
- Consider atrophic vaginitis and discuss possible oestrogen cream treatment if resident continues to suffer multiple UTIs.

Further reading

Howell, AB. 2007. Bioactive compounds in cranberries and their role in prevention of urinary tract infections. *Molecular Nutrition & Food Research* 51: 732–737.

Jepson RG, Mihaljevic L, Craig JC. 1998. Still waiting for evidence about whether cranberries are a useful treatment for urinary tract infections. *Cochrane Database of Systematic Reviews* 4: CD 001322.

Juthani-Mehta M. 2007. Asymptomatic bacteriuria and urinary tract infection in older adults. *Clinics in Geriatric Medicine* 23: 585–594.

Loeb M, Bentley DW, Bradley S, et al. 2001. Development of minimum criteria for the initiation of antibiotics in residents of long-term-care facilities: results of a consensus conference. *Infection Control & Hospital Epidemiology* 22: 120–124.

McGeer A, Campbell B, Emori TG et al. 1991. Definitions of infection for surveillance in long-term care facilities. *American Journal of Infection Control* 19: 1–7.

Section H

Procedures and Observations

Chapter 14

Specialised Procedures

14.1 Nasogastric (NG) and percutaneous endoscopic gastrostomy (PEG) tubes

Alison Cracknell

Leeds Teaching Hospitals NHS Trust, Leeds, UK

Key points

- Home enteral tube feeding is used to maintain adequate nutritional intake for selected residents.
- There is a significant risk of complications.
- Every healthcare professional involved in the management of residents receiving enteral feeding in care homes should have specialised training and access to expert advice and support at all times.

Home enteral tube feeding (HETF) should be used for residents who are unable to meet nutritional requirements through oral intake alone. It refers to the delivery of food directly into the gut via a tube.

Common reasons for enteral feeding include:

- dysphagia (see Chapter 5.2) caused by neurological disease (e.g. stroke, motor neurone disease, Parkinson's disease);
- gastrointestinal obstruction (for example from a tumour);
- after trauma;
- post surgery.

The types of enteral feeding most commonly used are nasogastric tubes (NG) and percutaneous endoscopic gastrostomy tubes (PEG).

PEG tubes are more commonly used in care homes and are generally easier to manage in the medium to long term.

NG tubes are generally used as a short-term option, but can be used long term where alternatives, such as PEG, are either not possible or the risks of the procedure are too great.

All residents receiving enteral feeding should have an individualised care plan and be supported by a multi-disciplinary team (typically involving a dietician; a care home nurse or district nurse; a pharmacist; and a speech and language therapist) (see Chapter 8.2).

Training of carers and management in care homes

Tubes should be inserted by appropriately trained staff. Most tubes are initially inserted in hospital. Before discharge from hospital, clear arrangements and clinical responsibility for ongoing management of enteral feeding must be in place.

Guidelines published by the UK National Institute for Health and Clinical Excellence (NICE) advise that patients and their carers should receive training from the multi-disciplinary team on:

- The management of the tube, delivery system and the regime (including setting up feeds, using feed pumps), methods for troubleshooting common problems and provision of an instruction manual.
- Routine and emergency telephone numbers to contact a healthcare professional who understands the needs and potential problems of HETF.
- The delivery of equipment and feed, with contact details of the home care company involved.

Percutaneous gastrostomy

Gastrostromy tubes are passed percutaneously through the abdominal wall directly into the stomach. These tubes are usually placed initially under local anaesthetic and light sedation with the use of an

The Care Home Handbook, First Edition. Edited by Graham Mulley, Clive Bowman, Michal Boyd and Sarah Stowe.
© 2015 John Wiley & Sons, Ltd. Published 2015 by John Wiley & Sons, Ltd.

endoscope (hence the name Percutaneous Endoscopic Gastrostomy) and the procedure involves a small incision in the abdominal wall.

Most PEG tubes need replacing every few years, but rather than undergoing further endoscopic placement, a standard gastrostomy tube can be fitted through the existing tract. Commonly these replacement gastrostomies are 'balloon' (where a balloon inflated with sterile water holds the tube in place) or 'button' devices. These tubes should be changed every few months.

Troubleshooting

Most complications can be reduced or even prevented by good care and maintenance, and it is essential to follow advice described in your local protocol.

- Blocked PEG tubes: This can be caused by delays in feeding and flushing. Should a tube block, there are several methods to unblock it, including flushing with warm water, fizzy drinks or pineapple juice.
- Accidental tube removal: *Prompt replacement is crucial to avoid closure of the tract.* If replacement tubes and trained staff are not immediately available, it is recommended that a similar French size Foley catheter is gently inserted into the tract to maintain patency.
- Redness and inflammation at the PEG site: These are common, and can be associated with infection. Daily cleansing with sterile water, swabs and systemic anti-microbial treatment may be necessary. It is also necessary to consider pressure necrosis if the bolster is held too tightly against the skin, and allergic reactions around the tube as causes of inflammation. Very rarely, necrotising fasciitis can occur around the site, usually evident 3–14 days after PEG insertion. It is characterised by fever, oedema and rapidly spreading cellulitis; *urgent medical attention is required.*
- Abdominal bloating, diarrhoea, nausea and vomiting are common side-effects:The rate or method of administration of the feed can be reviewed to reduce gastro-intestinal side-effects.
- Aspiration: The risk of aspiration (inhalation of the stomach contents) can be reduced by using intermittent or continuous feeding regimes rather than rapid boluses. *Residents receiving feeds while in bed should have the head of the bed raised to 35–45⁰ during feeding and for 1 hour afterwards.*

Nasogastric tubes

NG tubes are usually used for short-term enteral feeding. They are a less preferable option to PEG in the longer term, as the risks of misplacement or dislodgement are greater. The position of the tube also requires checking before each use. Fine bore 5–8 French Gauge tubes are used.

The UK National Patient Safety Agency (NPSA) has produced guidance and alerts following incidents of death and serious harm where NG tubes were placed in the respiratory tract rather than gastrointestinal tract. This had not been detected before commencement of feeding.

As well as misplacement upon insertion, NG tubes inserted correctly initially can move out of the stomach if the tube becomes dislodged (with similar unfortunate consequences).

It is essential to check position of NG tubes in the following situations:

- After initial insertion.
- Before starting each feed or giving medication.
- Once daily, during continuous feeds.
- Following vomiting, retching or coughing (in case of displacement).
- If the tape around the nose is loose, or the visible tube appears longer than previously documented.

How to check the position of an NG tube

It is essential that care home staff managing NG feeding have received appropriate training and have clear written local guidelines to follow.

Within the UK, guidelines are based on recommendations from the NPSA, which advises aspiration (withdrawal with a syringe) of gastric contents and pH testing of this aspirate using pH graded indicator paper that is CE marked (CE is a mark of quality).

A pH <5.5 is consistent with gastric placement and the tube can be used for feeding. The test and test result should be documented in the care plan.

What to do if the pH is >5.5

Reasons for an elevated pH in a correctly positioned tube include the feed itself and the use of antacid medications.

- Do not commence feeding.
- Wait 1 hour (with nothing running through the tube during this time) and take a further aspirate and test the pH.

- If pH remains >5.5, *do not feed and do seek advice* from the local nutritional team. It may be necessary to arrange for a chest x-ray.

What to do if you cannot aspirate the contents of the stomach

- *Do not commence feeding.*
- If possible, turn the resident onto their side and attempt syringe aspiration again.
- Try injecting 10–20 ml of air into the tube and wait 15 minutes before trying aspiration again.
- If you are still unable to obtain an aspirate, do not use the tube, and seek advice from the local nutritional team.
- A chest x-ray may be required, depending on the clinical situation.

Troubleshooting

- Nasal irritation and nose bleeding (epistaxis): Nasal damage and irritation are common. If persistent and problematic, alternative feeding options may need to be considered.
- Gastro-oesophageal reflux and aspiration: Aspiration remains a major risk with NG tubes (and is potentially greater than with percutaneous gastrostomy). Prokinetic drugs may be used and feeding rates reduced. If problems continue, alternative feeding options may need to be considered.
- Tube dislodgement: *If the tube has become dislodged or the tube position cannot be confirmed by aspiration of gastric contents, it must NOT be used.*
- Abdominal bloating, diarrhoea, nausea and vomiting are common side-effects: The rate or method of administration can be reviewed to reduce gastro-intestinal side-effects.

Further reading

National Collaborating Centre for Acute Care. 2006. Nutrition support for adults: Oral nutrition support, enteral tube feeding and parenteral nutrition. London, National Collaborating Centre for Acute Care (commissioned by National Institute for Health and Clinical Excellence).

National Patient Safety Agency. 2011. Reducing the harm caused by misplaced nasogastric feeding tubes in adults, children and infants. London, NPSA. Available at: http://www.nrls.npsa.nhs.uk/resources/?EntryId45=129640 [Accessed October 2013].

14.2 Tracheostomy

Caroline Kane[1] and Ronan Collins[2]

[1] Peamount Healthcare, Ireland
[2] Adelaide and Meath Hospital, Dublin, Ireland

Key points

- Tracheostomy is to protect or aid respiration.
- Not commonly encountered in care homes.
- Always seek expert advice if you are unsure about any aspect of tracheostomy management.
- Never apply suction when the inner tube is fenestrated.
- Always change tubes and ties with two people present.
- Always have replacement tubes, suctioning equipment and resuscitation equipment to hand when changing tubes.
- Always have manufacturer's quick reference guide available.

What is a tracheostomy?

- Tracheostomy is an incision into the trachea to form a temporary or permanent opening. The opening or 'hole' is called a stoma. The incision is usually vertical and runs from the second to the fourth tracheal ring (see Figure 14.2.1).
- A tube is inserted through the stoma to allow for passage of air and removal of secretions. Instead of breathing through the nose and mouth, the resident will now breathe through the tracheostomy tube.

Indications for a tracheostomy

- *To bypass* an airway obstruction at any level (from the nose to the trachea), and for any reason (trauma, infection, tumours, major head and neck surgery).
- *To protect* the lungs from aspiration.
- *To reduce* respiratory dead space and the effort required for breathing as indicated in acute and chronic neurological or neuromuscular diseases, for example Guillain-Barre syndrome, motor neurone disease.
- For positive pressure ventilation.
- *For tracheobronchial 'toilet'* to aid in secretion management.

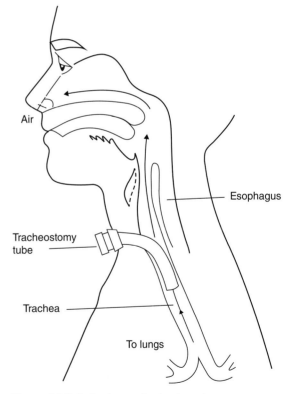

Figure 14.2.1 Anatomy of a tracheostomy.

The Care Home Handbook, First Edition. Edited by Graham Mulley, Clive Bowman, Michal Boyd and Sarah Stowe.
© 2015 John Wiley & Sons, Ltd. Published 2015 by John Wiley & Sons, Ltd.

Types and terminology of tracheostomy tubes

'Cuffed' : an air-inflated cuff around the inner tube to prevent penetration of secretions from mouth, pharynx and stomach. Most tracheostomy tubes in care homes will be non-cuffed

Indications for a cuffed tube:
- Immediately post-operatively – to prevent aspiration of blood or serous fluid from the wound.
- To seal the trachea during mechanical ventilation.
- To seal the trachea during hydrotherapy.
- To prevent aspiration of leakage from a tracheo-oesophageal fistula.
- To prevent aspiration due to laryngeal incompetence/absent gag reflex.
- *Should never* be used with speaking valves, as will obstruct breathing.

Outer tube types (Figures 14.2.2 and 14.2.3):
- Non-fenestrated : Outer tube with no hole.
- Fenestrated: Outer tube with a hole or multiple holes; which permits airflow through the larynx and oral/nasal pharynx.

Inner tubes:
- Fenestrated tube: 'holed' – may be used as an aid to weaning ventilation or assisting speech.
- *Should never* be used while suctioning as could damage the trachea wall.
- Non- fenestrated: not holed; *always* to be in place if patient is being suctioned

Complications

Long-term complications from the presence of a tracheostomy tube are mainly caused by tracheal scarring and erosion.

- **Stenosis**: narrowing of the trachea from scar tissue occurs in 5 to 15% of patients. Risk is increased by a history of endotracheal intubation and/or excessive tracheostomy tube cuff pressure.
- **Scarring**: can occur at the stoma, the tube cuff site, or at the point where the distal end of the tube presses on the tracheal wall. Can extend beyond the trachea, in web-like fashion, or appear as a localised granuloma.
- **Fistulas**: caused by pressure from a poorly fitted tracheostomy tube, overinflated cuffs, and/or a nasogastric feeding tube *in situ* which can all contribute to tissue necrosis, ulceration and ultimately fistula formation.

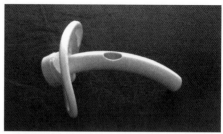

(a)

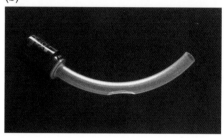

(b)

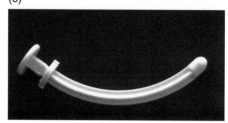

(c)

Figure 14.2.2 (a) Non-cuffed fenestrated tube. (b) Fenestrated inner cannula. (c) Obturator.

- ◦ A fistula can develop between trachea and oesophagus or erode into a major artery.
- ◦ *Aspiration* of gastric contents is the consequence of the first path erosion. *Haemorrhage* results from the other.

Care of tracheostomy

- Daily care of the tracheostomy stoma is needed to prevent infection and skin breakdown.
- The surrounding skin should be cleaned with normal saline or soap and water and dried.
- Use of dressings around the stoma site is not recommended. They may contribute to skin breakdown and a build up of bacteria.
- Change tracheostomy ties if needed (leave one finger space between ties and the resident's neck).

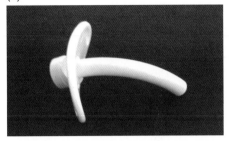

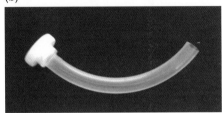

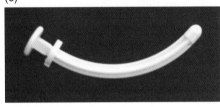

Figure 14.2.3 (a) Non-cuffed, non-fenestrated outer tube. (b) Non-fenestrated inner tube. (c) Obturator.

- *Always* have *two* people when changing tracheostomy ties – one person to hold the tube in position and second person to change the tie.

Care of the inner tube

- Whenever possible, have a double cannulated tube *in situ*, that is a disposable inner tube within the outer tube.
- Disposable inner tubes should be changed when needed, and disposed of in a yellow clinical waste bag.
- A non-fenestrated inner tube is always needed when suctioning.

What to have by the bedside

- Spare tubes: same size and one size smaller.
- Suction machine fitted with filter, suction tubing, suction catheters.
- Gloves – sterile and non-sterile.
- Bottle of sterile water and galley pot.
- Humidification equipment.
- Clinical waste bag.

Suctioning

- Suctioning should *only* be carried out when resident is unable to clear their own airway. It should *not be done routinely*.
- Always explain to the resident what you are going to do, as explanation helps ease the distress of suctioning.
- Appropriate sized single-use multi-eyed catheters are used. Calculate size by the formula:

Tracheostomy tube × 3 / 2 e.g. Size 8 tube × 3 = 24/2 = size 12 suction catheter

- Check the suction pressure. Should be maintained below 120 mmHg in adults.
- Maximum of three suction catheter insertions to avoid tissue trauma to the trachea and no longer than 15 seconds to avoid hypoxia
- If the resident is prone to dropping oxygen saturations during this procedure, administer a small amount of oxygen (e.g. 2–3 l/min) for 5 minutes before suctioning and immediately after. An oxygen saturation monitor is desirable to ensure good saturation (i.e. ≥95% before and after suctioning).
- There may be colonisation with resistant bacteria, so in order to limit contamination, use an aseptic technique, apron and gloves. Eye protection will increase safety. Dispose of contaminated tubes and clothing carefully afterwards.

Suctioning is probably required when there is/are

- Noisy breathing (the sound of air bubbling through secretions).
- Visible secretions at the tracheostomy tube opening.
- A cough with the sound of secretions in the tube.
- Restlessness, agitation, crying (crying also increases the amount of secretions).
- Increased respiratory rate.

How to do the procedure

- Wash hands before and after procedure.
- Don non-sterile gloves and one sterile glove on your dominant hand.

- Explain the procedure to the resident and apply suction, using sterile technique.
- Insert the suction catheter with no suction applied until resistance is met, then pull back about 1–2 cm before applying continuous suction as the catheter is smoothly withdrawn from airway.
- Never re-insert the catheter; dispose of it by wrapping the catheter in your sterile glove and placing in a yellow bag, don a new sterile glove and re-insert a new suction catheter if needed.

Humidification

- The natural ability to warm and humidify air during inspiration is bypassed with a tracheostomy *in situ*.
- Alternative methods are needed to avoid excessive drying of the mucosal lining and minimise the risk of thickened secretions and blocked tubes. This is mandatory where oxygen is used routinely by the patient. Examples include
- Nebulisers
- Buchanan bibs (Figure 14.2.4)

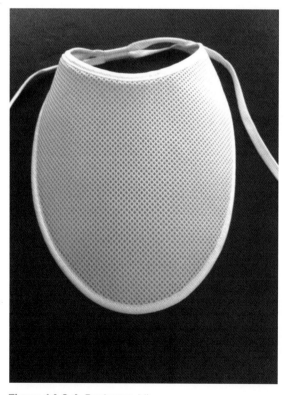

Figure 14.2.4 Buchanan bib.

- Swedish nose
- Heat and moisture exchangers.

Tracheostomy precautions

- Use extreme caution around water.
- Cover with waterproof bib in shower and prevent water splashing into tracheostomy.
- Check with doctor before applying any creams and so on near the stoma as these are not usually recommended. A barrier cream, for example Cavalon. may be used if skin breakdown occurs around the stoma site.
- *No* powder, talc, bleach, ammonia, aerosol sprays or perfume near the resident.
- *No* plastic bibs, fuzzy or furry stuffed toys.
- *No* smoking.

Troubleshooting

If the tube falls out

- Don't panic – if the tube has been in place for five days, the tract should be well formed.
- Reassure the resident and encourage them to breathe normally.
- Call for expert help (expert = any competent member of the multi-disciplinary team with experience in caring for patients with tracheostomy).
- Insert the spare tube (which you have at the bedside at all times!) or a smaller one.

Occlusion

Suspect if any of the following evident:

- Presence of respiratory distress – use of accessory muscles or increased respiratory rate.
- Increasing oxygen requirements or decreased SaO_2.
- Hypotension or tachycardia.
- Decreased level of consciousness.
- Noisy breathing.
- Difficulty removing secretions either by suctioning or asking the patient to expectorate. Visible sputum, tissue or blood in tracheostomy tube.
- Resident complains of shortness of breath.
- Resident is agitated.

Priorities:

- Is the tracheostomy tube patent?
- If patent, give the resident high flow oxygen via the tracheostomy tube.
- Is the resident appropriately monitored?

- Is help coming?
- Look for the causes of the problem and, where possible, resolve these.

Changing tracheostomy tubes

- Tracheostomy tubes with inner tubes should be changed according to manufacturer's instructions, for example at least every 29 days for a Shiley.
- The person changing the tracheostomy tube must be experienced and feel competent in carrying out the procedure.
- Two people are required usually.
- Dispose of all used tracheostomy equipment in yellow clinical waste bags.
- Wash hands thoroughly. Remove the new tracheostomy tube from the sterile pouch.
- Remove the inner tube (cannula) and insert the obturator into the outer tube.
- Attach the clean tracheostomy ties to the neck plate so that the ties will be able to attach around the neck.
- Lubricate the end of the tube and the obturator with a thin layer of water-soluble lubricant, such as KY-jelly. *Do not* use an oil-based lubricant.
- Untie the neck ties from the tracheotomy tube that is being replaced.
- With the thumb and forefinger, grasp the neck plate. Carefully remove the entire tube in a straight downward motion. *Do not* force the tube. If you are unable to remove it, contact the doctor.
- Immediately insert the new tracheostomy tube with gentle backwards pressure.

- Remove the obturator when the new tube is in place and allow air to flow in.
- Insert the new inner cannula.
- Secure the trachestomy ties around the neck leaving a good finger breadth of space).

Further reading

Russell C. 2005. Providing the nurse with a guide to tracheostomy care and management. *British Journal Nursing* 8:428–433.

St John RE, Malen JF. 2004. Contemporary issues in adult tracheostomy management. *Critical Care Nursing Clinical North America* 16: 413–430.

Edgtton-Winn M, Wright K. 2005. Tracheostomy: A guide to nursing care. *Australian Nursing Journal* 13: 17–20.

Paul F. 2010. Tracheostomy care and management in general wards and community settings: literature review. *Nursing in Critical Care* 1: 76–85.

Chulay M. 2010. Suctioning: endotracheal or tracheostomy tube. In: Wiegand DJ, Carlson KK, eds. *AACN Procedure Manual for Critical Care*. 6th edn. Philadelphia, PA: Elsevier Saunders, pp. 62–70.

Useful web sites

Health Care Improvement Scotland. Best Practice Statement. Caring for the patient with tracheostomy. Available at: https://www.evidence.nhs.uk/search?q=Tracheostomy%20 guidelines [Accessed October 2013]

Tracheostomy; The Guidelines – St James's Hospital. Available at: www.stjames.ie [Accessed October 2013]

Update on tracheostomy care. Available at: www.rn.com/ getpdf.php/615.pdf [Accessed October 2013]

14.3 Venepuncture

Sean Ninan

Yorkshire and the Humber Deanery, UK

Key points

- Ask the resident's permission before taking blood and explain the procedure to them.
- Wash your hands before taking blood.
- Venesection can be difficult in elderly patients: tips are given on how to improve the success rate of the procedure.
- Reminders are given on which sites to avoid.
- Remember to press on the venepuncture site for longer in residents who are taking warfarin.

Taking blood from a vein (venepuncture) is usually a straightforward procedure but can sometimes prove challenging in an elderly resident with fragile veins.

Equipment required

- Gloves.
- Tourniquet.
- Sharps bin and tray.
- Alcohol swab.
- Vacutainer (a sterile glass or plastic collection tube which draws up blood from a vein by creating a vacuum in the tube) or needle and syringe.
- Blood bottles (tubes).
- Cotton wool.
- Adhesive tape.

Procedure

- Explain the procedure to the resident.
- Identify a suitable vein. Veins in the antecubital fossa are usually the easiest to access for venepuncture. Alternative sites include the veins of the back of the hand or, more rarely, the foot (this can often be painful). A suitable vein can be identified by visual inspection and palpation. Clenching the fist or tapping gently over a vein may encourage venous distension.
- Position the resident's arm, for example by resting it on a pillow.
- Wash your hands thoroughly.
- Tie a tourniquet round the arm proximal to the site of venepuncture.
- Put on your gloves.
- Clean the site of infection using an alcohol swab. Allow to dry completely (note that there is no consensus on whether skin preparation with alcohol or other antiseptics is necessary before venepuncture).
- Do not touch the insertion site after cleaning the skin.
- Anchor the vein by tethering the skin below the vein with the thumb of your free hand. This will prevent the vein rolling when you insert the needle.
- Insert the needle at angle of around 30°. The exact angle will depend on the size of the vein and the depth of the vein from the skin (e.g. for a small superficial vein, a shallower angle may be required).
- When you have entered the vein, reduce the angle slightly and advance the needle, if required, so as to position the needle in the lumen of the vein. Attach the vacutainer tube.
- Release the tourniquet.
- Collect samples in the order recommended by the manufacturer.
- As you remove the needle, apply pressure over the insertion site with a cotton wool swab.
- Apply tape to secure the cotton wool.
- Label your tubes at the bedside.
- Safely discard unwanted material.

The Care Home Handbook, First Edition. Edited by Graham Mulley, Clive Bowman, Michal Boyd and Sarah Stowe.
© 2015 John Wiley & Sons, Ltd. Published 2015 by John Wiley & Sons, Ltd.

Sites to avoid

- The same side as a mastectomy.
- The same side as an arterio-venous fistula.
- The same side as a current blood transfusion.
- Sites above an IV infusion.
- A scarred area.
- An infected area.

Tips for difficult venepuncture

- Try applying a heat pack or immersing the limb in warm water for 10 minutes.
- A needle and syringe may be preferable to a vacu-tainer system as 'flashback' can be seen when the vein is entered.
- For small fragile veins, a smaller needle, and the smallest possible syringe, may improve success rates. For small superficial veins, a 'butterfly' needle may be easier to manipulate.

Other points

When leaving the resident, ensure that no equipment (particularly needles) is left lying around.

Warfarin procedures – apply pressure after the needle is withdrawn for a longer period of time (2–5 minutes), watch for bleeding and bruising at the area of the venpuncture.

Further reading

Dougherty L, Lister S. 2008. Venepuncture. In: *The Royal Marsden Hospital Manual of Clinical Nursing Procedures*. 7th edn. Wiley Blackwell, pp. 919–931.

Sutton CD, White SA, Edwards R, Lewis HH. 1999. A prospective controlled trial of the efficacy of isopropyl alcohol wipes before venesection in surgical patients *Annals of the Royal College of Surgeons England* 81: 183–186.

14.4 Fractures, casts and splints

Sadia Ismail

Leeds Teaching Hospitals NHS Trust, Leeds, UK

Key points

- Bone pain after a fall might indicate a fracture – especially if the limb is swollen, bruised, red or deformed and if the resident cannot bear weight on that limb.
- If a fracture is suspected, an x-ray is necessary.
- Casts and splints help to immobilise limbs: it is important to examine them frequently to ensure that there are no ulcers or signs of skin infection.

The most common problem caused by osteoporosis is a fracture: about 1 in 2 women over 50 will break a bone. Therefore, there are many older residents with fractures.

This section will deal with fractures of the limbs, not the back.

What to do if you suspect a limb fracture

If an older person falls and experiences pain as a result, a simple assessment can determine whether a fracture is likely (Table 14.4.1).

If these steps indicate a likely fracture, *the resident must have an x-ray and then possibly manipulation, immobilisation or an operation.*

Splints and casts

Many different types of splints (Figure 14.4.1) and casts (Figure 14.4.2) can be used to position a limb for optimal fracture healing (Table 14.4.2). Generally, *splints* are easily removable and can be custom-made or ready-made, whereas *casts* are not easily removable and are custom-made from fibreglass or plaster.

Table 14.4.1 Assessment to ascertain a limb fracture.

Inspect	Is the limb swollen? Bruised? Red? Deformed? Is there a visible injury? Is it being held at an odd angle?
Palpate	*Gently* touch the injured area – is there crepitus (a crunching sound/feeling)? Is it warm? Can you feel a pulse below the injury? Is it an abnormal shape when compared with the other side?
Sensation	Can they feel light touch on the injured side or is it numb?
Mobility	*Gently* assess for pain and the ability to move the area normally. In lower limb/pelvic fractures, the clue is usually severe pain and an inability to tolerate putting weight through the affected side. In this case ask the resident to *stop* any weight bearing as walking may worsen separation of the bones and affect healing of the fracture

The Care Home Handbook, First Edition. Edited by Graham Mulley, Clive Bowman, Michal Boyd and Sarah Stowe.
© 2015 John Wiley & Sons, Ltd. Published 2015 by John Wiley & Sons, Ltd.

(a) (b)

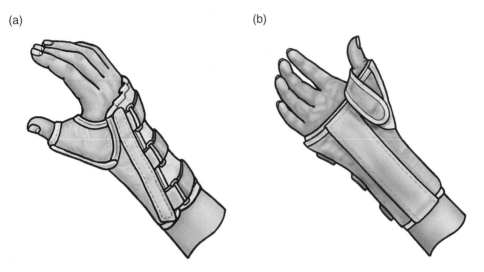

Figure 14.4.1 Wrist splint. Courtesy of Paul Brown, Medical Illustrator, Medical Illustrations Department, Leeds Teaching Hospitals Trust, UK.

(a) (b)

(c)

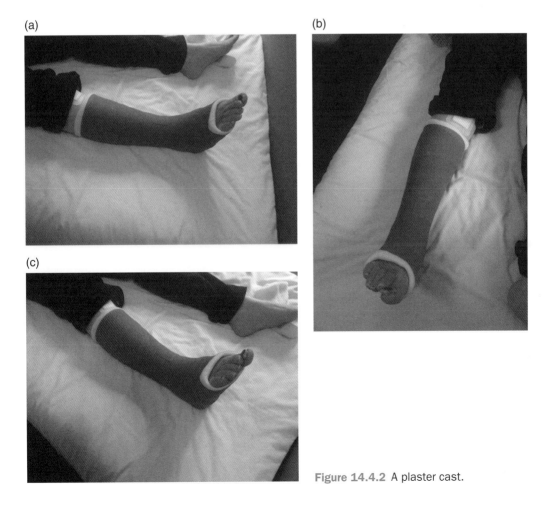

Figure 14.4.2 A plaster cast.

Table 14.4.2 Splints and casts.

Item	Used for	Advantages	Risks/problems
Splint	• Some fractures • Sprains • Tendon injuries • Injuries awaiting orthopaedic review or intervention	• Dynamic – can allow movement • Can be static • Fewer complications • Easier application and removal	⊗ Compliance ⊗ ↓ Range of movement ⊗ Cannot use if fracture potentially unstable
Cast	• Definitive management of many fractures • Soft tissue injuries unsuitable for splinting	• Better immobilisation • Allow better positioning and healing • Better compliance	⊗ More complications e.g. nerve compression ⊗ Technically difficult to apply

Common risks or complications of casts

- Swelling:
  - Leads to pressure effects such as nerve damage or blood vessel damage which can be permanent
- Non-union/malunion:
  - This is where the fracture does not heal properly.
  - Can be due to intrinsic poor healing.
  - Can be a result of weight-bearing on a broken leg, for example.
- Pain:
  - Due to the cast, the fracture or swelling of the affected area.
- DVT:
  - Common if mobility is reduced in people with fractures
  - Patient may complain of a red, hot, tender, swollen calf.
  - Measure both calves and *seek medical advice*.
- Cellulitis/skin irritation or infection:
  - If you see redness of the skin disappearing into the cast *seek medical advice* as the cast may need to be removed to inspect and treat the irritation or infection.

Conclusions

- Preventing falls prevents fractures (see Chapter 6.6).
- If a resident with a fracture or suspected fracture has persistent severe pain on using the limb in question, *stop* and *seek medical advice* as the fracture may be becoming unstable.
- Inspect skin under a splint and around the borders of a cast regularly in case of pressure areas, ulcers, skin infections or cellulitis.
- Ensure weight-bearing status is clarified and followed consistently.
- Remain alert for signs and symptoms of DVT.
- Encourage the resident to keep a cast dry, clean and not to scratch.

Acknowledgement

I wish to thank Carole Clifford for her helpful advice with this chapter.

Useful web sites

Managing falls and fractures in care homes for older people – good practice self assessment resource. Available at: www.scswis.com [Accessed October 2013]

Splints and Casts – Indications and Methods. Available at: www.aafp.org/afp/2009/0901/p491. html [Accessed October 2103]

Chapter 15

Clinical Measurement and Observations

15.1 The pulse

Claire Rushton[1] and Peter Crome[2]

[1]Keele University, Keele, UK
[2]Department of Primary Care and Population Health, University College London, London, UK

Key points

- The pulse rate can be fast, slow or irregular in healthy as well as ill residents.
- Determining whether the pulse is abnormal is very important.
- Always check the apex of a resident with atrial fibrillation before giving then Digoxin – if the apex is <60, omit the dose.
- Inform the doctor if the pulse is too fast, too slow or there is a change in pulse volume.

Measuring and recording a resident's pulse forms part of regular clinical assessment and provides nurses with important information in relation to cardiovascular health.

The pulse is initiated by the ejection of blood from the left ventricle of the heart. The blood flows into the aorta and to the rest of the arterial system and, as the arteries expand to accommodate the ejected blood, a pulse is formed.

A pulse will vary across individuals and within the same individual, according to a variety of circumstances, but recognition of both abnormal pulse signs and a change to a resident's normal pulse, can trigger early investigation and medical management of the resident.

Measuring the pulse

- A pulse can be detected wherever arterial blood flows close to the surface of the body and can be measured using a range of techniques, including automated blood pressure devices (see Chapter 15.2), cardiac monitors, stethoscopes or manually.
- Manual measurement can be the most useful method, as detailed information in relation to the rate, rhythm and volume of the pulse can be sought.
- The most common pulse points are the brachial and the radial points.
- Peripheral vascular disease can weaken or prevent the detection of pulses, particularly in areas that are most distal to the heart (such as the feet).

- The nurse uses two fingers placed over the pulse point, lightly pressing the artery over the bone and records the pulse for one minute. If the pulse point is pressed too firmly, this can reduce the blood flow and prevent an accurate reading.

Rate

- A normal heart rate is between 60 and 100 beats per minute (bpm). Less than 60 bpm is called bradycardia and more than 100 bpm is known as tachycardia (see Chapter 9.8).
- The heart rate is controlled by the nervous system and the rate naturally increases to meet cardiac demand during exercise, pain and anxiety. The heart rate in these circumstances would normally gradually increase and then reduce once the stimulus is removed.

For this reason, it is always best to record the resident's pulse when they are relaxed and rested.

- *Any sustained tachycardia should be documented in the nurse's notes and further investigation and referral considered.*
- It is normal for older people to have a slightly slower than normal heart rate because of changes in the conduction pathways in the heart during ageing. Providing that the pulse is regular and stable and the resident is not experiencing low blood pressure, falls or dizziness, then this will normally not need intervention.

The Care Home Handbook, First Edition. Edited by Graham Mulley, Clive Bowman, Michal Boyd and Sarah Stowe.
© 2015 John Wiley & Sons, Ltd. Published 2015 by John Wiley & Sons, Ltd.

However, progressive heart block leading to complete heart block can be well tolerated in some older people – even at rates as low as 25–40 bpm. Despite current tolerance of this rhythm, intervention (perhaps with a pacemaker) will be required.

Other causes of abnormal heart rates can be related to underlying disease processes and medication and will require individual assessment.

Whatever the rate abnormality, immediate attention should be given to investigating the impact of the heart rate on the resident's overall haemodynamic status and symptoms, such as whether the individual is experiencing dizziness.

Rhythm

* A normal pulse should be regular. An irregular pulse can be normal (sinus dysrhythmia) but may be a sign of conduction abnormalities and will require further investigation. Irregularity should be recorded in the nurse's notes and used as a trigger for further investigation and assessment. A 12-lead ECG where available should be recorded (see Chapter 15.7).
* The most common abnormal irregularity in old age is atrial fibrillation (AF) with around 10% of people over 80 years having this condition.

Atrial fibrillation

Early detection of AF is important, as it is a major predisposing factor for stroke. AF is a conduction defect where the natural pacemaker of the heart (the sinus node) is replaced by atrial conductions. These atrial electrical waves are discharged in a completely erratic manner, commonly up to 300–500 discharges per minute. Fortunately, most of these waves are blocked from being transmitted through to the ventricles by the atrio-ventricular node.

The electrical waves that are transmitted through to the ventricles will usually result in ventricular contractions that are irregular and vary in strength. The apex is totally irregular.

Depending on the strength of the ventricular contraction, the resulting pulse may or may not be palpable via the radial or brachial pulse point. It is better in this circumstance to measure the pulse rate at the apex point using a stethoscope.

It is useful to document the resident's apex and radial pulse to indicate what this deficit might be.

Using oxygen saturation machines and automated blood pressure devices can give an inaccurate heart rate for patients in AF. A common medication for patients in AF is Digoxin, which slows the heart rate. *This drug should not be given to patients with a heart rate of less than 60 bpm.* This needs to be recorded at the apex for an accurate reading given the unreliability of the brachial and radial pulse in these residents.

Volume

The volume of the pulse is determined by the amount of blood pumped out by the left ventricle in each contraction, the strength of the contraction and the resident's blood pressure. Again, this will normally vary in response to the body's demands.

Any change to the resident's pulse volume should be recorded and reported to medical staff.

A thin and thready or weak pulse can indicate atherosclerosis (reduced elasticity of the arteries) or low blood pressure, which may be a result of heart failure (weak contraction) or dehydration (low blood volume) or both. Likewise, a strong and bounding pulse may indicate that the heart is working harder than normal and may be a result of fluid overload. Table 15.1.1 summarises pulse abnormalities and what to do about them.

Table **15.1.1** Summary of pulse abnormalities and what to do about them.

Pulse	Normal	Abnormal	Indication	Action
Rate	60–100 bpm	Less than 60 bpm	Bradycardia. Could be related to dysrhythmias (e.g. heart block), morbidities (e.g. cardiac disease), metabolic disturbances (e.g. hypothyroidism), medication (e.g. beta blockers, digoxin)	(1) Is this new or normal for the patient? (2) Blood pressure recording – is the resident maintaining their normal blood pressure?

(Continued)

Table 15.1.1 (Continued)

Pulse	Normal	Abnormal	Indication	Action
		More than 100 bpm	Tachycardia. Could be related to dysrhythmias (e.g. atrial/ventricular tachycardia), morbidities (e.g. cardiac disease), metabolic disturbances (e.g. hyperthyroidism), electrolyte disturbances, medication (e.g. Theophylline), stimulants (e.g. caffeine, alcohol), infection, stress/anxiety	(3) Record 12-lead ECG if able (4) Review medications and medical history (5) Has the resident had electrolytes monitored in the previous month? (6) Document findings and report to medical staff any change to the resident's normal status (7) Communicate findings to the rest of the health and social care team as appropriate
Rhythm	Regular	Irregular	Dysrhythmia (e.g. AF, sick sinus syndrome), electrolyte disturbances	
Volume	Normal strength	Weak/thready	Low blood pressure (e.g. in dehydration, heart failure)	
		Strong bounding	High blood pressure (e.g. in hypervolemia)	

Further reading

Kannel W, Wolf P, Benjamin E, Levy D. 1998. Prevalence, incidence, prognosis, and predisposing conditions for atrial fibrillation: population-based estimates. *American Journal of Cardiology* 16 (82(8A)):2N–9N.

15.2 Blood pressure measurement: lying, standing, sitting

Lauren Ralston[1] and Lynda Dorsey[2]

[1] Bradford Teaching Hospital Foundation Trust, Bradford, UK
[2] Leeds Teaching Hospitals NHS Trust, Leeds, UK

Key points

- Always record the blood pressure in residents on entry to the care home.
- The technique of taking the blood pressure ensures accuracy: try to record it with the resident standing, wherever possible.
- Hypertension can be the result of anxiety and pain but is an important risk factor for stroke and heart attack.
- Hypotension is associated with falls. It is important to find the reason for low blood pressure (such as dehydration or drugs).

What is blood pressure?

Blood pressure (BP) refers to the pressure blood exerts against an artery wall as the heart beats. It is measured in millimetres of mercury (mmHg). Two values are recorded: the first is the systolic reading and the second is the lower diastolic reading

The systolic reading: This is the pressure against the artery wall whilst the heart contracts. This is the first and larger reading to be recorded.

The diastolic reading: This is the pressure against the artery wall whilst the heart is resting, that is between beats. This is the second and lower reading.

For example, if the systolic reading was 130 and the diastolic reading was 70 this would be denoted as 130/70.

Why measure blood pressure?

Blood pressure changes with age, the older population are prone to both hypertension (high blood pressure) and hypotension (low blood pressure) (Table 15.2.1). Hypertension is associated with an increased risk of strokes and heart attacks and can be exacerbated by stress, pain and anxiety. Hypotension is associated with symptoms such as dizziness, blurred vision and increased risk of falls and may be exacerbated by dehydration, infection and medications.

All new residents should have a blood pressure measurement documented on arrival in a care home to aid interpretation of future readings.

Table 15.2.1 Hypertension and hypotension

Low	Normal	High
<90/60 Risk of falls, injury and dizziness	<140/90 but >90/60	>140/90 Increased risk of heart attacks and strokes

Postural hypotension

Blood pressure is regulated by baroreceptors present in large vessels of the body; when an individual stands up, these sensors act to raise the heart rate and constrict blood vessels to maintain an adequate blood supply. In older people this mechanism can become impaired and may result in a drop in blood pressure on standing, which may lead to dizziness, blurred vision and falls. This problem may be exacerbated further by medications which lower the blood pressure, such as diuretics, anti-hypertensives, and some anti-depressants.

Postural hypotension is defined as a drop in systolic BP of >20 mmHg or a drop in diastolic BP greater than 10 mmHg on standing when compared to lying blood pressure values.

All patients entering care homes should have lying and standing (or lying and sitting) values documented. A postural drop in blood pressure is always significant and should trigger a GP assessment and medication review. In addition, conservative advice can be suggested:

- Rise from sitting to standing (or lying to sitting) slowly to allow BP stabilisation.
- Encourage individual to flex feet to increase blood flow.
- Ensure adequate hydration.

Measuring lying and standing blood pressure

Many care homes use automated blood pressure machines and all users should be trained in their use. Such machines are easy and safe to use, however, they require frequent calibration and may not be as accurate in individuals with an irregular pulse, for example atrial fibrillation. To measure lying and standing blood pressure:

1. Gain consent and explain the procedure to the person.
2. Ensure the individual is lying down and relaxed for at least 5 minutes.
3. Remove any tight clothing from their upper arm.
4. Select an appropriate sized cuff – Table 15.2.2. The bladder should surround approximately 80% of the upper arm.
5. Support the arm to be used at the level of the heart, for example with a pillow: Figure 15.2.1.
6. Place the cuff over the upper arm, aligning the centre of the cuff over the brachial artery (often indicated by the brachial artery indicator): Figure 15.2.2.

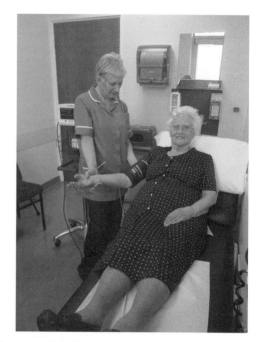

Figure 15.2.1 Support the arm to be used at the level of the heart, for example with a pillow.

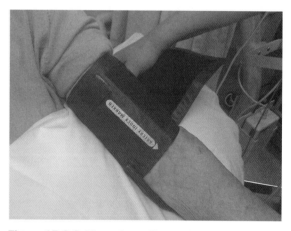

Figure 15.2.2 Place the cuff over the upper arm aligning the centre of the cuff over the brachial artery (often indicated by the brachial artery indicator).

7. Switch on the automated device and press start.
8. Document the systolic and diastolic readings.
9. Leave the cuff in place and ask the resident to stand, support as required.
10. Allow resident to stand for 1 minute.

Table 15.2.2 From BHS guidelines, 2006.

	Arm circumference (cm)	Bladder width and length (cm)
Small adult	<23	12×18
Standard adult	<33	12×26
Large adult	<50	12×40

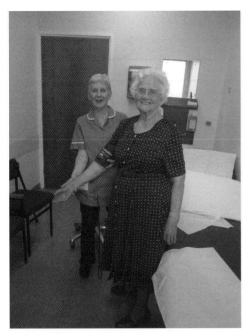

Figure 15.2.3 Supporting the arm at the level of the heart, press 'start'.

Documentation

- Record BP as systolic over diastolic, for example 120/80.
- If required, chart BP on a graph using dots or checkmarks, clearly marking lying and standing/sitting values.
- Document limb used and resident's position.
- Document person notified about BP result and any required action.

---

11. Supporting arm at the level of the heart, press 'start': Figure 15.2.3.
12. Help the individual to sit/lie down.
13. Document reading.
14. Switch off automated device, remove cuff.
15. Compare readings with previous blood pressure readings and inform nurse in charge.

Sources of error

Inappropriate cuff size: If the cuff size is too large the blood pressure will be underestimated. If the cuff size is too small the blood pressure will be overestimated.

Atrial fibrillation: Blood pressure readings in atrial fibrillation can be unreliable; the accuracy may be improved with repeat readings. Whilst mercury devices may provide more accurate readings, such devices are no longer found in care home settings.

Audit ideas in the care home setting

- Ensure all new residents have a lying and standing/sitting BP taken on arrival at the care home. If a significant drop is present, that is the patient has orthostatic hypotension, request a GP medication review. Audit the impact this has on falls in your care home.
- Audit the use of the appropriate cuff size by nursing staff to measure your resident's BP. If problems were identified you can then provide education to improve the practice and the accuracy of your readings.

15.3 Respiratory rate and oxygen saturation

Rachel Hepherd[1] and Claire Sissons[2]

[1] *Hull and East Yorkshire Hospitals NHS Trust, Hull, UK*
[2] *Highfield Nursing Home, Tadcaster, UK*

Key points

- The respiratory rate is the number of breaths per minute.
- It is part of the Early Warning Score.
- A rapid respiratory rate can be the first (and only) sign of a chest infection.
- There are several reasons for a rapid and a reduced respiratory rate. Advice is given on what to do if the breathing is abnormal.
- One cause of breathlessness is reduced oxygen saturation of blood – this can be measured by pulse oximetry.

Respiratory rate

The respiratory rate is arguably the most sensitive and easiest to measure of all clinical observations.

Measuring the respiratory rate can provide useful information on altered state of health from a variety of causes, including pain, underlying infection, underlying chronic lung disease or drug toxicity.

A rapid respiratory rate may be the first – and only – obvious sign of a potentially serious chest infection. It is therefore very important to measure the rate accurately at all times

How is it calculated and measured?

- Respiratory rate is the number of full breaths taken in one minute.
- The simplest way to measure respiratory rate is simply to count the number of breaths taken in one minute.
- To ensure your measurement is accurate, try not to allow the resident to become aware of what you are doing.
- Continuing to palpate the radial pulse while counting breaths often helps.

What is a normal respiratory rate?

According to most Early Warning Systems used in hospitals, normal respiratory rate is 9–14 breaths per minute (see Chapter 15.8).

Table 15.3.1 Possible causes of abnormal respiratory rates.

High respiratory rate (>14)	Low respiratory rate (<9)
Pain	Drug toxicity
Respiratory tract infections	Cheyne–Stokes
Underlying chronic lung disease	respiration*
Lung cancer	Spinal cord
Aspiration of foodstuffs/secretions	injury
Anxiety	
Cardiac causes (e.g. angina, heart failure)	
Sepsis/other systemic illness	

*Cheyne–Stokes respiration is a pattern of breathing associated with ischaemia to the brainstem and is seen frequently following a stroke or near the end of life. It can also occur in sleep and sometimes in apparently healthy old people. It is characterised by a period of apnoea (no breathing), followed by periods of rapid breathing.

The Care Home Handbook, First Edition. Edited by Graham Mulley, Clive Bowman, Michal Boyd and Sarah Stowe.
© 2015 John Wiley & Sons, Ltd. Published 2015 by John Wiley & Sons, Ltd.

What could cause an abnormal respiratory rate?

Possible causes of an abnormal respiratory rate are highlighted in Table 15.3.1.

What should I do if I identify an abnormal respiratory rate?

- Look at the resident.
- Ask if they are in pain, or if they are unable to speak, do they appear to be in pain? (See Chapter 8.6.) Simple analgesia may be all that is required.
- Are they anxious and do they just need the comfort of reassurance?
- Is this pattern of breathing normal for them, especially in cases of known underlying lung disease? Do they appear chesty or unwell? Could they have aspirated?
- *If you are in any doubt or are concerned then consult a doctor.*

Oxygen saturations

Oxygen saturations, (sometimes called pulse) is the proportion of oxygen bound to haemoglobin in the blood and is expressed as a percentage.

It is measured using a pulse oximeter, a device which is placed on the finger.

Why is it important to measure oxygen saturations?

Low oxygen saturations (low blood oxygen) can explain why a person becomes breathless. Normal oxygen saturations are generally regarded as 96–100%. In certain situations (such as chronic lung diseases), lower saturations can be a normal finding. However, because of the way in which oxygen binds to haemoglobin, a relatively small drop in saturation (e.g. to 92%) can mean a clinically significant fall in blood oxygen and therefore be indicative of a serious underlying problem that requires prompt medical assistance.

Further reading

Cretikos MA, Bellomo R, Hillman K, et al. 2008. Respiratory rate: the neglected physical sign. *Medical Journal of Australia* 188: 657–659.

Kenzaka T Okayama M, Kuroki S, et al. 2012. Importance of vital signs to the early diagnosis and severity of sepsis. *Internal Medicine* 51: 871–876.

15.4 Temperature

John Gladman[1] and Graham Mulley[2]

[1]*University of Nottingham, Nottingham, UK*
[2]*University of Leeds, Leeds, UK*

Key points

- Accurate temperature recording is a centrally important clinical skill.
- If a resident becomes non-specifically unwell, always check their temperature.
- Mercury thermometers are no longer in use and have been replaced by digital and chemical devices.
- The site for temperature taking varies with the individual resident, but tympanic measurements are now widely used.
- Hypothermia can be a sign of underlying infection.
- The cause of fever or low temperature must be determined – the GP should be informed.

Accurate temperature recording is an important nursing skill. Feeling the skin is not a reliable way of measuring temperature, so if someone is ill, it is worth measuring their temperature – even if they do not feel hot or cold. There are several types of thermometer and different sites for measuring body temperature.

Which thermometer?

- Mercury in glass: these are cheap, low-tech, reliable, portable and accurate but because of potential hazards (broken glass causing cuts; inhalation of mercury from broken thermometers; environmental hazards) are no longer available. They should not be used. However, some care homes still have them: they should be disposed of carefully (the pharmacist may be able to help).
- Gallium in glass: these have been found to be inadequate in old people.
- Electronic devices: these record temperatures rapidly. They have a flexible tip and are convenient for residents and staff. Some have a limited battery life.
- Chemical: small, flat devices with about 50 dots that change colour at specific temperatures. Disposable single use ones are useful if there is a suspicion of

C. difficile (see Chapter 13.4) as they reduce the risk of cross-infection. They do not register hypothermia accurately.
- Crystal: these liquid crystal strip thermometers have temperature-sensitive colour bars that change colour when held against the forehead.

Which site?

- Oral: may not record accurately if the mouth is dry. Agitated residents may damage their teeth on them.
- Axillary: it takes eight minutes to record peripheral temperature.
- Rectal: rarely measured, but useful when using a low-temperature thermometer to diagnose hypothermia.
- Forehead: crystal thermometers can be inaccurate if the resident is perspiring.
- Tympanic: gives a measure of deep body (or core) temperature. Sometimes difficult to insert because or different anatomy of the auditory canal, problems can arise because of soreness caused by in-ear hearing aids or by otitis media.
- Urinary: measuring the temperature of freshly voided urine is useful to confirm hypothermia.

The Care Home Handbook, First Edition. Edited by Graham Mulley, Clive Bowman, Michal Boyd and Sarah Stowe.
© 2015 John Wiley & Sons, Ltd. Published 2015 by John Wiley & Sons, Ltd.

Temperature in old age

Whereas younger people use a variety of metabolic and behavioural changes to keep cool when it is hot or keep warm when it is cold, frail older people are at risk of hypothermia or heatstroke.

Although heatstroke is easy to suspect, because it occurs only in heatwaves, hypothermia can occur at normal room temperatures even in warm climates and not just during winter freezes.

Hypothermia, a temperature of 35 °C (centigrade) or less, is a classic example of the 'loss of homeostasis' or vulnerability to environmental challenges that can occur in older people.

Hypothermia produces only subtle signs and can be a cause of a non-specific decline, so *measuring a resident's temperature should be one of the first simple things to do when assessing a person for a non-specific decline.*

The underlying changes that render frail old people liable to hypothermia mean that changes in the body temperature are not so consistently seen as in younger people, and this makes interpretation difficult. For example, a person can have a rampant infection and their temperature can be normal or even low; or run a low grade fever without any ill health (see Chapter 9.9).

If the temperature is low or high, the cause must be identified and treated – you should inform the resident's GP in the first place

Further reading

Fadzil FM, Choon D, Arumigan K. 2012. A comparison study on the accuracy of non-invasive thermometers. *Australia Family Physician* 39: 237–239.

Giantin V, Toffanello Ed, Enzi G, et al. 2008. Reliability of body temperature measurements in hospitalised older patients. *Journal of Clinical Nursing* 17: 1518–1525.

15.5 Pulmonary function tests

Natalia Gunaratna[1] and Sarah Morris[2]

[1]*Leeds Teaching Hospitals NHS Trust, Leeds, UK*
[2]*University College London Medical School, London, UK*

Key points

- Lung function tests can help to diagnose the cause of breathlessness and guide treatment.
- The simplest measure is how far a resident can walk in 6 minutes.
- A hand-held peak flow meter is easy to use; it measures the degree of airway obstruction.
- Spirometry usually requires a trip to hospital. It measures the amount and speed of air exhaled and requires the cooperation of the resident.
- More sophisticated tests (such as gas exchange) are always done in hospital.

Breathlessness is common in older residents. However, the signs and symptoms are often non-specific and there are many causes. Objective investigations can help in determining the underlying condition(s).

Pulmonary function tests (PFTs) are reproducible and validated measurements of breathing – simply: how *fast, forcefully* and how *much* air can be blown out.

- Full PFTs are recorded with a *spirometer* in hospital clinics. Spirometry means measuring the breath. This apparatus consists of a tube and a mouthpiece for breathing into which is attached to a device that interprets and records the airflow measurements.
- PFTs can also assess how well gases can pass across the lungs. They detect airflow disturbances and abnormal gas exchange patterns that can help diagnose respiratory causes of breathlessness and hence guide appropriate treatment.
- A far more common, home-based method of testing is via the *peak flow device*. This is a small hand-held cylinder, with an exhalation port and graduated measurement markings along its length. It is best used in a standing or seated position. A smaller low-flow device can be used for older residents, which is lighter to handle and more sensitive to small changes in airflow.
- The peak flow device measures the ability to breathe out air and reflects the degree of obstruction in the bronchi.

Box 15.5.1 How to prepare the resident before having pulmonary function testing in hospital

The resident should avoid:

- Eating a large meal for 2 hours
- Smoking for at least 1 hour
- Consuming alcohol for 40 minutes
- Performing vigorous exercise for 30 minutes

Record your resident's weight in kg and height in cm (without shoes), especially if they have difficulty mobilising.
Make sure the resident is not wearing tight-fitting clothes.
Leave well-fitting dentures in place.
The requesting doctor may leave instructions to hold off bronchodilating inhalers for a few hours – *check this*.
Ensure the resident or escort has a full list of doses of current and recent medications to hand.
Inform the technicians if the resident has:*

- Haemoptysis (coughing up blood)
- Bleeding gums
- Open sores on the mouth or lips
- Active pulmonary TB.

*Any of these will affect equipment cleaning, timing and location of testing. However, it is important to note that there is no direct evidence that routine PFTs pose an increased risk of infection.

- General assessments of exercise tolerance can also reflect lung function. Structured tests such as the 6-minute walk (recording the total distance travelled) are easy to conduct in any long corridor. However, results are influenced by several factors including height, age, gender, muscle strength, joint disease; and encouragement, making them less reliable as direct measures of lung function.

Indications

- The most frequent indication for PFTs is to confirm a clinical diagnosis of Chronic Obstructive Pulmonary Disease (COPD) or to help distinguish COPD from asthma. These diseases result in an *obstructive* pattern of breathing (slowed flow from narrow airways and destruction of lung tissue from smoking and chronic inflammation).
- The second most frequent indication is in suspected lung fibrosis, which shows a *restrictive* pattern of airflow (small lung volumes).
- PFTs are also sometimes required to help overall lung capacity, which may determine an individual's suitability to undergo serious surgery.

Where possible, it is best practice to help confirm a suspected diagnosis of COPD with spirometry. Although diagnosis relies on complex clinical assessment and requires more than PFTs alone, it is important that older people do not miss out on the potential diagnostic benefits of testing. These practical suggestions are aimed at helping you facilitate safe and optimal testing for your resident.

The tests

The resident will be asked to breathe through tubing with a microbial filter, into the spirometer (Figure 15.5.1) and will wear a nose clip to stop air leak.

They will take a full breath in; breathe out once slowly and fully; and again fast and forcefully. This may be repeated to check consistency of the readings or repeated after administering bronchodilator inhalers.

The tests are usually well tolerated but can be physically demanding for some individuals. The resident is required to:

- Be seated *or* standing for about 30 minutes (they can be in a wheelchair).
- Be able to cooperate with verbal instructions.
- Be able to seal their lips well around tubing.
- Tolerate enclosure in a sealed box (so ask about claustrophobia).

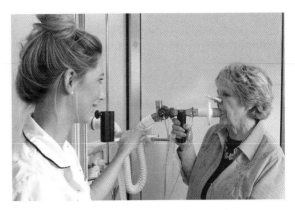

Figure 15.5.1 Measuring PFTs using a spirometer in hospital.

Box 15.5.2 Risks of undergoing PFTs

Blowing hard can increase the pressure in the resident's eyes, abdomen and chest. There are a few conditions which make spirometry less safe:

- Unstable angina

Recent:

- Pneumothorax ('collapsed lung')
- Heart attack
- Stroke
- Haemoptysis (coughing blood) without known cause
- Eye or abdominal surgery

Results may be inaccurate if the resident:

- Has chest or abdominal pain of any cause
- Has oral or facial pain
- Suffers from stress urinary incontinence
- Has cognitive impairment
- Is obese and cannot stand
- Has ill-fitting dentures (these should be temporarily removed)

Check with the requesting doctor if you are concerned about any of these.

Results

The results are reported as forced expiration over time. This is expressed as the proportion of the amount of breath that can be blown out in 1 second over the total amount of air that can be blown out in one breath. Lung disease severity is based on the resident's spirometry results compared to what would be predicted for a person of the same age. The results do not give an absolute diagnosis, but are valuable in informing clinical assessment and helping guide treatment and may be repeated in future follow up.

Further reading

Cooper K, Mitchell P. 2003. Procedure for the assessment of lung function with spirometry. *Nursing Times* 99(23): 57.

Levy M, Quanjer PH, Booker R, et al. 2009. Diagnostic Spirometry in Primary Care: Proposed standards for general practice compliant with American Thoracic Society and European Respiratory Society recommendations. *Primary Care Respiratory Journal* **18**(3): 130–147.

National Institute for Clinical Excellence. 2010. *Management of Adults with Chronic Obstructive Lung Disease in Primary and Secondary Care*. London, NICE.

Pearce L. 2011. Understanding spirometry. *Nursing Times* 107: 422.

15.6 Head injury observations

Angela Juby[1] and Sandra Kavanagh[2]

[1]University of Alberta, Edmonton, Alberta, Canada
[2]South Terrace Continuing Care Centre, Edmonton, Alberta, Canada

Key points

- In all cases of head injury, inform the GP and the family.
- Unless the resident has previously stipulated otherwise, arrange urgent transport of the unconscious resident (or one with fluctuating consciousness) to hospital.
- Assessment and documentation should include lacerations and bruises, eye movements, pupil inequality, motor responses, gait pattern and speech, as well as vital signs and blood glucose.
- Contact the resident's family and physician immediately in all circumstances.
- Examine for scalp lacerations or bruises. Dress any scalp wounds as needed.
- The circumstances of the fall may also be helpful in determining the possibility of injury.

The unconscious head injured resident needs assessment in hospital, and transfer should be arranged – unless this is against the advance directives (see Chapter 16.1) of the resident. Always check the blood glucose as a priority.

In cases where there is an altered level of consciousness as the result of a head injury, again transfer to hospital should be considered – if this is in accordance with the resident's and their family's wishes. Discuss the situation with the GP or nurse practitioner. Again, you must check the blood glucose.

If the decision is for the resident to remain at the care home, then a member of staff has to take responsibility for monitoring them.

- Ensure that the altered level of consciousness happened after the fall/injury and not before so as to rule our pre-existing conditions (see Chapter 10.2). When in doubt, assume they are delirious too and complete the necessary evaluation/investigations to identify treatable causes of this.
- Measure vital signs (blood pressure, pulse rate, oxygen saturations, respiratory rate) (see Chapter 15.8) and document the presence of nausea and pain every 4 hours for the first 24 hours, then reassess the frequency of evaluations. Inform their physician if these measures are different from baseline.
- Check the blood glucose with a glucometer, and repeat if abnormal. Inform the physician if the readings are abnormal.
- Examine the pupils of the eyes. Check to see if they are the same or if one is bigger than the other. Shine a light in their eyes and see if both the pupils contract. Note that in many elderly patients who have had eye surgery, the pupils can be misshapen or asymmetrical.
- If they are mobile, assess their walking pattern and note any changes, for example, one-sided weakness of the arm or leg. Similarly, if they are talking, assess their speech to see if it is slowed or slurred in comparison to before the fall. Contact the physician if abnormalities are noted (see Chapter 8.1).

The Glasgow Coma Scale (see Appendix 1.2) is a reliable, objective neurological scale which grades best eye, verbal and motor responses and scores these. (The lower the score, the more serious the head injury.) This should be used initially and when continuing to monitor the injured resident.

A simpler scale is the abbreviated AVPU coma scale: **a**lert; responds to **v**ocal stimuli; responds to **p**ain; **u**nresponsive

The Care Home Handbook, First Edition. Edited by Graham Mulley, Clive Bowman, Michal Boyd and Sarah Stowe.
© 2015 John Wiley & Sons, Ltd. Published 2015 by John Wiley & Sons, Ltd.

What is most important in these situations, is that the resident is assessed and monitored by a care provider who has previous knowledge of them, their behaviour, their breathing pattern and their gait. Ensure that your assessment findings and monitoring details are clearly documented in the resident's case notes.

Further reading

Teasdale G, Jennet B. 1974. Assessment of coma and impaired consciousness. A practical scale. Lancet 2: 81–84.

15.7 Electrocardiogram (ECG) and ambulatory ECG

Tajammal Zahoor[1] and Mahwesh Rafique[2]

[1]Edinburgh Royal Infirmary, Edinburgh, UK
[2]Pinderfield's Hospital, Wakefield, UK

Key points

- The standard ECG is a machine which produces a paper record of the electrical activity of the heart.
- It is a useful investigation in the diagnosis of rhythm disorders of the heart, such as atrial fibrillation.
- The ECG can also be helpful in diagnosing a range of conditions, such as blackouts, chest pain, seizures and electrolyte abnormalities.
- The ECG may be normal but the resident might still have important heart disease.

Electrocardiogram (ECG)

Figure 15.7.1 shows the trace of a normal electrocardiogram.

What is the resting ECG used for?

Indications for electrocardiography include:

- Chest pain.
- Syncope or collapse.
- Seizures.
- Suspected cardiac dysrhythmias.
- Cardiac murmurs.
- To assess patients with systemic disease as well as monitoring during anesthesia; and monitoring critically ill patients.
- To see the effects of mineral abnormalities (such as low potassium levels).

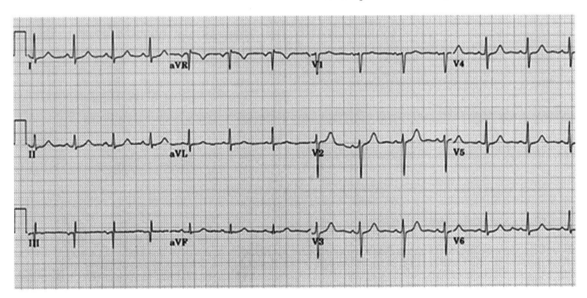

Figure 15.7.1 Example trace of normal electrocardiogram.

The Care Home Handbook, First Edition. Edited by Graham Mulley, Clive Bowman, Michal Boyd and Sarah Stowe.
© 2015 John Wiley & Sons, Ltd. Published 2015 by John Wiley & Sons, Ltd.

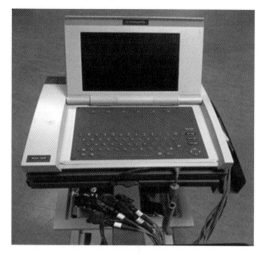

Figure 15.7.2 ECG machine with its leads.

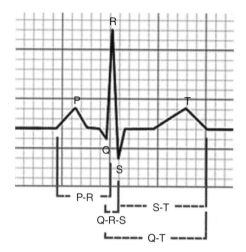

Figure 15.7.3 Waves and intervals.

How is an ECG performed?

- Up to 12 self-adhesive electrodes are attached to selected locations of the skin on the arms, legs and chest.
- I, II, III are bipolar limb leads. avR, avL , avF are unipolar limb leads and V1–V6 are the chest leads. Each of these 12 leads represents a particular orientation in space in relation to heart's electrical activity.
- Limb leads are attached as: red to right arm, yellow to left arm, green to left foot, black to right foot. All the chest leads are attached as indicated in Figure 15.7.2.
- Modern machine's electrodes indicate the position where electrodes should be attached.
- Areas where the electrodes are placed may need to be shaved.

The test is completely painless and takes less than a minute to perform once the leads are in position. The machine detects and amplifies the electrical impulses that occur at each heartbeat and records them on paper.

Waves and intervals

- *P wave*: represents the sequential activation (depolarisation) of the right and left atria (Figure 15.7.3).
- *QRS complex*: right and left ventricular depolarisation (normally the ventricles are activated simultaneously).
- *ST-T wave*: ventricular repolarisation.
- *PR interval*: time interval from onset of atrial depolarisation (P wave) to onset of ventricular depolarisation (QRS complex).

- *QRS duration*: duration of ventricular muscle depolarisation.
- *QT interval*: duration of ventricular depolarisation and repolarisation.
- *RR interval*: duration of ventricular cardiac cycle (an indicator of ventricular rate).

How to interpret the ECG

Principles of interpretation of ECG and examples of ECG patterns in different heart conditions are beyond the scope of this book and can be found for interested readers at www.ecglibrary.com and other sources listed in Further reading. Common abnormalities on ECG are atrial fibrillation, myocardial infarction, supra-ventricular tachycardia, bundle branch blocks (right and left) and atrio-ventricular blocks.

- Sinus rhythm: Every P wave should be followed by QRS complex, RR interval should be regular. Heart rate range should be 60–100 minute.
- Sinus tachycardia: Heart rate more than 100 per minute.
- Sinus bradycardia: Heart rate less than 60 per minute.

Limitations of the electrocardiogram

An ECG is a simple and valuable test, which can frequently diagnose a heart problem.

However, a normal ECG does not rule out serious heart disease.

Specialised ECG recordings, like exercise tolerance test or ambulatory ECG, sometimes help to overcome some limitations like angina or irregular heart beat where the recording can be normal between episodes.

Ambulatory ECG

- In ambulatory ECG the patient wears a small holter monitor. This records the electrical activity of heart when the resident is walking about (ambulatory) and doing their normal activities.
- It aims to detect abnormal heart rhythms that may come and go. The electrical activity is usually recorded for 24–48 hours. It is often used to rule out cardiac rhythm problem associated with syncope, dizziness and palpitations.
- The more sophisticated devices, like the event recorder or loop recorder, can record more infrequently occurring episodes when activated by the patient.

Further reading

British Columbia Guidelines and Protocols. 2004. Ambulatory ECG Monitoring (Holter Monitor and Patient-Activated Event Recorder) (revised 2007).

Hampton, JR. 2013. *The ECG Made Easy*, 8th Edn. Nottingham, Churchill Livingstone.

Society for Cardiological Science & Technology. 2010. Consensus guideline for recording a 12-lead ECG.

Useful web site

Alan E, Lindsay ECG learning center in cyberspace. Available at: http://library.med.utah.edu/kw/ecg [Accessed October 2013].

15.8 Modified Early Warning Score (MEWS)

Tajammal Zahoor[1] and Mahwesh Rafique[2]

[1]*Edinburgh Royal Infirmary, Edinburgh, UK*
[2]*Pinderfield Hospital, Wakefield, UK*

Key points

- The Modified Early Warning Score (MEWS) is a simple bedside scoring system for the assessment of unwell residents.
- It is based on physiological measurements that should be recorded at an initial assessment of all residents and again if they become unwell.
- These simple observations detect when a sick resident requires more frequent observations and further investigations in order to reduce the risks of cardiac arrest, admission to hospital (including a high dependency unit) and death.

All residents should have their vital signs routinely recorded on admission to the care home as a baseline score.

If the resident's condition suddenly deteriorates, reassessment of their vital signs can provide an indication of their physiological status, warranting medical review by either a senior nurse and/or the GP.

The Modified Early Warning (or MEWS, Figure 15.8.1) score is a record of the resident's physiological state. It is a good predictor of clinical decline and adverse outcomes: those with high MEWS scores are more likely to deteriorate, have a cardiac arrest, be admitted to critical care and die. They may benefit from more intensive medical input.

There are different versions of this score used in different countries. The basic score is based on four physiological observations (systolic blood pressure, heart rate, respiratory rate and temperature; and a clinical observation – the level of consciousness).

Here we describe a MEWS score which also includes urine output, oxygen saturations and pain (see Chapters 15.2, 15.2, 15.3, 15.4, Appendices 1.2 and 1.3).

All medical and nursing staff should receive information, instruction and training on the MEWS system. They should be comfortable with the scoring system and its documentation.

NB: The AVPU is a simplified version of the Glasgow Coma Scale. It is useful for recording the level of consciousness.

V is response to your voice (which might be by eye movement, speaking or vocalizing (e.g. by grunting or moaning) or moving).

P is for pain response.

Once vital signs have been measured, they are converted into numbers.

The higher the number, the more abnormal the vital signs.

MEWS 1–2: Observe the resident and repeat observations as directed in care plan or following discussion with the senior nurse or GP, if required.

Document all discussions and actions taken in the care home resident's records.

MEWS 3–4: Continue to carry out observations and consider increasing the frequency of observations.

Inform the nurse in charge and the GP about the health status of the resident, who may require a GP visit if the medical condition deteriorates.

MEWS 5 or above: Monitor observations frequently (every 30 minutes or so).

Contact the senior nurse and the GP to request an urgent visit to review the resident because of deterioration in the resident's condition.

If there is no improvement, discuss with the resident and their family the possibility of hospital admission.

If their condition deteriorates, consider calling for an emergency ambulance.

Use of a Modified Early Warning Scoring system can:

The Care Home Handbook, First Edition. Edited by Graham Mulley, Clive Bowman, Michal Boyd and Sarah Stowe.
© 2015 John Wiley & Sons, Ltd. Published 2015 by John Wiley & Sons, Ltd.

Score	3	2	1	0	1	2	3
Systolic BP	<45% e.g. 45–70 mmHg	<30% e.g. 70–89 mmHg	15% down e.g. 90–99 mmHg	Normal for resident e.g. 100–140 mmHg	15% up e.g. 140– 160 mmHg	30% up 160– 200 mmHg	>45% >200 mmHg
Heart rate (BPM)	<40	—	40–50	51–100	101– 110	111– 130	>130
Respiratory rate (RPM)	<8	—	8–11	12–20	21–25	26–30	>30
Oxygen saturations (%)	<85	>85	>90	>94	—	—	—
AVPU	—	—	—	Alert (A)	Voice (V)	Pain (P)	Unconscious (U)
Urine output (ml)	<80	80–119	120– 200	>200	>800	—	—
Pain score	Severe	Moderate	Mild	None	—	—	—

NB: The AVPU is a simplified version of the Glasgow coma scale. It is useful for
recording the level of consciousness.

V is response to your voice (which might be by eye movement, speaking or
vocalizing (e.g. by grunting or moaning) or moving).

P is for pain response.

Figure 15.8.1 Modified Early Warning Score (MEWS) chart. Reproduced from Burch et al. (2008) with permission from Elsevier.

- Improve the quality of monitoring.
- Improve communication within the multi-disciplinary team.
- Allow timely admissions to hospital, if appropriate.
- Support good medical judgement.
- Aid in securing appropriate assistance for sick residents.

However, the MEWS is not:

- A predictor of outcome.
- A comprehensive clinical assessment tool.
- A replacement for clinical judgement (though it is better than a general clinical assessment).

Who requires MEWS

In all high-risk residents, it is a good practice to monitor MEWS. They include:

- Unstable residents.
- Those who have stepped down from a higher level of care (e.g. recently transferred from hospital).
- Selected residents who are failing to progress.

In residents who are terminally ill, the use of MEWS scoring is inappropriate.

Where the responsible doctor decides that MEWS scoring is not appropriate, then this should be clearly written on the front of the observation chart.

Further reading

Burch VC, Tarr G, Morroni C. 2008. Modified early warning score predicts the need for hospital admission and in-hospital mortality. *Emergency Medicine Journal* 25: 674–678. doi: 10.1136/emj.2007.057661

National Institute for Health and Clinical Excellence. 2007. Acutely ill patients in hospital: Recognition of and response to acute illness in adults in hospital. Available at: www.nice.org.uk [Accessed October 2013]

National Patient Safety Agency. 2007. Recognizing and responding appropriately to early signs of deterioration in hospitalized patients. Available at: www.npsa.nhs.uk [Accessed October 2013]

Section I
The End of Life

Chapter 16

Dying and Death

16.1 Advance directives and end of life planning

Eileen Burns

Leeds Teaching Hospitals NHS Trust, Leeds, UK

Key points

- An advance directive states what treatment the resident would *not* want, should they lack capacity to make this decision in the future.
- It cannot be used to specify which treatment *should* be given.
- Discussions on end of life care should take place as soon as possible after the person is admitted to the care home.
- Each resident's preferences and priorities can be determined by such tools as the Gold Standards Framework.

What is an advance directive?

- An *advance directive* is a statement explaining what medical treatment the individual would *not* want in the future, should that individual 'lack capacity' (as defined in the UK by the Mental Capacity Act 2005) (see Chapter 4.6).
- Moreover, it can relate to *all* future treatment, not just that which may be immediately life-saving.
- An advance directive is legally binding in England and Wales.
- Except in the case where the individual decides to refuse life-saving treatment, it does not have to be written down – although most are, and a written document is less likely to be challenged.

The advantage of having an advanced directive is that it allows an individual to make decisions about their care should they lose capacity in the future.

An advanced directive cannot be used to request a specific medical intervention or to make an illegal request, for example assisted suicide.

It does not allow an individual to select another individual to make decisions on their behalf (this would require a Lasting (or Enduring) Power of Attorney.

An advance directive cannot be used to refuse treatment for mental health conditions.

To ensure validation a directive must be:

- signed,
- witnessed and
- freely written without coercion.

There must be no doubt about the person's capacity at the time of writing.

End of life care planning

End of life care planning allows an individual to express their views, preferences and wishes for their future care at the end of life.

The discussion should be between the health care worker and the individual but could also include family, friends, other health and social care workers.

- Care planning: is the first step in making care and treatment decisions for a person with a life-limiting illness, irrespective of their capacity to participate or to decide.
- Ideally, an end of life care plan should be introduced soon after the resident enters a care home.

The English national end of life care programme advocates the use of 'the preferred priorities of care' document (see Useful web sites)

The use of this document can allow an individual to express their wishes on resuscitation, religious/spiritual beliefs (see Chapter 16.8) or any specific instructions at time of death – for example, who they want to be with them, or what music is to be played.

It also includes their right to choose their place of death.

The Care Home Handbook, First Edition. Edited by Graham Mulley, Clive Bowman, Michal Boyd and Sarah Stowe.
© 2015 John Wiley & Sons, Ltd. Published 2015 by John Wiley & Sons, Ltd.

Box 16.1.1 Example of an end of life plan document

End of life care plan

Your preferences and priorities

In relation to your health, what has been happening to you?

> I have had a bad chest for a long time. My breathing is getting worse, I have had a lot of chest infections, I'm not eating and I am losing weight. I keep having to go into hospital but I have been told there is nothing more they can do for me.

What are your preferences and priorities for your future care?

I am afraid I will die gasping for breath and would like to die in my sleep.

I would like my daughter to be with me when I die but don't want my grandchildren to see me.

I have discussed with my carer that I do not want to be revived if my heart stops.

I also want to carry on smoking.

Where would you like to be cared for in the future?

I don't want to go into hospital again. I would like to die here.

Signature   Date

Please record any changes to your preferences and priorities here.

The Gold Standards Framework

- Initiation of these conversations is difficult but, if not undertaken, it is impossible to ascertain people's wishes and needs and therefore to plan appropriately.
- The Gold Standards Framework is a systematic, evidence-based approach to optimising care for residents nearing end of life and enables care homes to provide quality care for all residents.
- Holding regular Gold Standard Framework meetings can help build confidence in communication about end of life planning with residents and families with support and advice from the palliative care team.
- The plan should be kept in a prominent position and each care home should have a consistent system so that all staff can find a care plan whenever it may be needed.

See Box 16.1.1 for an example of a completed end of life care plan using The Preferred Priorities of Care document.

Box 16.1.2 Case study

Mr H, an 87 year old was admitted to a care home for palliative care following a diagnosis of lung cancer.

His condition rapidly deteriorated one morning. He became confused, distressed and very agitated. Staff attempted to do baseline observations, which included a blood glucose level which was found to be 2.1 mml. Following this, paramedics were called. While waiting for paramedics, an attempt was made to give Mr H oral glucose (Mr H was not diabetic).

The paramedics attempted resuscitation without success. In line with paramedic policy, this was deemed an 'unexpected death' and therefore the police were called. At this point the family arrived and were asked not to enter the room until the police had finished their investigations. The family later expressed how angry and distressed they were about the whole experience.

Exercise

Read the case study in Box 16.1.2.

Reflect on the events and consider how care planning could have improved the end of life experience for Mr H, his family and care workers.

Useful web sites

For information on Advanced Directives: www.patient.co.uk [Accessed October 2013]

For information on Lasting Powers of Attorney: www.justice.gov.uk [Accessed October 2013]

For preferred priorities of care (National end of life programme): http://www.endoflifecare.nhs.uk/ [Accessed October 2013]

For details of the Gold Standards Framework: www.goldstandardsframework.org.uk [Accessed October 2013]

16.2 Prognosis: when to stop observations and interventions

Julie Spencer[1] and Cath Gilpin[2]

[1]Armley Moor Health Centre, Leeds, UK
[2]Pudsey Health Centre, Leeds, UK

Key points

- When a resident is coming to the end of their life, there is no need to do many standard observations and procedures.
- The emphasis should switch to those practices which improve symptoms and comfort.
- Medications should be reviewed and, if possible, simplified or stopped.
- Looking for signs of distress is central to good care.
- Use a check list to ensure that nothing is overlooked.

Recognition of imminent death is important (see Chapter 16.4)

When a resident is nearing the end of life, changes to observations and interventions should be made.

- Consider the relevance or benefits of completing usual observations, such as blood pressure, temperature, blood glucose monitoring and so on. These observations should be stopped.
- Assessment of symptoms or signs of distress should be made more closely and frequently, for example pain, agitation, nausea, skin damage, breathlessness and other reasons for discomfort.
- Nursing interventions such as mouth care (see Chapter 5.7), pressure area care (see Chapter 5.6), and continence care (see Chapter 5.4) are now the priorities and should be carried out using a regular systematic approach.
- A standardised end of life pathway for the dying focuses on the last hours or days of life. This type of document can enhance a systematic approach.
- A medication review should be undertaken. With the support of the GP, all unnecessary medication should be discontinued. Symptom management medication only should be continued.
- Plans should be made to have anticipatory medications prescribed and available. These should include anti-emetics, analgesia, sedation, anti-secretory medications.

Check list to support good end of life care

- Early discussion with resident and relatives about wishes for future care.
- Complete an end of life care plan.
- Ensure everyone is aware that care plan exists and where to find it.
- Ensure 'Do not attempt resuscitation' document is completed and everyone is aware it exists and where to find it.
- Ensure anticipatory drugs are prescribed and unnecessary medication is discontinued.
- Discontinue unnecessary observations, and closely observe for distressing symptoms.
- Implement a systematic approach to symptom management.
- Ensure the GP reviews the resident every 14 days (in the UK) to ensure in due course that a death certificate will be accepted by the coroner's office.

Effective communication and open and honest discussions will improve the resident's and family's experience at the end of life.

The Care Home Handbook, First Edition. Edited by Graham Mulley, Clive Bowman, Michal Boyd and Sarah Stowe.
© 2015 John Wiley & Sons, Ltd. Published 2015 by John Wiley & Sons, Ltd.

Further reading

Clark J, Marshall B, Skeward K, Allan S. 2012. Staff perceptions of the impact of the Liverpool care pathway in aged residential care in New Zealand. *International Journal of Palliative Nursing* 18: 171–178.

Kinley J, Froggat K, Bennet MI. 2012. The effect of policy on end-of-life care practice within nursing care homes: A systematic review. *Palliative Nurse* 28(3): 164–168.

16.3 Resuscitation

Eileen Burns

Leeds Teaching Hospitals NHS Trust, Leeds, UK

Key points

- Cardio-pulmonary resuscitation is rarely effective in frail old people.
- Ideally, the individual's attitude to CPR should be ascertained and documented.
- Information on a resident's wishes should be shared with others when a resident is re-located (such as a hospital admission).
- Some residents do not have the capacity to make an informed decision on CPR. A medical decision on the resident's 'best interests' should then be made by the doctor.

What is cardio-pulmonary resuscitation?

- Cardio-pulmonary resuscitation (CPR) is a process intended to maintain the body's circulation and oxygenation of the blood so that essential functions of the body are sustained while measures are instituted to attempt to restore normal function of the heart or of the lungs.
- The process of CPR can appear brutal, and observation of a CPR attempt can be traumatic; the process involves vigorous chest wall compressions, which can fracture the ribs of a frail older person. Attempts to gain venous access, especially if via a large vein, can be distressing for relatives or other residents. Thus, wherever possible, privacy should be allowed.
- However, it also needs to be borne in mind that some resident's relatives do wish to observe CPR attempts.

Cardio-pulmonary resuscitation (CPR) is an emotive topic, and sometimes residents or their carers hold views which may not always be fully informed.

Role of nurses and doctors

- The role of care home staff along with other staff (such as GPs, community nurses or hospital staff where relevant) is to help residents and their families understand the rationales for CPR decisions and, where appropriate, participate in the process of decision-making.

- In general, doctors have a duty to offer patients the treatments from which they believe their patients are likely to benefit. Patients (and their families) have no right (in law) to require a doctor to institute any treatment which the doctor believes to have no significant chance of helping the patient and which therefore s/he believes to be futile.

Capacity to decide on CPR

- Residents have a right to accept or refuse the advice of their doctor, and the doctor must respect the resident's wishes, whether or not the doctor believes the resident's acceptance or refusal to be sensible. The exception to this is when the resident is assessed as lacking the capacity to make the decision (see Chapter 4.6).
- CPR is a treatment and the decision to offer this treatment or withhold it is a medical one, based upon a careful assessment of the likelihood that the recipient of the CPR will benefit from the treatment.
- If the medical assessment is that the resident may benefit from CPR, then the treatment should be instituted if the person suffers a failure of the cardiac or respiratory systems – unless the resident has indicated that they do not wish to be treated. Clearly, when someone has collapsed and is extremely unwell it is inappropriate to begin conversations about their wishes; thus decision-making on this topic needs to take place in a planned way, rather than in a crisis, wherever possible.

The Care Home Handbook, First Edition. Edited by Graham Mulley, Clive Bowman, Michal Boyd and Sarah Stowe.
© 2015 John Wiley & Sons, Ltd. Published 2015 by John Wiley & Sons, Ltd.

Decision-making

- Often a resident's views regarding CPR are elicited as part of a broader discussion about advance care planning (see Chapter 16.1).
- If a resident is unable to express their views, then all possible steps should be taken to maximise their ability to do so. For example, hearing loss or difficulty with speech should be addressed. Can an amplification device be used to allow the resident to participate in conversation? (see Chapter 7.2). Can a resident who has hearing or speaking difficulties communicate by written word?
- Sometimes it will be apparent to those who know the resident well that a discussion would be distressing for the resident.
- Sometimes it will be impossible for the resident to express their views – perhaps as a result of loss of capacity due to dementia. In this situation, it may be inappropriate to embark upon discussions with the resident, and the duty of the doctor is to attempt to identify what the views of the resident might be, based on information which those who know the resident best might hold, if there are any such informants.

The family's perspective

Unless a resident has taken out a lasting (enduring) power of attorney, a relative or friend has no right in law to insist upon or refuse a treatment on a resident's behalf; however, it is usually regarded as good practice to involve relatives in discussions. They may have had previous discussions with their loved one about their wishes in such a situation, and thus be able to offer the clinician information which is helpful in gauging what the resident's views may be, had they been able to express their view.

Futility

In a situation in which the main problem is not with cardiac function or with pulmonary function, an attempt at cardiopulmonary resuscitation will be unsuccessful and thus would be futile.

Another medical reason for a decision that CPR would be futile is when the clinician believes that the heart or lungs have suffered an overwhelming injury (either as a single event or as a series of illnesses) so that there is no realistic prospect of their recovery.

There is no obligation to perform or offer to a resident a treatment which a clinician believes to be futile and thus CPR should not be offered those residents. It is regarded as good practice to compassionately communicate to residents, where appropriate (or to their relatives), that such a decision has been taken, and the rationale for this decision.

Documentation of CPR decisions

It is important to communicate CPR directives when a resident moves between different locations (for example, when a resident is admitted to or discharged from an acute hospital). Common forms are available so that community-based staff, ambulance crews and acute hospital staff are all aware of decisions which have been made, and the basis on which such decisions have taken.

Likelihood of a successful outcome

Knowledge of the likelihood of success of CPR can be helpful in discussions with families of residents. Even in hospital, CPR attempts are successful in only about 12% (about 1 in 8) people. This statistic refers to all age groups, including those patients who are in facilities like coronary care units where access to treatment is immediate (and therefore potential for a good outcome is maximised).

The outcome data for frail older people outside of hospital are much lower, though exact figures are hard to find. Common estimates are that about 1 in 20 attempts at resuscitation in care homes will be successful but, of those who survive, at least a third will have suffered brain damage.

Factors such as suffering from more than one long-term condition (such as heart disease, chronic obstructive airways disease (COPD) and diabetes) reduce the likelihood of a successful outcome. For most residents of nursing homes, resuscitation is very unlikely to be successful.

Further reading

Benkendorf RSR, Jackson R, Rivera-Rivera EJ, Demrick A. 1997. Outcomes of cardiac arrest in the nursing home: destiny or futility? *Prehospital Emergency Care* 1: 68–72.

16.4 Recognising dying

Katie Athorn

Hull and East Yorkshire Hospitals NHS Trust, Hull, UK

Key points

- Most deaths in care homes follow a period of slow decline.
- Prediction of when death will occur is often inaccurate.
- Some of the signs of impending death may be caused by other conditions, which might be treatable. Examples are oesophageal thrush causing dysphagia, irregular heart beat in pneumonia and reduced urine output in dehydration.
- Changes in skin colour and temperature and the 'death rattle' (caused by difficulty clearing oral secretions) usually mean that death is imminent.

Dying in care home residents can vary greatly in its pattern. A sudden and unpredicted event may occur, such as a heart attack or brain haemorrhage. At other times, death follows a period of relentless decline, for example in a resident with advanced cancer.

However, most care home residents slowly deteriorate and this is often associated with features of underlying diseases or conditions (for example, dementia and frailty). In the last few months and weeks of life, there are often physical changes that can alert carers to an increasing possibility of the dying process. If recognised, these signs can help carers and relatives to understand the changes occurring and prepare them for impending death.

Note that some of these changes can occur in people who are not about to die. Prediction of death – even by experienced clinicians – is often imprecise

Changes in the last few months and weeks

These usually depend on the underlying disease or condition (Table 16.4.1)

Changes in the last few days

These can apply to most residents, regardless of their underlying medical condition (Figure 16.4.1). The changes tend to follow a 'common pathway'.

Table 16.4.1 Changes in the last few months and weeks.

Dementia	Inability to walk
	Speech difficult to understand
Chronic lung disease	Loss of muscle bulk
	Muscle weakness
	New ankle swelling
Chronic heart failure	Low blood pressure
	Light headedness
	Weak, thready pulse

- NB: The resident may not eat because of oral thrush or a sore tongue – always check for treatable mouth problems.
- Dysphagia can be caused by thrush in the oesophagus, which is easily treatable.
- An irregular breathing pattern can occur in heart failure, pneumonia and other conditions – which might be treatable.
- Low urine output may be the result of dehydration – check the axillae for dryness (see Chapter 5.3)

Other signs – changes in behaviour

See Figure 16.4.2.

The Care Home Handbook, First Edition. Edited by Graham Mulley, Clive Bowman, Michal Boyd and Sarah Stowe.
© 2015 John Wiley & Sons, Ltd. Published 2015 by John Wiley & Sons, Ltd.

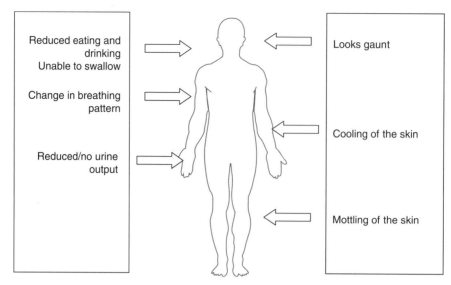

Figure 16.4.1 Changes in the last few days.

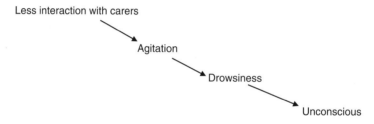

Figure 16.4.2 Changes in behaviour.

Specific changes in the last few hours

Mottling

This is a colour change producing a dappled appearance (Figure 16.4.3). It usually starts in the extremities and over bony prominences, such as the knees. This occurs because the blood pressure is low and the heart has slowed, resulting in under-perfusion of tissues and skin.

Cooling of the skin

This is also the result of reduced blood flow through the tissues and can be a sign of impending death.

Change in breathing with 'death rattle'

Periodic breathing (Cheyne–Stokes respirations) occurs because the part of the brain that normally controls the breathing rate and rhythm is no longer responding. The pattern produced is shallow

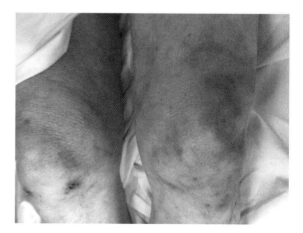

Figure 16.4.3 Mottling.

breathing interspersed with periods when the breathing stops for up to 30 seconds (see Chapter 15.3).

The 'death rattle' is the loud gurgling sound as air passes through secretions in the back of the throat that the resident is no longer able to clear. This can be upsetting for carers and for families sitting with the resident. Simple measures, such as repositioning, raising the head of the bed and suction, can help. Medications can also reduce the amount of secretions produced – ask the GP.

Some of these changes can be easily identified by families and carers as signs of impending death (e.g. skin colour, skin temperature and breathing pattern changes). They are all useful prompts to trigger arrangements to be made, others to be contacted, and help those present to understand, know what to expect and have time to prepare.

Further reading

Coventry PA, Grande GE, Richards DA, et al. 2005. Prediction of appropriate timing of palliative care for older adults with non-malignant life threatening disease: A systematic review. *Age Ageing* 34: 218–227.

Morita T, Ichiki T, Tsunoda J, et al. 1998. A prospective study on the dying process in terminally ill cancer patients. *American Journal of Hospice and Palliative Care* 15: 217–222.

National Council for Hospice and Specialist Palliative Care Services. 2006. Changing Gear - Guidelines for Managing the Last Days of Life in Adults. London, National Council for Hospice and Specialist Palliative Care Services.

Pitorak E. 2003. Care at the Time of Death: How nurses can make the last hours of life a richer, more comfortable experience. *American Journal of Nursing* 103: 42–52.

16.5 Signs of death

Katie Athorn

Hull and East Yorkshire Hospitals NHS Trust, Hull, UK

Key points

There are five checks which should be done to confirm that a resident has died:

- No response to stimuli.
- No pulses palpable.
- No heart sounds for 3 minutes
- No breath sounds for 3 minutes
- Pupils are fixed and dilated.

At the moment of death, the breathing stops, following moments to minutes later by the heart stopping.

This can occasionally be associated with a sigh or possibly a vomit.

There are five main checks to carry out to confirm death (Box 16.5.1).

In the presence of all the above signs, death can be verified and documented in the care plan.

Box 16.5.1 Five main checks to confirm death.

	1. No response to stimuli
Checked with	Firm squeezing of earlobe Firm pressure on eyebrow ridge Firm pressure on fingernail Rubbing your knuckles on sternum
Potential pitfalls	If the patient is unconscious but still alive, they will not respond to the above measures

	2. No pulses felt
Checked with	Feeling over the carotid artery for a pulse for 3 minutes
Potential pitfalls	If the blood pressure is very low, you may not be able to feel the pulses – even though they are still present

	3. No heart sounds for 3 minutes
Checked with	Listening over the heart for 3 minutes with a stethoscope for any heart sounds
Potential pitfalls	Stethoscope may not be working or be of poor quality so it is difficult to hear heart sounds Noisy environment can make it difficult to hear

The Care Home Handbook, First Edition. Edited by Graham Mulley, Clive Bowman, Michal Boyd and Sarah Stowe.
© 2015 John Wiley & Sons, Ltd. Published 2015 by John Wiley & Sons, Ltd.

4. No breath sounds for 3 minutes

Checked with	Listening over the lungs for 3 minutes with a stethoscope
	Feeling the chest wall for any movement
Potential pitfalls	Breathing pattern is irregular with periods where the breathing stops for short periods but then restarts
	Stethoscope may not working or of poor quality
	Noisy environment

5. Pupils fixed and dilated

Checked with	No change in pupil size when a light is shone into the eye
	Pupils large in diameter (Figure 16.5.1)

(a)   (b)

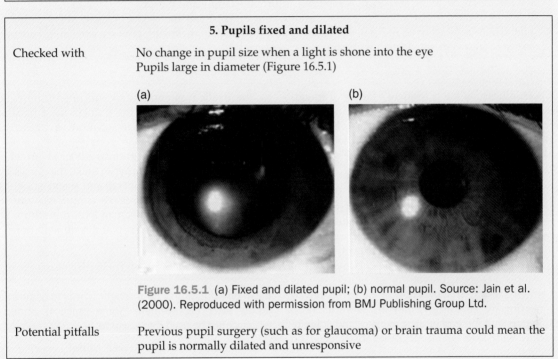

Figure 16.5.1 (a) Fixed and dilated pupil; (b) normal pupil. Source: Jain et al. (2000). Reproduced with permission from BMJ Publishing Group Ltd.

Potential pitfalls	Previous pupil surgery (such as for glaucoma) or brain trauma could mean the pupil is normally dilated and unresponsive

The acknowledgement of the lack of vital signs to the family at the bedside can wait until they appear ready to receive it.

Reference

Jain R, Assi A, Murdoch IE. 2000. Urrets-Zavalia syndrome following trabeculectomy. *British Journal of Ophthalmology* 84(3): 338–389.

Further reading

Albarran-Sotelo R, Flint L, Kelly-Thomas K. 1988. *Healthcare Provider's Manual for Basic Life Support* (1st Edn., digitized 2008). American Heart Association.

Pitorak E. 2003. Care at the Time of Death: How nurses can make the last hours of life a richer, more comfortable experience. *American Journal of Nursing* 103: 42–52.

16.6 What to do and what to say to carers and relatives when someone dies

Eileen Burns

Leeds Teaching Hospitals NHS Trust, Leeds, UK

Key points

- If a resident is declining and death is expected, inform the family and the GP.
- Be aware of the different preferences and customs concerning dying and seeing the body after death.
- Phone calls from relatives after a death are an opportunity to help them with grieving and should not be seen as a sign of dissatisfaction with care.

Opportunities to talk to a resident's family or friends about the gravity of a resident's illness can help to prepare them for bereavement and should be used wherever possible. It is unusual (though not unknown) for a care home resident to die suddenly, without warning.

- It is a responsibility of care home staff who observe a slow deterioration to talk to family members, as well as involving a GP in discussions about end of life care.
- When relatives knows what to expect, they are often grateful to the staff for care and less likely to complain – even if some minor aspects of care aren't perfect. If they know their loved one is nearing the end of life, they are more likely to understand the end of life processes and collaborate with staff about decisions that focus on comfort.

Formal and informal carers who have known a resident for some time will also suffer bereavement when a resident passes away, though staff over time realise that such events are inevitable as part of a caring role for frail older people.

Family members will often want to be with their relative when they are in the final stages of their illness and may want to stay and spend time with the body after death. There are different religious or cultural practices that are important to try to accommodate (as far as possible) to avoid causing additional grief or distress (see Chapters 2.2 and 16.8).

- If a resident has died alone, relatives will often want to hear something of the mode of death. If the death was anticipated and opportunities to ensure the comfort of the resident were maximised, this can provide comfort to grieving families.
- Families will require practical advice about what to do after a death in order to make the necessary arrangements for a funeral and disposal of the body. Care home staff have a responsibility to ensure that they are aware of local procedures so that families can be helped at this difficult time.

Helpful phrases after a death

It can be difficult to find the right words to comfort a family after bereavement. Some practical phrases which could be used may include:

- Do you want to sit with your Mum?
- She/He didn't suffer.
- It was a pleasure and privilege to nurse your mum/care for them/know them.
- I know you will miss them terribly.

Unhelpful phrases include: 'She/He isn't suffering anymore', or ' She/He is in heaven', or 'Everything happens for a reason' – bereaved relatives have expressed that they often do not find these phrases comforting.

The most commonly expressed view of bereaved relatives is that they need something to be said to acknowledge their loss. However clumsily expressed, this is far preferable to avoiding the subject.

Sometimes a family member may contact a care home a little while after a bereavement, to ask more about the death. This is not an indication that there is

The Care Home Handbook, First Edition. Edited by Graham Mulley, Clive Bowman, Michal Boyd and Sarah Stowe.
© 2015 John Wiley & Sons, Ltd. Published 2015 by John Wiley & Sons, Ltd.

dissatisfaction with care, and it is important not to be defensive in this situation. Often the need to know more can help a relative in the grieving process.

It can be helpful to have contact details for organisations which can help bereaved spouses and other family members (such as Cruse in the UK).

Useful web sites

www.crusebereavementcare.org.uk [Accessed October 2013]
dyingmatters.org.uk [Accessed October 2013]
www.grief.com [Accessed October 2013]

16.7 Removal of pacemakers and implantable defibrillators

Aidan Dunphy and Simon Conroy

University Hospitals of Leicester NHS Trust, Leicester, UK

Key points

- Implanted pacemakers and defibrillators must be removed after death to avoid distressing and potentially dangerous explosions during cremation.
- These devices continue to work after death and the shocks that they can cause can be distressing to families.

Implanted pacemakers provide a regular electrical impulse to maintain a steady rate (pacing). This is particularly useful for:

- a heart with conduction problems that cause it to run too slow (see Chapter 9.8) or
- difficulty with synchronisation, such as heart failure.

Internal cardiac defibrillators (ICDs) can pace and give a small shock to the heart if an abnormal rhythm is detected (cardioversion). In the absence of a rhythm, they will give a larger shock (defibrillate). They are generally provided for those who have had a life threatening rhythm problem or those who may be at risk from genetic disorders.

Pacemakers and ICDs can explode during cremation, causing damage and distress. It is therefore very important that these devices are removed before the body is cremated.

Care is needed with removal to avoid upsetting the resident's family.

Cremation

Defibrillators and pacemakers continue to work even after death. These devices can be turned off by technicians, though in practice seeking their involvement is generally restricted to residents being fitted with a defibrillator.

Handling of ICDs after death requires the deactivation of the defibrillator function. Devices *must* be removed before cremation.

The data in the device may sometimes be required by the coroner (see Chapter 17.12) to aid clarification of the cause of death.

Considerations at the end of life

1. Before the terminal phase, a discussion should be held with the resident to understand their wishes about deactivation of the defibrillator.
2. During the terminal phase of life, listen carefully to the resident. At this point they may have autonomy to choose to have the device switched off remotely. Both residents and family should be aware that the ICD in itself does not sustain life.
3. The sustained shocks in the last moments of life and post mortem may be both distressing and painful both physically and emotionally to the resident and their loved ones.

Considerations after death

1. If there is a concern about the ICD emitting a shock post mortem, this function may be temporarily disabled by placing a magnet over the device. This may be necessary following a traumatic injury, such as a fall.
2. ICDs and pacemakers must be removed before cremation as the lithium battery will explode if exposed to heat. This is *not* the responsibility of care home staff.
3. It is important to know the nature of the device: a pacemaker will not shock mortuary staff, but will still need to be removed before cremation.
4. Depending on local policy, the undertaker or mortuary staff will need to contact the local cardiology centre to ask if a technician is available to

The Care Home Handbook, First Edition. Edited by Graham Mulley, Clive Bowman, Michal Boyd and Sarah Stowe.
© 2015 John Wiley & Sons, Ltd. Published 2015 by John Wiley & Sons, Ltd.

attend to disable the ICD. It can then be safely removed.

You need to be aware of your local policy in advance; your local undertaker or mortuary department may be a good source of information.

Useful web sites

http://www.bhf.org.uk/heart-health/treatment/implantable-cardioverter-defib.aspx [Accessed October 2013]

http://www.improvement.nhs.uk/LinkClick.aspx?fileticket=KBUUEsR0mms=&tabid=56 [Accessed October 2013]

http://www.mhra.gov.uk/home/groups/dts-bs/documents/medicaldevicealert/con025836.pdf [Accessed October 2013]

16.8 Care for the dying for people of different faiths

Anne Forbes

RC Diocese of Leeds, Leeds, UK

Key points

- Societies are becoming increasingly diverse.
- The number of faiths of residents and care home staff make it ever more difficult to prepare appropriately for the wide range of faiths encountered.
- If it's not clear what care is expected for a dying resident, make sure that family, friends (and of course religious priests or chaplains or whoever can provide guidance) are asked.

The wider context

Many countries have become increasingly multicultural and multifaith. For example, in the UK, the population has long been diverse. Immigration in the twentieth century brought new people from many different countries, especially those of the Commonwealth. According to the 2001 UK Census, 72% of the population at that time were Christians, 3% Muslims, 1% Hindus, 0.5% Jewish, 0.3% Buddhists and 15% had no religion.

Irrespective of their cultural and religious background, everyone in due course comes to the moment of preparation for life's close, and will need appropriate care at this special time.

The main faith groups found in the UK at present are listed below.

1. Christianity, within which there are different branches, for example Protestantism (Anglicans, Methodists, United Reformed, Baptists etc.); Roman Catholicism and the Orthodox Church
2. Judaism
3. Islam
4. Hinduism
5. Sikhism
6. Buddhism
7. Chinese beliefs and customs
8. Japanese beliefs and customs.

In addition, there is another relevant category of people: Humanists. Although they don't describe themselves as a faith group, they have beliefs and practices that need to be understood at the time of preparation for death.

Aspects of care for consideration

This major topic cannot be condensed into a short chapter. However, there is a growing body of literature that is relevant to the care home population, of which Julia Neuberger's excellent book *Caring for Dying People of Different Faiths* is probably the best known. The key aspects of care of dying residents highlighted by Neuberger are listed below.

1. Finding out about the resident's beliefs. Often a person's own beliefs and practices may not correspond to the formal doctrine of their particular faith; for example, with regard to diet.
2. Recognising the resident's needs. Neuberger writes:

   'The fact that someone has bothered to ask whether it would be helpful to have a Bhagavad Gita or a pair of Jewish Sabbath candlesticks, or a Koran or a few drops of Ganges water brought in, makes all the difference to the individual who feels that he is in unfamiliar surroundings, and is often in pain of discomfort.' (Neuberger, 2007: 3).

3. Recognising the different forms of each religion. A well-known example is Islam, where there are Shi'ite and Sunni Muslims, as well as Ismaili Muslims and Ahmaddiya. Family members and the resident may be only too willing to clarify the situation.
4. Areas for examination. These include the Last Rites, beliefs regarding immortality of the soul and the afterlife, prayers, and who can touch the body.

The Care Home Handbook, First Edition. Edited by Graham Mulley, Clive Bowman, Michal Boyd and Sarah Stowe.
© 2015 John Wiley & Sons, Ltd. Published 2015 by John Wiley & Sons, Ltd.

The importance of recognising spiritual needs

Attention paid to the cultural and religious needs of the resident adds considerably to care which addresses purely physical needs; in fact, they complement each other.

If you are aware of spiritual needs, then it will have a number of benefits to the resident. These include emotional stability, acceptance of what is happening and an opportunity to make their peace with God with family and friends.

For residents who are terminally ill, familiar rituals, beliefs and customs can take on great importance for the residents and their families.

Local contacts for faith communities

Details can usually be found in the local telephone directory under the heading 'Churches and Other Places of Worship'. If in doubt, contact the principal Anglican minister, the local hospital chaplain or an ecumenical group (such as Churches Together in the UK) for information.

Reference

Neuberger, J. 2007. *Caring for Dying People of Different Faiths*, 3rd Edn. Radcliffe Medical Press.

Further reading

Henley A, Schott J. 1999. *Culture, Religion and Patient Care in a Multi-Ethnic Society. A Handbook for Professionals*. Age Concern England.

Contacting Other Professionals

Chapter 17

Referrals and Template Letters to Colleagues

17.1 Referral to the geriatrician

John Gladman[1] and Verity Hallam[2]

[1]*University of Nottingham, Nottingham, UK*
[2]*The Byars Nursing Home, Nottingham, UK*

Key points

- Geriatricians are physicians in elderly care who have a broad view of the medical, psychological, social and rehabilitation needs of old people.
- The geriatrician will usually become involved at the request of the family doctor (general practitioner or GP), who has overall responsibility for the resident's care.
- Geriatricians are particularly skilled at evaluating complex problems, determining the causes of unsolved or uncontrolled symptoms, simplifying multiple medications, helping with end of life care and assisting in resolving conflicts between residents, carers and others.
- If you feel that a resident might benefit from seeing a geriatrician, do not hesitate to suggest this to the GP. Your observations and concerns will often help the consultant to find the best ways of managing the resident's problems.

The community geriatrician

Recent years have witnessed an expansion in the provision of community geriatricians, who now make assessments of patients in care homes rather than expecting them to travel to a hospital clinic.

In the UK, NHS geriatricians are usually not directly available to care home staff: they consult patients at the request of their general practitioners, who have the primary medical responsibility for residents of care homes. General practitioners can delegate the responsibility for referral to other members of the primary care team, but only where there are unusually close arrangements between the health, social and private sectors can referrals be made directly by care home staff to NHS geriatricians.

Even when referred, geriatricians (in the UK) do not provide the primary care for care home residents: they advise the general practitioner and primary care team.

The expertise of general practitioners in the management of the medical problems seen in care home residents varies, but all general practitioners will have been trained in the care of older people and be responsible for many of them either in care homes in their own homes.

Geriatricians have particular expertise in the management of complex problems that are sometimes difficult for general practitioners, such as those associated with multiple medications or apparently inexplicable symptoms.

When to consider referral

Even though care home staff cannot directly refer to geriatricians in the UK, they are not without influence, and can suggest to the general practitioner when such a referral might be helpful. The type of indicators that might suggest the need for referral would include:

- unexplained symptoms
- uncontrolled symptoms
- ethical dilemmas
- uncertainty over end of life plans
- uncertainty about how to reduce a complex medication regime
- conflict between staff, agencies or families.

Care home staff may feel uncomfortable about suggesting referral to a geriatrician to the general practitioner for fear of undermining a relationship or

The Care Home Handbook, First Edition. Edited by Graham Mulley, Clive Bowman, Michal Boyd and Sarah Stowe.
© 2015 John Wiley & Sons, Ltd. Published 2015 by John Wiley & Sons, Ltd.

appearing to be critical. However, it is reasonable for the care home staff to ask for clear instructions about medical management of the residents for whose care they are responsible. Just as a relative of a vulnerable person may ask whether a further opinion should be gathered, so should care home staff feel equally empowered.

If asked to consult, geriatricians will make a thorough assessment, and care home staff are vital in ensuring that this is fully informed.

Information which can help the geriatrician

Details of the medical history and prescribed treatment will be provided by the general practitioner, but the care home team's day-to-day observations and perspectives are vital. For example, eye witness accounts of 'funny turns' or falls are often essential for any sense to be made of such complaints. The care home team often will have made critical observations, such as the relationship of symptoms to medications, but may feel reluctant to voice such views, fearing that it is not their job to say so or that it will appear critical to do so. But it is essential, especially as many care home residents will not have the mental capacity to say so for themselves.

Capacity

Geriatricians not only assess patients, but help to formulate management plans. Where possible, the resident will be involved in making choices on these plans. But often they do not have the mental capacity to do so, or perhaps the confidence (see Chapter 4.6). Care home staff are well placed to know the views and preferences of residents who lack mental capacity and to speak up for them, and can be the only people to do so for those who have no relatives or friends. Such information is vital if actions are to be taken in the best interests of the resident lacking mental capacity. Care home staff should expect to be consulted about such matters and should take steps to anticipate such questions by listening to their residents and recording relevant views and preferences that emerge during day-to-day care giving.

Although, formally, the geriatrician consults at the request of the general practitioner, the day-to-day management of the residents falls to staff to deal with, so it is important for the care team to not only to act on behalf of the resident, but to raise their own concerns and their questions at the consultation. For example, it is often helpful for staff to gain explicit directives about how to use PRN medication, or when to omit prescribed medication such as diuretics. Also, care home staff are also expected to provide information to residents' families, and so should expect to be well informed.

17.2 Referral to the old age psychiatry services

John Wattis and Steven Curran

University of Huddersfield, Huddersfield, UK

Key points

- Mental illnesses are common in care home residents but they are often not recognised.
- Depression is easy to miss, but can be improved by treatment.
- Your observations (for example about mood, suicidal ideas, fluid and food intake and concordance with medication) can be most helpful in assisting the old age psychiatrist to evaluate and treat the resident's problems.
- It is helpful to inform the old age psychiatry services about the urgency of the referral – urgent (within 4 hours) or routine (within 14 days).
- If in doubt about any aspect of mental health care, phone the local old age psychiatry service.

Most old age psychiatry services in the UK only accept referrals from health and social care professionals, such as GPs, psychologists and social services.

- Mental illness in older people is common in care homes and depression in particular is frequently missed (see Chapter 10.3).
- In most cases, referral to old age psychiatry services should be via the local GP. The GP has an important overview of the resident's medical history. S/he may be able to intervene directly and to distinguish physical problems from those which need help from specialist mental health services.
- Before making a referral, the resident's consent should be sought.
- For residents who lack capacity, referral should be made if it is judged to be in their best interests (see Chapter 4.6).

Staff in care homes can:

- Provide the GP with a clear description of the problem, for example low mood, suicidal thoughts as well as the duration of problems, their severity and impact on the person.
- Highlight any risks to self or others.
- Give information about fluid intake, nutrition and compliance with medication.

Other useful information includes past and current physical health, drug history, social functioning and activities of daily living.

This information can be combined with that available to the GP to produce a comprehensive but succinct referral letter to local services. This would typically be processed through a single point of access.

It is important to be clear how quickly the resident needs to be seen and to be aware of local definitions of 'urgent' and 'routine' ('urgent' might be defined as 'within 4 hours' and routine 'within 14 days').

- If in doubt, contact your local old age psychiatry service for advice.
- Many services in the UK now have a care homes liaison service (CHLS). These have been set up to support residents with mental health problems in care homes. If your service has a CHLS, you could contact them informally for information. They are usually able to see residents quickly and may provide care as well as advice, training and support for staff.
- Some services now do regular clinics in care homes, allowing problems to be dealt with at an early stage. Make contact with your local service and understand what they can provide so that when you need to make a referral, you can access support quickly and efficiently.

The Care Home Handbook, First Edition. Edited by Graham Mulley, Clive Bowman, Michal Boyd and Sarah Stowe.
© 2015 John Wiley & Sons, Ltd. Published 2015 by John Wiley & Sons, Ltd.

17.3 Referral to the emergency department

John Gladman[1] and Verity Hallam[2]

[1] University of Nottingham, Nottingham, UK
[2] The Byars Nursing Home, Nottingham, UK

> ### Key points
>
> - It is good practice to formulate an advance care plan for every resident before an emergency arises. This is best done after discussions between the care home staff, the resident, the family and the family doctor (GP).
> - Try to contact the GP at the onset of a medical emergency.
> - If necessary and appropriate, phone the emergency services.
> - Write a brief, yet comprehensive, referral letter, which should include details of diagnoses, recent medical problems, medications, capabilities, advance care plans and the ability of the home to provide palliative or other specialist care. Send this to hospital emergency department with the resident. Keep a copy of this letter.
> - Monitor all emergency referrals and discuss them as part of quality improvement.

Raising an emergency (such as a 999 or 911 call) from a care home often poses a quandary for staff. Should they wait and see or react immediately to the crisis? For residents who lack capacity to make such decisions themselves, what would the resident want them to do? Care home staff know that emergency care can sometimes help, but can also sometimes disrupt the finely tuned care they have been striving to achieve.

Furthermore, they are aware that emergency departments are generally not conducive and are often seen as hostile to care home residents. The role of emergency departments is to assess if patients need urgent medical treatment. They 'triage' people into those who do not need emergency treatment and who can go home, those who need treatment there and then, and those that need to be referred on to ward admission. Emergency department staff are expected to do this quickly, yet communication takes time. They find assessing complex patients, such as those in care homes, difficult.

Escorting residents to the emergency department

Worse still, it is usually not feasible for a member of care home staff to escort the resident to the department without compromising the staffing of the home. There is usually little time to write anything other than a brief letter to accompany the resident. It is not easy to telephone the emergency department and relay useful information and, sadly, care home staff often report that they are not listened to anyway. It is easy to see why problems that require careful and protracted analysis and negotiation are best not dealt with by the emergency department.

The ambulance team

Fortunately, emergency (999 in the UK) calls usually bring helpful, well-trained ambulance staff who are often able to provide urgent assessment, intervention, advice and reassurance without the need to transfer the resident to the emergency department. Although some admissions are preventable, some are appropriate (such as to check for a fracture after a fall). But the ease of access makes dialling 999 (or equivalent) tempting, and can become a knee jerk reaction.

'Stop and think' notices by the phones may help stop such reflex actions.

Contacting the GP

To make the best use of the alternatives, negotiations with the general practitioner who provides primary care for the residents should be undertaken to ensure

The Care Home Handbook, First Edition. Edited by Graham Mulley, Clive Bowman, Michal Boyd and Sarah Stowe.
© 2015 John Wiley & Sons, Ltd. Published 2015 by John Wiley & Sons, Ltd.

that arrangements for emergency and near-emergency care are in place, covering office hours and out-of-office hours. It is often better to get help and a clear plan from a general practitioner for an impending crisis during the working day, rather than wait until the evening or weekend.

The decision to make an emergency call depends not only upon the seriousness and urgency of the emergency, but also upon previous care planning. The early development of an Advance Care Plan (ACP), and familiarity with its content, will enable the duty staff to deal with a crisis with knowledge of the resident's preferences for care. Most residents in care homes will suffer their final illness in the care home so, for all residents, some sort of decline will occur. Such declines cannot be prevented or their timing known but they must be anticipated and plans made for a range of events.

The care home team, general practitioner, resident and family should jointly develop plans for urgent situations and write them down.

Information to accompany the resident to the emergency department

For those who are transferred to the emergency department, it is good practice to prepare an up-to-date summary of information that lists

- the details of each resident's diagnoses,
- their current medications,
- recent medical history and
- the gist of their advance care plan.

The summary should also give a brief indication of the care home's health care capabilities, such as its ability to provide terminal care, or the visiting arrangements of the general practitioner. Remember that many hospital staff do not know the difference between a care home with nursing and one without, and some even expect care homes with nursing to be mini-hospitals. This summary should be concise, on one side of a brightly coloured A4 page. It won't be returned, *so copies should also be kept for future use.*

Many people seen in an emergency department return swiftly to the care home, usually with little feedback or information. Sometimes the underlying problem remains unresolved. For example, a resident who has fallen may return with a report that no bones are broken, but may be more immobile than usual. This is another opportunity for contacting the primary care team.

Quality assurance

Care homes should monitor emergency referrals as part of quality assurance and periodically reflect upon them with the primary care team. This can be used to reaffirm the correct processes to be used, and can identify whether improvements can be made.

17.4 Referral to the hospital ward

John Gladman[1] and Verity Hallam[2]

[1] University of Nottingham, Nottingham, UK
[2] The Byars Nursing Home, Nottingham, UK

Key points

- Many staff in hospital have not worked in care homes and their knowledge and understanding of your capabilities and skills – as well as elderly care generally – may be incomplete.
- Hospital ward staff will benefit from timely information about a resident's medical condition in the care home and details of how to communicate with, feed and mobilise the resident, and manage their incontinence.
- As well as sending a letter with the resident to hospital, always fax the medical summary to the receiving ward at the earliest opportunity.
- It is good practice for a senior nurse at the care home to keep in close contact with the ward and help to optimise discharge arrangements.
- The ward team should ideally give a copy of the hospital discharge letter to the resident.
- Regular reflective reviews of hospital admissions can help improve the quality of care in the care home.

Many residents who are on hospital wards have entered the hospital via the emergency department. This means that the hospital ward may have little information about the resident. But ward staff need to know how to communicate with, feed, mobilise and maintain the continence of their patient. Care home staff will know this intimately.

Sometimes the information sent with the resident to hospital is already lost. Copies of the resident's medical summary can be faxed to the hospital ward. This is best done as soon as possible and as a routine process whenever a resident is admitted.

The Advance Care Plan is particularly important.

It is important to recognise the limitations of hospital wards, especially those that do not specialise in the care of older people.

Many hospital staff do not know what sort of care is possible in care homes, and the capabilities of homes and their primary care support varies enormously in the UK.

Many hospital staff assume that care homes are mini-hospitals. So they might wish to discharge patients with care needs that cannot be met in the home.

They are often unaware of the role of care home staff and assume that they only need to communicate with the GP, and may even appear dismissive towards care home staff and their enquiries.

Hospital staff may think that care home staff are trying to prevent residents returning home – even though care home staff are usually desperate to have their residents back, they are simply trying to establish their care needs and make arrangements for meeting them.

Wherever possible, it is helpful for a senior member of the care home staff to make contact with the hospital ward on a regular basis, mindful of the communication failures that might ensue, and attempt to engage in discharge planning. Many UK hospitals have discharge coordinators with whom constructive relationships can be built.

Many care home staff will have formed relationships with the residents' families, and may find themselves providing advice, solace and support to them during a hospital admission.

Early discharge schemes are now common in the UK, but operate differently from place to place. It is important for care home staff to be aware of such services that are available locally and to be prepared to work with them, and this may allow their residents to come home sooner than would otherwise be possible. By being involved in discharge planning, care home staff can also alert the general practitioner so that the hospital discharge is as safe as possible. But be careful not to be over-optimistic of your ability to meet the resident's needs.

The Care Home Handbook, First Edition. Edited by Graham Mulley, Clive Bowman, Michal Boyd and Sarah Stowe.
© 2015 John Wiley & Sons, Ltd. Published 2015 by John Wiley & Sons, Ltd.

It is now considered best practice for all hospital correspondence about a patient to be copied to the patient. Sometimes doctors and others will not think to send a copy for care home residents, but it is important for staff, residents or their families to request that a copy of the hospital discharge summary is also sent to the patient, and these can be kept securely and confidentially on their behalf by the care home staff. In the event of further problems, they are also helpful for the GP when visiting, who often does not have access to the computer system on which records are usually stored.

Care homes should monitor hospital admissions as part of quality assurance and periodically reflect upon them with the primary care team. This can be used to reaffirm the correct processes to be used, and can identify whether improvements can be made.

17.5 Referral to the dentist

Rachel Hepherd[1], Katherine Sage[1] and Claire Sissons[2]

[1]Hull and East Yorkshire Hospitals NHS Trust, Hull, UK
[2]Highfield Nursing Home, Tadcaster, UK

Key points

- Oral care is central to a resident's well-being.
- Provision and access to dentistry differs between countries.
- The main oral problems that should prompt you to consider requesting a dental opinion include loose or broken teeth; loose, ill fitting or lost dentures; gum disease; infections and suspicious lesions in the mouth.
- A template referral letter to the community dentist is provided.

Dental health is important to maintaining well-being, especially in the care home. Poor dentition and oral hygiene can be the cause of health problems such as low mood, under-nutrition and weight loss. Common dental health problems affecting care home residents may include the following:

- loose teeth
- caries/decay
- infections/abscesses
- broken teeth or dentures
- ill-fitting dentures
- lost dentures/replacement sets.

How to arrange an appointment with a dentist

If a resident is registered with a dentist, then with their permission, appointments can usually be made over the telephone.

If a resident is unable to make an informed decision, then the decision to arrange an appointment with their dentist should be made in their best interests, with the aid of a relative or appointed deputy (e.g. Lasting or Enduring Power of Attorney).

What to do if your resident is not registered with a dentist/dental practice

The situation varies from country to country. In England and Wales, finding NHS dental treatment can often be difficult and time-consuming. NHS Choices in England and Wales (www.nhs.uk) is a useful resource and can provide a list of dentists within your local area.

In Scotland, Scottish Dental (www.scottishdental.org) provides a similar resource.

In other countries, dentistry is often not covered through the public health system. However, there is increasing concern about oral health for older people in care homes and a recognition of the lack of available dentistry services. Private dentistry is currently the only option, and therefore the care home staff must work closely with family to arrange for these services.

What if urgent dental treatment is needed?

If urgent out-of-hours dental treatment is needed, then help and advice can be obtained by either of the following ways:

By telephone:

Contact the resident's usual dental practice. There is often a recorded message explaining how to access urgent dental treatment.

NHS Direct Dental Helpline (England and Wales) 0845 600 3249

NHS24 (Scotland) 08454 242424

Via the internet:

NHS Choices in England and Wales (www.nhs.uk), and NHS24 in Scotland (www.nhs24.com), provide regional links to emergency dental care facilities in your area.

What if your resident is immobile and cannot gain access to a dentist?

Being housebound does not exclude a resident from accessing dental care should they require it. Most general dental practitioners no longer make domiciliary visits, but residents can be referred to a community dentist instead. Community dentists specialise in providing treatment to those who cannot gain access to an ordinary dental surgery.

In the UK, community dentists deal with the same problems as a general dental practitioner, but provide the service at the patient's home or other residence. This includes screening, education and prevention, fillings, extractions, scale and polishes and making dentures.

Community dental services can be found in the same way as a regular dentist, but unlike a regular dentist, residents cannot self-refer. Referrals to a community dentist must be made by another health care professional.

Below is an example of a referral letter to a community dentist about a resident with severe dental pain (assuming that they do not provide their own referral proforma).

Again, if the resident does not have capacity to decide about dental treatment, then the contact details of a relative or appointed deputy should be included in the letter.

[Care Home]
[Address]
[Telephone no]
[Date]

[Name of Community Dentist]
[Dental Service Address]

Re [Resident's Name] [Date of Birth]

Dear [Community Dentist]

I am writing to refer [Resident] as they are no longer able to leave the care home because of severe frailty and ill-health. [Resident] is aware of this referral and has given their consent for me to request dental advice on their behalf.

Over the last few days, [Resident] has complained of significant pain from one of their back teeth, which seems to be constant and severe, despite analgesia. I am especially concerned as they are waking at night with pain and are reluctant to eat for fear of the pain being made worse.

If there is any further information that you require then please do not hesitate to contact me on the above telephone number.

Many thanks for your help in this matter.

Yours sincerely

[Care Home Manager]

17.6 Referral to the pharmacist

Adam Gordon

Nottingham University Hospitals NHS Trust, Nottingham, UK

Key points

- Letters to the pharmacist should include an updated summary of medical conditions.
- Also include a full list of medications (preferably their generic names), with details of dose, time of administration, route and frequency, as well as allergies. (This should ideally be on the Medicine Administration Record, which should be attached to the letter.)
- Address your letter to a named pharmacist. State your query clearly and state what you would like the pharmacist to do.
- Follow up your letter with a phone call at an agreed time and day.
- A template letter for referral to a pharmacist is provided.

Template letter for referral to a pharmacist

A Care Home
Main Street
Anyborough
Tel: (0123) 123 4567
Email: the.manager@acarehome.co.uk

Dear Mr Smith, ← If possible, phone ahead and find out the name of your pharmacist. Address the letter directly to them, this will improve your chances of getting a response.

Re.: Mr John Brown – Date of Birth 01/01/1910

Current health conditions:

List all of the resident's current health conditions here; if these haven't been updated in the care record in the last six months, obtain an up-to-date list from the resident's GP.

1. Alzheimer's Dementia
2. Ischaemic Heart Disease
3. Type 2 diabetes
4. Hypertension
5. Gout

The Care Home Handbook, First Edition. Edited by Graham Mulley, Clive Bowman, Michal Boyd and Sarah Stowe.
© 2015 John Wiley & Sons, Ltd. Published 2015 by John Wiley & Sons, Ltd.

Current medications:

> It is preferable to attach the Medicines Administration Record (MAR) (see Chapter 11.1), since this contains all relevant information for the pharmacist on drug dose, timing, allergies, as well as administration. If it is not possible to attach a MAR sheet, then list the medications to include: drug name (use the generic, rather than trade, name where possible); dose; route and frequency.

MAR sheet attached (YES/NO)

1. Donepezil 5 mg po od
2. Aspirin 75 mg po od
3. Mixtard 18 units sc bd
4. Bendroflumethiazide 2.5 mg po od
5. Allopurinol 100 mg po od

> Possible abbreviations are as follows:
>
> Route
> po = by mouth (per os in Latin)
> sc = subcutaneous
> im = intramuscular
> iv = intravenous
> pr = by rectum (per rectum in Latin)
> pv = by vagina (per vaginam in Latin)
> inh = inhaled
> neb = nebulised
>
> Frequency
> od = once daily (omne in die, in Latin)
> bd = twice daily (bis in die, in Latin)
> tds = three times daily (ter die sumendum, in Latin)
> qid = four times daily (quattuor in die, in Latin)
> mane = taken in the morning
> nocte = taken at night

Known drug allergies and sensitivities:

> If a MAR sheet is attached, this is not necessary.
> If it is not possible to attach a MAR, list any allergies/sensitivities and if possible the type of allergy (rash/breathing difficulties/diarrhoea); if none is known, write 'none known'.

ALLERGIC TO PENICILLIN (RASH AND BREATHING DIFFICULTIES); AND OMEPRAZOLE (DIARRHOEA).

Specific questions:

We would like your help and advice with the following aspects of Mr Brown's medication:

> Be very explicit here. State the question, the medication you are asking the question about and what you expect the pharmacist to do about it.

- Can Donepezil be mixed with food and drink – telephone advice required.
- Can Aspirin be administered via PEG – written advice required.
- Is a liquid preparation of bendrofluazide available, or can it be crushed – telephone advice required.

- Can you assist us with a multi-disciplinary review of Mr Brown's medications – attendance at MDT meeting at the care home would be required.

I will phone to follow up this letter on 1st November 2013.

Yours sincerely,

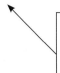

> If possible, always follow up the letter with a phone call, to ensure it has been received and to build a relationship with the pharmacist. Specify a date for your call and be sure to keep your promise!

Mrs Jane Doe
Care Home Manager

17.7 Referral to a physiotherapist

Baldeep Sagu

Riverside GP Vocational Training Scheme, London, UK

Key points

- Physiotherapists can help the resident who has mobility problems, pain, infectious chest diseases and incontinence, as well as those whose function is declining.
- Their advice on positioning and handling stroke residents can be particularly helpful.
- Referrals are usually via the GP but the physiotherapist may be a member of the care home team, and receive informal referrals.
- The physiotherapist should be aware of the resident's cognitive state.
- A check list of other important information is provided.

Physiotherapists are primarily concerned with the remediation of disability and the promotion of mobility, functional ability and quality of life through assessment, diagnosis and physical intervention.

A physiotherapist can provide advice and assistance with:

- factors concerning mobility and function;
- musculoskeletal problems, such as back and joint pain;
- management of incontinence;
- chest physiotherapy.

Acute medical illness in elderly residents is often accompanied by a decline in physical strength and mobility, and early intervention from a physiotherapist should be considered to help optimise their recovery.

Mobility assessments

A physiotherapist can conduct a mobility assessment in the care home. This involves observing how an individual stands from a chair, walks and turns through 180 degrees and, if appropriate, climbs stairs. By doing this, the therapist is able to:

- Gain important information about the resident's gait and balance.

- Develop a treatment plan.
- Determine whether a walking aid is required.

Physiotherapy input is also useful to help residents to perform functional tasks and other activities of daily living. This is achieved by improving and maintaining muscle strength, often through a tailored exercise regime that the resident must practise daily. Furthermore, some physiotherapists are involved in providing group 'keep fit' classes in care homes.

Musculoskeletal problems

Physiotherapists can assess, treat and provide advice about many musculoskeletal complaints once medical causes, such as fractures, have been addressed. For example, they are often involved in the management of chronic low back pain and postural complaints, and are able to recommend non-pharmacological methods to control pain, such as the use of TENS and acupuncture. In residents who have sustained any type of limb injury or neurological insult, such as a stroke, a physiotherapist can assist and offer advice on positioning with the use of cushions and aids in the chair or bed to increase comfort and reduce the risk of contractures.

The Care Home Handbook, First Edition. Edited by Graham Mulley, Clive Bowman, Michal Boyd and Sarah Stowe.
© 2015 John Wiley & Sons, Ltd. Published 2015 by John Wiley & Sons, Ltd.

Women's health

Some physiotherapists are trained in the area of women's health, which deals predominantly with the management of urinary and/or faecal incontinence due to muscular weakness within the pelvis. They can provide advice and tailored exercises to help with these problems.

Suitable residents are usually referred for such treatment by their GP once a medical assessment has been carried out, and other causes of incontinence have been excluded and treated (see Chapter 5.4).

Chest physiotherapy

Physiotherapy can be useful in some residents with chest complaints, particularly those with recurrent chest infections or chronic lung diseases.

The therapist can offer airway clearance advice and teach breathing exercises, which can be used to clear the lungs of phlegm and maintain the strength of the chest wall muscles. Many residents with chronic respiratory illnesses can also be taught breathing techniques to help reduce the anxiety associated with the sensation of severe breathlessness.

Cognitive impairment

In all exercise-based physiotherapy, residents must be able to understand and follow instructions, and then remember these in order to progress with treatment. This can often present a challenge if they have cognitive impairment.

Making a referral

When making a referral for expert physiotherapy assessment and intervention, the therapist will require the following details:

- Resident's name.
- Primary reason for referral (such as reduced mobility, pain or the need for a walking aid).
- Medical history and the findings of medical assessments from either the resident's GP or a hospital doctor.
- Current medication history.
- Details of the resident's baseline function – what is their normal level of activity, what can they do at present?

Access to the community physiotherapy team is usually coordinated through the resident's GP.

17.8 Referral to the adult protection team

Dagmar Long[1] and Louise Taylor[2]

[1]Leeds Community Healthcare NHS Trust, Leeds, UK
[2]Park Lodge Care Home, Leeds, UK

Key points

- All care home staff should be aware of the features that might suggest abuse.
- Report any concerns about abuse promptly to the adult protection team, following your local procedures.
- Keep a written record of any concerns raised and action taken.
- A template for the documentation of important aspects of suspected abuse is provided. This includes full details of the type of abuse, where it took place, and information of the alleged perpetrator.
- Do remember to print and sign your name and add the date that the report was written.

- This form is designed to support good practice when making a referral to the adult protection team for a resident who is suspected or alleged to have been abused and to assist with the monitoring of any reported incidents.
- It is very important that *all* staff in the care home understand the physical signs or behavioural changes that may indicate that the resident has been subjected to abuse and the ways in which vulnerable residents can be placed at risk.
- In addition, *all* staff must be aware of their personal responsibility to report any concerns immediately, either to the care home manager or directly to the adult protection team.
- Your area may have its own policies and procedures to be followed when reporting such incidents – these should be readily available to all members of staff with emergency contact numbers clearly displayed.
- *It is important to keep a careful record of the concerns raised and any actions taken, as this information may be required at a later date in legal or disciplinary proceedings.*

Details of Resident

Full name: _____

Preferred name: _____

Address: _____

_____

_____

Previous address: _____

(if relevant) _____

_____

Key worker: _____

Date of birth: _____

The Care Home Handbook, First Edition. Edited by Graham Mulley, Clive Bowman, Michal Boyd and Sarah Stowe.
© 2015 John Wiley & Sons, Ltd. Published 2015 by John Wiley & Sons, Ltd.

Details of Alerter (the person who brings the concern to your attention)

Alerter name: _____

Relationship to resident: _____

Alerter contact number: _____

Nature of abuse (indicate one or more that apply)

Discriminatory ☐   Physical ☐   Sexual ☐

Psychological ☐   Financial ☐   Neglect ☐

Details of incident (provide a description of the alleged abuse)

Location: _____

Date & time of incident: _____

What happened? _____

_____

_____

_____

Did anyone witness the incident?   **YES / NO**

If yes, please give details: _____

_____

_____

Were there any triggers for the incident?   **YES / NO**

If yes, please give details: _____

_____

_____

_____

What was the resident's reaction to the incident? _____

_____

_____

What would the resident like to be done? (Please state if the resident is unable to express their wishes) ___

_____

Is there a history of any previous incidents with this resident? (Please give details if known)   **YES / NO**

_____

_____

_____

Is the resident able to give consent to this referral being made?   **YES / NO**

Best Interests Decision details (if applicable): _____

_____

_____

Has a body map detailing any marks, bruises, etc. been completed? **YES / NO**

Has medical attention been sought? If yes, please specify who has been contacted. **YES / NO**

_____

_____

Have you taken any action to avoid immediate risk because of an emergency situation? If yes, please give details (e.g. calling police, moving resident to different part of home). **YES / NO**

_____

_____

Is Power of Attorney held by one or more people? If yes, please give details. **YES / NO / not known**

_____

_____

Details of alleged perpetrator (as far as is known)

Full Name: _____

Address: _____

_____

_____

_____

Date of Birth: _____

Occupation:

Relationship to Service user: _____

_____

Does the alleged perpetrator know that an allegation has been made against them?

☐ YES   ☐ NO   ☐ Don't know

Any additional information relevant to the alert (advice taken from a safeguarding team, senior staff, GP or other agencies involved)

_____

_____

_____

_____

_____

_____

_____

_____

Completed by:

Full Name: _____

Position / relationship: _____

_____

Contact number: _____

Date: _____

17.9 Referral to the continence advisor

Adrian Wagg

University of Alberta Edmonton, Alberta, Canada

Key points

- All cases of urinary incontinence should be assessed in detail in order to find the underlying cause(s) – which may be reversible or modifiable.
- Involving a continence advisor is often helpful in diagnosing and treating incontinence.
- A template referral letter is provided, which will help the continence advisor in their assessment.
- Do try to include details of the type of incontinence, urinalysis , post-void residual urine and current management whenever possible.

Template letter to continence advisor

Dear

Re:

I should be most grateful if you would see this xx-year old man/woman who is a care home resident with urinary incontinence.

He/She has symptoms of [state storage symptoms/voiding symptoms].

A urinalysis shows [insert findings].

The post-voiding residual volume (if available) is [insert volume in ml].

We made a preliminary symptomatic diagnosis of [insert most likely condition, based upon symptomatic diagnosis] and have begun to [insert current management care plan].

Since this time … [state exact problem requiring specialist referral].

We should be grateful of your further advice and input.

Yours faithfully

The Care Home Handbook, First Edition. Edited by Graham Mulley, Clive Bowman, Michal Boyd and Sarah Stowe.
© 2015 John Wiley & Sons, Ltd. Published 2015 by John Wiley & Sons, Ltd.

17.10 Referral to the optometrist

Dagmar Long[1] and Louise Taylor[2]

[1] Leeds Community Healthcare NHS Trust, Leeds, UK
[2] Park Lodge Care Home, Leeds, UK

Key points

- Sudden loss of vision (in one or both eyes) is a medical emergency and you should contact the doctor right away.
- Other reasons for urgent medical referral include inability to tolerate light (photophobia), pain in, or around, the eye, pain in the side of the scalp or in the jaws when chewing, a rash near the eye, a red eye or recent trauma to the eye.
- Gradual loss of vision may manifest itself by falls, disorientation, agitation or social withdrawal.
- A template letter for the optometrist is provided, which includes the details of the change in vision and a full ophthalmic, drug, allergy and medical history.

Visual impairment in older people is often undetected (see Chapter 7.1). All residents should be asked about their vision and encouraged to see an optometrist regularly. In the UK, eye tests are free to people aged over 60 – this includes a domiciliary assessment, if necessary. Nurses and other carers should be alert to symptoms suggesting a deterioration in visual acuity – new visual impairment in a resident should be considered if falls become more frequent, if there is new visuospatial disorientation, or if there is a change in mood with agitation (see Chapter 10.3) or social withdrawal.

Loss of vision will require *urgent* (same day) review by the general practitioner in the following circumstances:

- Sudden loss of vision in one or both eyes,
- Pain – in the eye, around the eye, or adjacent headache.
- Pain on chewing or tenderness of the adjacent scalp.
- Photophobia.
- Redness of eye.
- Discharge from eye.
- Rash over the face adjacent to the eye (e.g. shingles rash).
- History of trauma (e.g. damage from fingernail, chemicals).
- If there is not an acute problem requiring medical attention, then a referral to an optometrist should be made. It will be helpful for the optometrist to have details of the resident's history and current medication, as outlined in the template referral letter.

Template referral letter

Dear Colleague	
Re: Name	**Date of birth**
Address	**NHS number**
Telephone	
GP Name	Telephone
Address	

The Care Home Handbook, First Edition. Edited by Graham Mulley, Clive Bowman, Michal Boyd and Sarah Stowe.
© 2015 John Wiley & Sons, Ltd. Published 2015 by John Wiley & Sons, Ltd.

Contact details of family member (if applicable)

Thank you for your help with the further assessment of this lady's/gentleman's symptoms. I would be grateful if s/he could be offered an urgent/routine appointment for review. S/he is a care home resident who will not be able to attend your practice and a domiciliary visit will be necessary (delete if not applicable).

Define the presenting problem

Visual loss – describe if in one eye or both, complete or partial loss of sight, reading or peripheral vision most affected

Is there distortion of vision, for example straight lines do not appear straight?

Are there flashing lights or floaters?

Duration of symptom

Give length of history of current symptoms. State whether there was a sudden change or whether symptoms have evolved over time.

Ophthalmic history – is the resident known to have any of these conditions:

Glaucoma

Cataracts (whether there has been previous surgery or not)

Treatment for diabetic retinopathy

Macular degeneration

Complete visual loss for another reason (e.g. trauma in younger adulthood)

Is the person registered partially sighted or registered blind?

Is there only one eye with useful vision?

Medical history

High blood pressure

Diabetes

Chronic obstructive airways disease (COPD) treated with inhalers or nebulisers

Dementia – will the person find it easy to cooperate during treatment?

Is there medication which cannot be omitted (e.g. insulin or treatment for Parkinson's disease)?

Indicate mobility problems if these will affect the examination

Current medication

(including eye drops, inhalers or nebulisers, prednisolone, warfarin)

Allergies

With thanks for your help

Name

Title

17.11 Referral to an audiologist

Evelyn Tan

Leeds Teaching Hospitals NHS Trust, Leeds, UK

Key points

- Hearing impairment can cause social isolation and distress. The underlying cause must be sought, as the deafness might be treatable (e.g. blockage of the auditory canal by ear wax or a flat battery in the hearing aid).
- If deafness occurs suddenly or is associated with other symptoms, contact a doctor right away.
- If the resident has a hearing aid, check that it is switched on, that the ear piece is not blocked with wax and that the battery is working. If the hearing aid is working properly, consider referral to the audiologist.
- Other reasons for referral to an audiologist include ear pain or discharge, tinnitus and vertigo.
- A validated questionnaire is provided, which will help identify the resident's ear problems.
- A template letter for the audiologist is also provided.

If a resident is suspected of having hearing difficulties, a hearing assessment should be considered.

Box 17.11.1 is a validated questionnaire which can be used to assess whether the resident has hearing loss and would benefit from hearing aids.

Occasionally, deafness occurs relatively quickly or occurs together with other signs and symptoms. In such cases, referral to audiology is not appropriate.

If any of the answer to the questions is yes, then the resident should be referred to either a GP, the emergency department or an ENT specialist.

Box 17.11.2 is a check list which can be used to assess appropriateness of referral to audiology. For those

- who already use a hearing aid, but still seem to have hearing difficulty and
- who do not have any other signs and symptoms (such as those listed in the table above),

Do not refer to audiology until the following have been checked:

1. The hearing aid is at the 'on' position and the volume is turned up.
2. The hearing aid is on the correct programme.
3. The battery is working – check this by using a battery tester. Also check that the battery is the

Box 17.11.1 Questionnaire

Q1 Do you have any difficulty with your hearing? No/Yes

Q2 Do you find it **very difficult** to follow a conversation if there is background noise (such as TV, radio, children playing)? No/Yes

Q3 How well do you hear someone talking to you when that person is sitting on your RIGHT SIDE in a quiet room?
With no difficulty
With **SLIGHT** difficulty
With **MODERATE** difficulty
With **GREAT** difficulty
Cannot hear at all

Q4 How well do you hear someone talking to you when that person is sitting on your LEFT SIDE in a quiet room?
With no difficulty
With **SLIGHT** difficulty
With **MODERATE** difficulty
With **GREAT** difficulty
Cannot hear at all

If the answer to Q1 or Q2 is yes, and the response to both Q3 and Q4 are at least with slight difficulty, then hearing aids might be of benefit.

The Care Home Handbook, First Edition. Edited by Graham Mulley, Clive Bowman, Michal Boyd and Sarah Stowe.
© 2015 John Wiley & Sons, Ltd. Published 2015 by John Wiley & Sons, Ltd.

Box 17.11.2 Check list

History

Persistent pain affecting either ear (defined as earache lasting more than 7 days in the past 90 days)	Yes / No
History of discharge (other than wax) from either ear within the last 90 days	Yes / No
Sudden loss or sudden deterioration of hearing (sudden = within 1 week, in which case send to emergency department or urgent care ENT clinic)	Yes / No
Rapid loss or rapid deterioration of hearing (rapid = 90 days or less)	Yes / No
Fluctuating hearing loss, other than associated with colds	Yes / No
Unilateral or asymmetrical, or pulsatile or distressing tinnitus (ringing in the ears) lasting more than 5 minutes at a time	Yes / No
Troublesome tinnitus which may lead to sleep disturbance or be associated with symptoms of anxiety or depression	Yes / No
Abnormal auditory perceptions	Yes / No
Vertigo, including dizziness, swaying or floating sensations	Yes / No
Normal peripheral hearing but with abnormal difficulty hearing in noisy backgrounds; possibly having problems with sound localisation, or difficulty following complex auditory directions	Yes / No

Ear examination

Complete or partial obstruction of the external auditory canal preventing proper examination of the eardrum and/or proper taking of an aural impression	Yes / No
Abnormal appearance of the outer ear and/or the eardrum (e.g. inflammation of the external auditory canal, perforated eardrum; active discharge)	Yes / No

correct size and that it is inserted properly into the hearing aid with the battery sticker removed.

4. If the battery or the hearing aid is cold, allow them to gradually return to room temperature.
5. Inspect all the openings of the hearing aid and ear mould to make sure that they are not plugged with earwax.
6. The ear mould tubing does not have moisture in it.
7. If the hearing aid is a body worn type, check that the cord is connected at both ends.
8. Make sure that the hearing aid is attached to the ear mould properly.
9. Check that there is no excessive ear wax in the resident's ear.

If all of the above checks prove negative, then there is either a problem with the hearing aid itself or the resident's hearing has deteriorated further.

A referral to audiology should then be done.

Referral letter

See on following page.

Useful web site

For further information on hearing aids: http://www.action onhearingloss.org.uk/your-hearing/need-hearing-aids/looking-after-your-hearing-aids/common-problems-with-hearing-aids-and-solutions.aspx [Accessed October 2013]

Resident's name
DOB
Address
Telephone
GP name and address

Never had hearing aid	Yes/No
Hearing aid in left ear	Yes/No
Hearing aid in right ear	Yes/No
Persistent pain affecting either ear (defined as earache lasting more than 7 days in the past 90 days)	Yes/No
History of discharge other than wax from either ear within the last 90 days	Yes/No
Sudden loss or sudden deterioration of hearing (sudden = within 1 week, in which case send to emergecy department or urgent care ENT clinic)	Yes/No
Rapid loss or rapid deterioration of hearing (rapid = 90 days or less)	Yes/No
Fluctuating hearing loss, other than associated with colds	Yes/No
Unilateral or asymmetrical, or pulsatile or distressing tinnitus lasting more than 5 minutes at a time	Yes/No
Troublesome tinnitus which may lead to sleep disturbance or be associated with symptoms of anxiety or depression	Yes/No
Abnormal auditory perceptions	Yes/No
Vertigo including dizziness, swaying or floating sensations	Yes/No
Normal peripheral hearing but with abnormal difficulty hearing in noisy backgrounds; possibly having problems with sound localisation, or difficulty following complex auditory directions.	Yes/No
Complete or partial obstruction of the external auditory canal preventing proper examination of the eardrum	Yes/No
Abnormal appearance of the outer ear and/or the eardrum (e.g. inflammation of the external auditory canal, perforated eardrum; active discharge).	Yes/No

Reason for referral:

With thanks for your help

Name:
Name and title of nurse making the referral:

Date: _____

17.12 Contacting the Coroner

Dagmar Long[1] and Louise Taylor[2]

[1]Leeds Community Healthcare NHS Trust, Leeds, UK
[2]Park Lodge Care Home, Leeds, UK

Key points

- The Coroner and his team establish the facts about death in specific circumstances: for example, where the cause is unknown; concerns about neglect; where there has been violence or other injury; when the death has been because of a medical intervention or the result of an industrial injury.
- The Coroner should be informed if a resident dies without having been seen by a doctor in the preceding 14 days. If the resident is expected to die in the near future, ask the GP to visit every 14 days to help prevent an unnecessary referral to the Coroner.
- If there is to be a Coroner's inquest, inform the family that there may be a delay in issuing the death certificate and that a post mortem may take place.
- If there is a complaint about a deceased's death, do not remove any cannulae, catheters or endo-tracheal tubes.
- A check list is provided, which will help in reporting a death to the Coroner.
- Remember to give facts, not opinions.

In the UK, a Coroner is an independent judicial officer who must be a lawyer or a doctor, and in some cases is both. The Coroner is supported by a deputy and a team of Coroner's officers who work under the direction of the Coroner and liaise with bereaved families, the police, doctors, witnesses and funeral directors.

The Coroner's officers receive the initial reports of deaths and make inquiries under the direction of the Coroner. These inquiries may result in the holding of an inquest – this is to establish who the deceased was and how, when and where the person died.

The Coroner's inquest is not allowed to determine civil or criminal liability, though the death may be referred on to the police or another organisation (such as, in England and Wales, the Care Quality Commission) for further investigation.

It is not unusual for the Coroner to be involved: 47% of all deaths in England and Wales were reported to the Coroner in 2010. It is important to be aware which deaths need to be reported so that the family can be informed that there may be a delay in the death certificate being issued and that a post mortem examination may be required.

Circumstances in which a death must be reported to the Coroner include when:

- The cause of death is unknown.
  - The deceased has not been reviewed by a doctor in the 14 days before death or the doctor(s) involved cannot be contacted. *If death is expected, it is crucial that the GP is asked to review the person regularly (at least every 14 days). This is important from a care point of view and to allow a death certificate to be issued without involving the Coroner.*
- The death may have been caused by violence, trauma or physical injury, whether intentional or otherwise.
- The death may have been caused by poisoning.
- The death may be the result of intentional self-harm.
- The death may be the result of neglect or failure of care (safeguarding issues may only become apparent after death) (see Chapter 4.3).
- The death may be related to a medical procedure or treatment.

- The death may be due to an injury or disease received in the course of employment (e.g. mesothelioma from asbestos exposure, or pulmonary fibrosis from inhalation of coal dust).

If the case is being referred to the Coroner, care must be taken not to interfere with anything that might be relevant to establishing the cause of death or lead to contamination of forensic evidence. On the very rare occasions (about 3% of cases) when a special forensic post mortem is required, the family can only view the body with the agreement of the Coroner and police. Where there is any complaint about the care of the resident, or the circumstances surrounding the death give rise to suspicion requiring forensic investigation, any cannulae, catheters or endo-tracheal tubes should be left *in situ* and the body should not be washed or be given mouth care in case evidence is destroyed.

This check list gives the details that are required when reporting a death to the Coroner (or equivalent officer). This may be over the telephone to one of the Coroner's officers or in a written statement.

1. The reporting professional's name and telephone number.
2. The deceased person's name, address, date of birth and GP details.
3. Family members' names, contact details and relationship to the deceased person.
4. Date and time of death.
5. Details of anyone present at the time of death.
6. The location and position of the deceased when discovered (if death not witnessed).
7. Details of the person who certified the death.
8. Details of what happened leading up to the death.
9. Details of medical history, usual medication and when last seen by GP.

10. Whether the deceased was on a palliative care pathway Liverpool Care Pathway has been withdrawn.

All information must be given as clearly stated *facts* rather than *opinion*. Actions must be described in the first person singular: for example, '*I observed* that the resident was not breathing and *I administered* oxygen' rather than 'oxygen was administered'. Enquiries by the Coroner's officers are to establish the facts of the case and not to apportion blame. At some point, you will be asked specifically whether you have any concerns about the deceased person's care.

The information above refers to the coronial system in England and Wales. The procedure varies in other countries – for example, in Scotland referrals are taken by the Procurator Fiscal and in some American states the role is undertaken by an elected official. The reasons for reporting a death are broadly similar in all countries but there are variations and practitioners need to be to be aware of their own legal requirements. Of note, Northern Ireland differs from the rest of the UK in that the death must be reported if the deceased has not been reviewed by a doctor within the previous 28 days.

Further reading

Coroners and Burials Division, Ministry of Justice. 2010. A Guide to Coroners and Inquests.

National Nurse Consultant Group (Palliative Care), National End of Life Care Programme. 2011. Guidance for staff responsible for care after death (last offices).

UK Ministry of Justice. 2010. Coroners' statistics England and Wales 2010. www.justice.gov.uk/downloads/publications/statistics-and-data/mojstats/coroners-bulletin-2010.pdf [Accessed October 2013]

17.13 Contacting the police

David Cowley[1] and Dagmar Long[2]

[1]West Yorkshire Police, Leeds District Safeguarding Unit, Leeds, UK
[2]Leeds Community Healthcare NHS Trust, Leeds, UK

Key points

- It is rare for the police to be involved with residents of care homes.
- If there is a serious incident or allegation, contact the police right away. If in doubt, phone them for advice.
- You should contact the police if there is a suspicion that poor care has contributed to a resident's death.
- If you suspect that a crime has been committed, ask the victim if they want the police to be involved. There are circumstances when the victim's wishes might be over-ridden.
- Ensure that any evidence is preserved and that the scene of the suspected crime is not disturbed.
- Keep a written record of all your decisions and actions.

There are many situations in which involvement of the police might be necessary, although these occur infrequently.

If you are unsure whether to involve the police, or you do not know what precautions are required, the incident should be discussed promptly with local police officers before any action is taken.

With serious allegations or incidents, it is important that a report is made straight away. It may not be advisable to wait until the morning if serious incidents occur outside working hours. If in doubt, the police will be able to advise you.

In this section, we outline important considerations at the time of an incident, including the preservation of evidence.

The first priority is to ensure the safety and welfare of the victim and any other person at risk. A decision can then be made whether to refer to the police.

The police must be notified of any sudden and unexpected deaths – particularly where an aspect of the care given to the resident may have contributed to the death.

If you believe a crime has been committed (depending on the seriousness of the incident), the victim should be asked whether they wish the matter to be reported. There may be circumstances when it is appropriate to act contrary to the victim's wishes, for example where:

- Other adults are at risk of a crime being committed against them.
- The victim lacks mental capacity to consent and it

is assessed as being in their best interests for the allegation or concern to be reported to the police (Mental Capacity Act 2005 – see Chapter 4.6).
- A resident has been unduly influenced or intimidated to the extent that they are unable to give consent.

If a serious crime has occurred and a person with mental capacity does not wish this to be reported, seek advice from your line manager and if necessary consult the police.

It is important that you record all your actions and decisions so that there is an audit trail that can be reviewed later. This is for your own protection as well as that of the resident at risk.

Forensic and investigative considerations

It is important that you take advice on preservation of evidence. Initial advice can be given over the phone by a detective. Depending on the allegation, the most common considerations are:

- Discourage the victim and suspect from washing or bathing.
- Do not handle items which may hold DNA or fingerprint evidence.
- Preserve any bedding or clothing which has been removed or significant items that have been given

The Care Home Handbook, First Edition. Edited by Graham Mulley, Clive Bowman, Michal Boyd and Sarah Stowe.
© 2015 John Wiley & Sons, Ltd. Published 2015 by John Wiley & Sons, Ltd.

to you (e.g. an item that has been used as a weapon) in a safe dry place.

- Do not disturb the 'scene of crime' until advice has been sought from the police.
- Prevent others from entering that 'scene' where practical.
- Do not alert the person alleged to have caused harm.
- Do not conduct your own interviews, as this may prejudice aspects of the police investigation.

Once again, take care to document your actions and decisions.

Care home managers are required to have safeguarding procedures and training in place to guide staff in dealing with such incidents (see Chapter 17.8). Advice can be obtained through local authority adult social care teams. Alternatively, all police forces will have 'vulnerable victims' or 'safeguarding' teams who will be able to offer advice and guidance.

17.14 Referral to the podiatrist

Pauline Bailey

Newcastle University Medicine, Johor, Malaysia

Key points

- Foot and leg care are important components of well-being in elderly residents.
- Podiatrists have a range of skills, including assessment of gait and footwear, provision of orthoses, relief of foot pain and treatment of wounds and infections, nail problems, corns and callouses.
- Referrals to podiatrists should include information on diabetes, stroke, peripheral vascular disease and arthritis.

The aim of podiatry is to improve foot health by assessing, diagnosing and managing common and complex foot and lower limb problems.

The main reasons older people visit podiatrists is for treatment of nail problems, corns and callouses and toe deformities. However, podiatrists can also perform minor surgery under local anaesthetic, assess and prescribe or manufacture orthoses and carry out complex wound care.

It may be necessary to refer someone to a podiatrist for pain relief, footwear advice, treatment of infection and soft tissue problems.

They also have a role to play in the prevention of falls. The relief of foot pain and the assessment of footwear may significantly reduce the risk of further falls.

Podiatrists can also assist with wound management by assessing the wound, tissue viability and vascular and neurological status. They can also provide orthoses or footwear that can improve gait and promote comfort.

Biomechanical assessment is concerned with the function of the foot and resulting abnormalities in gait. The assessment is carried out with the aim to provide corrective measures such as orthotic devices/insoles.

Podiatry referral form

See on following page.

Further reading

Orchard S, Ahearn DJ, Bhat S, Baker P. 2011. What to expect from a general podiatry service. *CME Journal Geriatric Medicine* 13: 54–55.

Patient Details

Name - ....

Address - ....

....

....

NHS Number - ....

Date of Birth - ....

Contact number - ....

Main spoken language - ....

Needs interpreter – Y/N

Ethnicity - ....

Smoker – Y/N

Mobility –   Independent

      With walking aid

      Transfers independently

      Needs assistance to transfer

      Chair/bedbound

GP Details

Name

Address

Contact Number

Can attend clinic – Y/N   Needs transport – Y/N

Needs home visit – Y/N

Long term conditions -   Diabetes   Peripheral Arterial disease   Stroke

                           Osteoarthritis   Rheumatoid Arthritis

             Other ....

History of memory impairment – Y/N

Medication (or attach separate list) ....

....

Foot conditions

Corns/callouses ☐

Nail problems (ingrown, thickened, deformed) ☐

Orthotics/insoles ☐

Wound management ☐

Biomechanical assessment ☐

Further detail - ....

        ....

        ....

Tel number and name of referring nurse

        ....

        ....

17.15 Referral to the palliative care team

Desmond O'Neill[1] and Suzanne Green[2]

[1]*Trinity College Dublin, Dublin, Ireland*
[2]*Tallaght Hospital, Dublin, Ireland*

Key points

- Palliative care involves controlling symptoms in those who are approaching the end of life.
- Control of pain and other distressing symptoms is not always easy.
- Members of the palliative care team can assist with relieving symptoms and improving the experience of dying.
- A template letter is included that you might wish to use when making a referral. This includes diagnoses, medical and nursing problems, the resident's awareness of their situation and spiritual needs, use of a care pathway, equipment as well as information given to the next of kin.

Template letter for making a referral
to the palliative care team

Family Name
First (given) Name
Date of Birth
Next-of-kin:
Relationship:
Contact details:

Date

Dear Palliative Care Team,

We would be grateful for your expert input to the care of Mr/Mrs/Ms _____ who has been a resident in our care home under the medical care of Dr. _____ since __/__/__.

The following is a summary of Mr/Mrs Y's current active medical problems and treatments:

Medical

Diagnosis	Active problems	Treatment
Pain		

Communication and Insight

The [primary presenting disorder] was diagnosed in _____, _____ (Month/Year) and the resident *has/has not* been informed of her condition and its prognosis. The next of kin *has/has not* been informed of her condition and its prognosis.

The resident's insight into the prognosis is *full/incomplete*. The next of kin's insight into the prognosis is full/incomplete.

The resident *has/has not* been informed of a request for palliative care to become involved with his/her care. The next of kin *has/has not* been informed of a request for palliative care to become involved with care. Cardiac resuscitation *has/has not* been discussed with the resident, and the current status is: .

The Liverpool or _____ care pathway has/has not been initiated with this the resident.

Mr/Mrs X *has/has not any* spiritual preferences:

Nursing and Multi-disciplinary Needs

Activity	Level of Function
Pain	Site(s) Pain Score Severity: 0 1 2 3 4 5 6 7 8 9 10
Cognitive impairment	None/mild/moderate/severe
Hearing impairment	None/mild/moderate/severe
Visual impairment	None/mild/moderate/severe
Mobility	Independent/Assistance with appliance/Assistance with 1–2/Wheelchair
Transfers	Independent/Assistance with appliance/Assistance with 1–2/Wheelchair
Feeding	Independent/Assistance/Tube Feeding
Urinary Incontinence	Yes/No/Catheter
Faecal Incontinence	Yes/No/Stoma
Dressing	Independent/Assistance
Skin care	Intact/Other – Please illustrate on diagram below:

Additional helpful information, including equipment (pressure-relieving, seating, transfers, syringe drivers, etc), dietary needs, etc:

Thank you for your assistance,

Name:_____Title: _____

Telephone number:

17.16 Contacting chaplaincy services and other sources of spiritual/religious help

John Wattis, Steven Curran and Melanie Rogers

University of Huddersfield, Huddersfield,UK

> **Key points**
> - Residents may wish to see a chaplain or another person who provides religious or religious help.
> - This can be particularly important towards the end of life.
> - It is good practice to ascertain whether such help might be wanted when the resident first enters the care home.
> - If a resident lacks capacity to request this help, check whether the next of kin has enduring (or lasting) power of attorney.
> - Referrals to spiritual advisors are usually verbal. If a request is in writing, the resident might wish to be involved in composing the referral letter.

Confidentiality and autonomy

Residents who have the mental capacity to do so, have a right to request (or refuse) access to a spiritual or religious advisor or chaplain (hereafter 'spiritual or religious advisor'). They also have a right to determine what confidential information the advisor can see.

For residents who have been determined to lack capacity (see Chapter 4.6), the obligation on staff is to act in the resident's best interest. This may include supporting the resident to keep in touch with other members of their faith group, or occasionally putting them in touch with a specific chaplaincy service.

Local practice

Each organisation should have its own policies and practice in this area and access to formal chaplaincy services is likely to be variable. There should be clear policies and procedures for getting in touch with spiritual advisors when this is requested by the resident.

In addition, consideration should be given to ascertaining in advance whether the resident wants a spiritual or religious guide and which advisor is to be called in particular circumstances. This particularly applies to end of life care, when it is important for staff to know whether and when the resident wants an advisor to be called in. This knowledge of the resident's wishes can also be useful in circumstances where they subsequently lack capacity, including the ability to communicate their wishes.

Similar consideration should be given to involving spiritual or religious advisors in formulating end of life care plans for people who lack capacity. Again, the standard to be applied is, bearing in mind the resident's previous history and information from relatives and friends, what is likely to be in the resident's best interest?

Occasionally, a friend or relative may have a lasting or enduring power of attorney, donated by the resident while they were still competent, that gives them power to act on the resident's behalf in these matters.

Most referrals to spiritual or religious advisors will be verbal, often over the phone, at the resident's request, and they should be documented appropriately. A formal referral note may occasionally be needed. *Competent residents should normally be assisted to write their own note.*

When acting in the best interest of a resident who lacks capacity, the referral should be confined to the need for the spiritual advisor to attend, the degree of urgency appropriate and the reason for the request.

The Care Home Handbook, First Edition. Edited by Graham Mulley, Clive Bowman, Michal Boyd and Sarah Stowe.
© 2015 John Wiley & Sons, Ltd. Published 2015 by John Wiley & Sons, Ltd.

Section K

What if ...

Chapter 18

Dealing with Challenging Problems

18.1 What if … you are contacted by the press?

Clive Bowman

City University, London, UK

Key points

- Be careful and sensible when the press contact you and take care not to break confidences about residents' health details.
- If your care home has a press officer or communications team, involve them as soon as possible.
- When talking to the press, use the checklist provided.

Press coverage of care homes is heavily weighted to negative stories and it is all too easy to be unthinkingly critical. Investigating reporters tend to be highly intelligent, but that does not mean they know everything about care homes. Once said, statements can be very difficult to retract; 'I didn't mean that' will be followed by the question, 'so what did you mean?' Not easy to answer in the heat of the moment.

Large care home companies often have communications or press offices and, where these exist, the best thing to do is make sure you refer press inquiries to them.

- Get the name and a contact number of the journalist.
- Ascertain who they are working for (which newspaper, radio or other media).
- Ask them what they are interested in and why.

If you have communications people, they will almost certainly want to quiz you about the topics that the journalist is interested in – so think carefully about what you know not what you think! so a proper response can be formulated.

It is very tempting and easy to be drawn into detailed discussions and, before you are aware of it, you may break confidences about residents (past or present).

Most journalists are reputable professionals who have a legitimate role in investigating and reporting news of public interest. Most, but not all – and from a few seemingly innocent inquiries, it is impossible to differentiate easily whether the journalist is behaving professionally.

If you are in a home without a communication service and you are either asked by your management or have an overwhelming desire to talk to an inquiring journalist, do try and follow this careful checklist.

1. Ask the journalist who they are working for and what story they are investigating.
2. Ask them why they want information from you and who else they are speaking to.
3. Ask how many questions they have or for how long they want to interview you.
4. Most journalists work to deadlines. It is quite reasonable to ask what their deadline is and to suggest that you will return their call. This gives you a chance to be clear in your own mind what you can and cannot say.

Before returning a journalists call, consider the following very carefully:

1. Why have they contacted me now? Be clear it is not likely to be because you are seen as famous or so expert that you are the most obvious person. It is more likely that they have got your name and are hopeful they can strike gold on a story that may be very uncertain. Are you really the person who should be speaking to them? Will the best course of action be to refer them to someone else?
2. What are they investigating? If they want information about specific residents, you have a duty of confidentiality. Beware open questions, such as 'What do you think about …', because, unless you have carefully thought about that subject, it is quite likely your response (however well intentioned) may divulge something you did not intend.

The Care Home Handbook, First Edition. Edited by Graham Mulley, Clive Bowman, Michal Boyd and Sarah Stowe.
© 2015 John Wiley & Sons, Ltd. Published 2015 by John Wiley & Sons, Ltd.

Further reading

Mebane F. 2001. Want to understand how Americans viewed long term care in 1998? Start with media coverage. *Gerontologist* 41: 24–37.

Nazarko L. 1994. Nursing home: past, present and future. *Nursing Standards* 8: 36–39.

Vere-Jones, E. 2006. Care homes hit back at bad press. *Nursing Times* 102–112.

18.2 What if … the GP refuses to visit?

Helen Slater

Leeds Teaching Hospitals NHS Trust, Leeds, UK

Key points

- The GP should never refuse to see a resident whose medical condition is causing concern to care home staff.
- However, there are times when assessment at the surgery or emergency admission to hospital may be more appropriate.
- A check list is provided in order to inform the GP of the seriousness and nature of the resident's medical state.

Ideally, the GP should never refuse a request to visit a resident at a care home, though there may be occasions when the GP feels that the review would be more appropriate in a GP surgery, hospital clinic or hospital ward.

- Care homes and GPs should develop a symbiotic relationship to optimise residents' care.
- There are times when it is more appropriate for a resident to be seen at the surgery and other times when it is most appropriate for a resident to be sent straight to hospital without waiting to see a GP.
- There are simple measures that can be undertaken and recorded before calling the GP to allow them to decide on urgency of the visit and give advice to managing the resident review.

If a resident is not seriously ill or very disabled, and is able to visit the GP's surgery, this may be more appropriate as there are may be specialist items of equipment and drugs at the surgery.

Red flags for calling an ambulance rather than referring to the GP are:

- severe respiratory distress
- major trauma
- chest pain
- head injury
- loss of consciousness
- broken bones
- severe bleeding
- severe burns or scalds

- drug overdose
- severe abdominal pain.

(For those in the UK: if in doubt call NHS Direct.)
(One exception to some of the above is if the resident is being given palliative care only, when it is important to discuss this with the GP.) (See Chapters 16.4 and 17.15.)

Information to have available when calling the GP:

1. Up-to-date observations.
2. The drug chart.
3. Medical history.
4. Resident's level of consciousness (see Appendix 1.2). The simplest recording for this is A V P U:
   Alert
   Responding to **V**oice
   Responding to **P**ain
   Unresponsive to the above
5. Blood glucose (see Chapter 8.4).
   Other considerations:
6. If concerned about dehydration: fluid intake that day.
   Urine output for the day (see Chapter 5.3).
7. Not eating and drinking: weigh the resident and have a previous weight to compare (see Chapter 5.1). Make a food chart of the proceeding days.
8. Breathlessness – make sure to sit the resident upright and ensure that they have had all necessary inhalers or nebulisers.
9. Constipation: the date and consistency of their last bowel motion.

The Care Home Handbook, First Edition. Edited by Graham Mulley, Clive Bowman, Michal Boyd and Sarah Stowe.
© 2015 John Wiley & Sons, Ltd. Published 2015 by John Wiley & Sons, Ltd.

Further reading

Bluemel MK, Traweger C, Kinzl JF, et al. 2011. Expectations of nurses and physicians in geriatric nursing home emergencies. *Emergency Medicine* 28: 283–286.

Corroon-Sweeney E, Murphy C, Collins DR. 2009. Caring for nursing home patients: a primary care perspective. *Irish Medical Journal* 102: 317–320.

18.3 What if ... a resident absconds?

Amy Illsley[1] and Sarah Stowe[2]

[1] Yorkshire and the Humber Deanery, Bradford, UK
[2] Airedale NHS Foundation Trust, Keighley, UK

Key points

- A resident who has absconded from a care home may have intentionally chosen to leave or may have unintentionally wandered from the premises.
- A risk of absconding assessment is done on admission for each resident.
- In the UK, all care homes are required by the Care Quality Commission (CQC) to have a protocol to follow in the event that a resident absconds, and similar policies are also required internationally.
- Care homes should have an analysis of the event after a resident absconds so that lessons can be learnt to prevent further episodes.

The UK Care Homes Regulation 2001 legislation states that 'the registered person shall give notice to the Commission without delay of the occurrence of any event in the care home which adversely affects the well-being or safety of any service user' and that they must have on site 'a statement of the procedure to be followed in the event of accidents or in the event of a service user becoming missing'.

It is important that staff are aware of local and national resident health and safety policies in their location.

Factors which may increase the risk of absconding are:

- Confusion (consider the use of scales such as CAM, MMSE or AMTS to identify residents with dementia or delirium; see Appendix 1.7).
- High suicide risk.
- Physical discomfort, such as pain, hunger, thirst, need to use the toilet.
- Physical barriers to wandering in residents with dementia.

- Previous attempts at absconding or a history of wandering (consider screening with the Dewing tool for wandering).
- Substance misuse.
- Emotional stress.

In all incidents of absconding, an assessment of the resident's mental capacity to decide to leave the care home should be made upon them being found and subsequent actions based on their wishes, if deemed to have capacity to make this decision, or in their best interests if capacity is not present.

Service providers should learn 'from adverse events, incidents, errors and near misses that have occurred within the service so that the risk of these being repeated is reduced to a minimum'.

Care home staff should perform an event analysis after each episode of absconding so lessons can be learnt and appropriate changes to procedure or environment made to reduce the risk in future. Figure 18.3.1 highlights what you should do if you believe a resident has absconded.

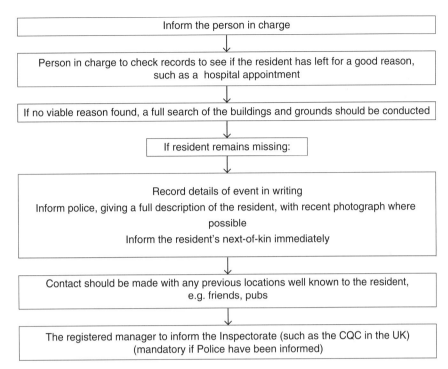

Figure 18.3.1 Suggested procedure if you believe a resident has absconded.

Useful web site

www.wanderingnetwork.co.uk [Accessed October 2013]

18.4 What if … a regulatory inspector or other authorities such as the police call unannounced?

Clive Bowman

City University, London, UK

Key points

- Unexpected or unfamiliar visitors to a home should have their credentials checked. Are they who they say they are?
- Try to establish what they are investigating or wish to inspect.
- Records of residents in the home are necessary for ongoing care and should not be removed without proper authority and the provision of copies to ensure continuity.
- Make sure your home manager or more senior manager is aware of the presence of unexpected visitors.
- Provide open and honest answers to questions. You cannot be expected to know everything. If you are asked something that you cannot answer, make clear whom you would contact or where you would go to get the information.

Regulators and other authorities have an important role in setting and monitoring standards in care homes.

While many visits will be planned, others will not be expected. If an unexpected visit occurs and the visitor is unknown to you, it is important to check their identity. Ask to see their identification; do not be shy or abrupt but professional. If you are not satisfied or no identification is offered, you should firmly indicate that you need to ask a senior manager before allowing the visitor access to the home. You have a duty of care which includes maintaining the privacy of your residents.

Having established the legitimacy of the visiting officials, ask why they are there they should (spontaneously offer this information).

In most homes, there are clear policies for informing a senior manager. If a senior manager is not in the home at that moment, contact the most senior person you can.

Do not be defensive. Answer questions to the best of your ability and answer them honestly. If you are unsure or do not know the answer, say so – but indicate how you would try to find the answer in the home. Who would you ask? Just saying that you do not know is not very professional.

On occasion, the matters being investigated may be very serious and authorities may wish to remove records. First, it is crucial that current records for existing residents are maintained, so that care can continue. Second, if such records are being sought, it would be normal for copies to be taken. Larger companies may have in-house legal advice or hotlines for legal support.

Your first responsibility is the safety and well-being of the residents remaining in the home and you should not be afraid to make that clear.

Further reading

Rickwood D, Braithwaite J. 1994. Why openness with health inspectors pays. *Australian Journal of Public Health* 18: 165–169.

18.5 What if ... you are confronted by a difficult or dysfunctional family?

Clive Bowman

City University, London, UK

Key points

- Most families are very helpful in aiding with the care of their relative in a care home.
- Occasionally, relatives can be 'difficult'. This may be because of unrealistic expectations of recovery.
- Family caregivers are often very experienced in understanding the resident's needs: their observations and experiences should form part of the care plan.

Residents' families may have strong views on how care should be provided. Often a spouse or main carer will have supported an individual successfully for a long period, and they may well be truly expert in preferences and the best way to administer various aspects of care. This can be particularly helpful in residents with mental impairment. It is essential that their knowledge and expertise is used in the development of a care plan and that the plan should involve them.

While most families and friends may participate actively and helpfully in their family member's care, there are occasions when this is not the case.

Typically, there will be relatives who may not be particularly close geographically or emotionally to the resident, and who may have widely differing perceptions of their family member's health and well-being.

Accordingly, they may have very different expectations about the care that is needed and what it can achieve.

The following considerations may be helpful:

1. Most care home residents are admitted to the home from hospital wards where, in a well-meaning manner, one or more staff members may have suggested that 'things will be much better in the care home'. Some will hear this as a clear expectation that their family member's health will improve and that everything will be just fine. The reality may be that, while the resident may recover from an acute illness, the likelihood is that their underlying conditions will continue to deteriorate. It is therefore essential to be both realistic about the future yet positive about what care can be delivered. If there is a lack of understanding or non-acceptance of the reality of the resident's state, it may be constructive to seek medical advice and opinion.

2. Communicating with a large, distressed and sometimes dysfunctional family can be very difficult. Slight differences in communication by different members can lead to wildly differing understanding and opinions. Experienced home managers will seek agreed lines of communication often with one or two family leaders and make sure staff understand the importance of good communication. Good practice must include the offer of update sessions with family members.

Occasionally, family members will interfere with the delivery of care, sometimes maliciously. The care home's responsibility is the safety and well-being of the resident, and if serious concerns are raised police or other appropriate external agencies such as adult safeguarding should be contacted.

Further reading

Sollins HL. 2007. Handling difficult family situations: practical approaches. *Geriatric Nursing* 28: 80–82.

Wewman K, Fagerberg I. 2006. Registered nurses working together with family members of older people. *Journal of Clinical Nursing* 15: 281–289.

18.6 What if ... you are asked to witness a resident's signature on a legal document?

Clive Bowman

City University, London, UK

Key points

- Residents who are asked to sign legal documents must have the capacity to do so.
- As a rule, you should not witness signatures on legal documents.
- Refer all requests for witnessing documents to your manager.

Care home staff can be asked to witness the signing of documents by a resident. This may be absolutely reasonable – but it also may not be.

It is best to be cautious to avoid being an accessory to malicious behaviour that is for personal gain.

Before legal documents are signed, everyone concerned must be sure that the resident has the capacity to sign the document (see Chapter 4.6).

Good practice would be that any document signing is planned in advance and that the signing has been agreed by the resident's family and/or the legal advocate.

Generally, care home staff should decline to witness signatures.

All legal representatives should be referred to the care home manager.

Further reading

Hayley DC, Cassel CK, Snyder L, Rudberg MA. 1996. Ethical and legal issues in nursing home care. *Archives of Internal Medicine* 156: 249–256.

Spears R, Drinka PJ, Voeks SK. 1993. Obtaining a durable power of attorney for health care from nursing home residents. *Journal of Family Practice* 36: 409–413.

18.7 What if ... you are asked to provide a resident's records to a third party?

Clive Bowman

City University, London, UK

Key points

- Sharing health information on residents can help improve care – but it is important to respect each individual's privacy.
- Use the flow chart to help you decide if it is appropriate to share personal details.
- Never allow the case notes to be taken away from the care home.
- If information is to be shared, make a photocopy.

In order to protect a resident's privacy, information about them should only be shared with others if several important criteria are fulfilled.

The flow chart (see Figure 18.7.1) is intended to help you to decide whether or not to allow third parties to see or take away written information concerning a resident.

This is intended as a general guide, not as definitive advice. If in doubt, discuss the request with a senior member of staff.

Further reading

Anderson MA, Helms LB. 1998. Comparison of continuing care communication. *Image the Journal of Nursing Scholarship* 30: 255–260.

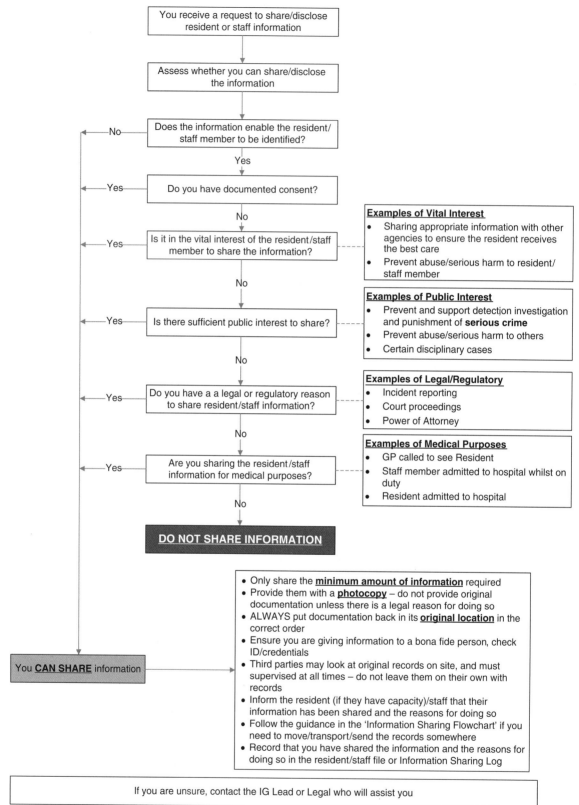

Figure 18.7.1 'Keeping information safe' flowchart.

18.8 What if ... you have to manage unreasonable complainants?

Clive Bowman

City University, London, UK

Key points

- As a general rule, complaints about care homes are understandable and should always be taken seriously.
- Occasionally, the person making the complaint might be unreasonable. In extreme cases, this can lead to a breakdown in relationships between the complainant and the care home staff.
- Guidelines are offered on how to manage difficult behaviour in complainants.

Complaints that are sympathetically received and attentively managed will satisfy most complainants.

However, there are regrettable exceptions, particularly when complaints relate to either major failings or serious harm.

In these instances, well-managed care home organisations will be as keen to identify and remedy faults transparently and with whatever official external investigation that is necessary.

Good complaints management treats all complaints fairly and impartially and should be capable of acknowledging errors and making clear what actions will be taken in an attempt to prevent further occurrences.

However, there is a rare but very difficult problem where the persistence of a complainant and/or their frequency of contact with the home become unreasonable. In such instances, it is crucial to seek agreement over the substance of the complaint(s) and to have a clear process with documented reporting schedule to which you can consistently refer.

No care home staff should have to accept abusive, offensive, deceitful, threatening or other forms of unacceptable behaviour from complainants.

If such behaviour should occur, staff should politely but firmly state that the complainant's behaviour is unreasonable and state that the meeting/phone call has ended. Immediately after such an episode, the care worker, nurses or home manager should report the event to their senior colleague and document what occurred. Very often, emotions run high because of one or more factors, which may include genuine anger over matters (proven or unproven) regarding care, guilt about a family member being in care and, on occasion, the complainants own mental state.

A small group of complainants become utterly fixated on their complaint(s). Their behaviour can be seriously disruptive to the safe running of a home. Homes with strong leadership will get the most senior manager available:

- To explain to the complainant why their behaviour is considered unreasonable.
- To confirm the details of the complaint under investigation.
- To reaffirm the timetable.
- To politely but firmly request a change in behaviour.
- To warn the complainant that if their behaviour continues, action will be taken to restrict their contact with the home.

If behaviour is so extreme that it threatens the immediate safety and welfare of staff, the matter should be urgently reported to the police. In these rare instances, the home manager might consider taking legal action. In such cases, the complainant may not be made aware of these intended actions.

In these rare events when relationships have broken, further contact with the care home should be

---

The Care Home Handbook, First Edition. Edited by Graham Mulley, Clive Bowman, Michal Boyd and Sarah Stowe.
© 2015 John Wiley & Sons, Ltd. Published 2015 by John Wiley & Sons, Ltd.

formalised and restricted to bring some order to what can become a chaotic situation. The sort of restrictions could include (but are not restricted to) the following:

- Limiting contact to one form only and limiting frequency (for example, a maximum of one letter a week).
- Limiting contact to take place with one named person within the organisation.
- Restricting telephone calls to specified days and times.
- Requiring the complainant to enter into an agreement about their behaviour before their case proceeds any further.
- Managing contact with the help of an independent advocate.

Other options may be considered, depending on the specific nature of the case.

The complainant will also be advised of the length of time that the restriction will apply for before it is reconsidered and will explain how this decision can be challenged.

If the care home staff have gone to these extraordinary lengths, and the complainant persistently breaches the restrictions that have been put in place, a home may decide to terminate contact with them and discontinue the complaint investigation. If matters have deteriorated to this point, it is likely that the complainant will have involved other agencies (including regulatory bodies) and the home may breathe a sigh of relief that the investigation is to be taken over.

If new evidence about the complaint is provided, this decision may be reviewed.

New complaints from a person who has previously displayed unreasonable behaviour will be treated separately. Any restrictions imposed previously will not automatically be applied to a new complaint.

Further reading

Majerovitz SD, Mollott RJ, Rudder C. 2009. We're on the same side: improving communication between nursing home and family. *Health Communication* 24: 12–20.

Stevenson DG. 2006. Nursing home complaints and quality of care: a national view. *Medical Care Research and Review* 63: 347–368.

Appendix 1

Rating Scales

Appendix 1.1 Pressure ulcers

Sarah Stowe[1] and Amy Illsley[2]

[1] *Airedale NHS Foundation Trust, Keighley, UK*
[2] *Yorkshire and the Humber Deanery, Bradford, UK*

Key points

- It is good practice to risk assess residents for pressure ulcer prevention (see Chapter 5.6) and tools can aid clinical judgement in identifying high risk individuals so that preventative strategies can be implemented.
- Several different tools are available for this.

Norton and her colleagues proposed the first pressure ulcer risk assessment tool. This was specifically designed for predicting pressure ulcers in older people in hospital and five factors were taken into account: mobility, incontinence, mental state, activity and physical condition. Scores ranged from 5–20 with a score of 14 or less indicating an individual is at risk. The lower a score, the higher the risk of developing a pressure ulcer.

The *Modified Norton Scale* (MNS) assesses residents across seven indicators of risk, each scoring between 1 to 4 as shown in Figure A1.1.1. A score below 25 identifies those at risk, with a lower score being higher risk. The Norton scale was subsequently superseded by more complex tools, which considered preventative strategies in addition to identifying high risk individuals.

Judy Waterlow created a risk assessment tool with seven main risk factors, including appetite and nutrition, underlying tissue pathology, surgical procedures and medications. This was updated in 2005 and is in widespread use today as shown in Figure A1.1.2. *Waterlow scores* range from 4 to 40, with a higher score implying higher risk. A score of 10 or more identifies an individual at risk with 20 or more equating very high risk.

The *Braden scale* predicts pressure sore risk by considering six domains, including sensory perception, activity, mobility, moisture, friction and nutrition, as shown in Figure A1.1.3. Residents can score between 6 and 23 points using the scale, with a lower score equating to higher risk. At risk individuals score 16 points or less.

A. Mental condition	4 = fully orientated
	3 = occasionally confused
	2 = cannot answer adequately
	1 = no contact
B. Activity	4 = ambulant
	3 = walks with help
	2 = chairbound
	1 = bedridden
C. Mobility	4 = full
	3 = slightly limited
	2 = very limited
	1 = immobile
D. Food intake	4 = normal
	3 = insufficient
	2 = parenteral
	1 = no intake
E. Fluid intake	4 = normal
	3 = insufficient
	2 = parenteral
	1 = no intake
F. Incontinence	4 = not
	3 = occasional
	2 = usually urine
	1 = double
G. General physical condition	4 = good
	3 = fair
	2 = poor
	1 = very bad

Figure A1.1.1 The Norton Scale. Reproduced from Ek and Bjurulf (1987) with permission from John Wiley & Sons, Ltd.

The Care Home Handbook, First Edition. Edited by Graham Mulley, Clive Bowman, Michal Boyd and Sarah Stowe.
© 2015 John Wiley & Sons, Ltd. Published 2015 by John Wiley & Sons, Ltd.

(a)

Waterlow pressure ulcer prevention/treatment policy
Ring scores in table, add total more than 1 score/category can be used

Build/weight for height	◆	Skin type visual risk areas	◆	Sex age	◆	Malnutrition screening tool (MST) (Nutrition vol.15, No.6 1999 - Australia)		
Average BMI = 20-24.9	0	Healthy	0	Male	1	A - Has patient lost weight recently		B - Weight loss score
		Tissue paper	1	Female	2			0.5 - 5kg = 1
Above average BMI = 25-29.9	1	Dry	1	14 - 49	1	Yes - Go to B		5 - 10kg = 2
		Oedematous	1	50 - 64	2	No - Go to C		10 - 15kg = 3
OBESE BMI > 30	2	Clammy, pyrexia	1	65 - 74	3	Unsure - Go to C and score 2		> 15kg = 4
		Discoloured grade 1	2	75 - 80	4			unsure = 2
Below average BMI < 20	3	Broken/sports grade 2-4	3	81 +	5	C- Patient eating poorly Or lack of appetite 'No' = 0; 'Yes' score = 1		Nutrition score If > 2 refer nutrition assessement/ intervention
BMI = Wt(Kg)/Ht (m)³								

Continence	◆	Mobility	◆	Special risk				
Complete/ catheterised	0	Fully	0	**Tissue malnutrition**	◆	**Neurological deficit**		◆
Urine incont.	1	Restless/fidgety	1	Terminal cachexia	8	Diabetes, MS, CVA		4-5
Faecal incont.	2	Apathetic	2	Multiple organ failure	8	Motor/sensory		4-6
Urinary + faecal incontinence	3	Restricted	3	Single organ failure (resp, renal, cardiac)	5	Paraplegia (max of 6)		4-6
		Bedbound e.g. Traction	4	Peripheral vascular disease	5	**Major surgery or trauma**		
		Chairbound e.g. Wheelchair	5	Anaemia (Hb < 8)	2	Orthopaedic/spinal		5
				Smoking	1	On table > 2 HR#		5
						On table > 6 HR#		8

Score

10+ at risk

15+ high risk

20+ very high risk

Medication - cytotoxics, long term/high dose steroids, anti-inflammatory   max of 4

\# Scores can be discounted after 48 hours provided patient is recovering normally

(b)

PREVENTION

Pressure Reducing Aids

Special Mattress/beds: 10+ Overlays or specialist foam mattresses.
15+ Alternating pressure overlays, mattresses and bed systems
20+ Bed systems: Fluidized bead, low air loss and alternating pressure mattresses
Note: Preventative aids cover a wide spectrum of specialist features. Efficacy should be judged, if possible, on the basis of independent evidence.

Cushions: No person should sit in a wheelchair without some form of cushioning. If nothing else is available - use the person's own pillow. (Consider infection risk)
10+ 100mm foam cushion
15+ Specialist gell and/or foam cushion
20+ Specialised cushion, adjustable to individual person.

Bed clothing Avoid plastic draw sheets, inco pads and tightly tucked in sheet/sheetcovers, especially when using specialist bed and mattress overlay systems.
Use duvet - plus vapour permeable membrane.

NURSING CARE

General Hand washing, frequent changes of position, lying, sitting, use of pillows

Pain Appropriate pain control

Nutrition High protein, vitamins and minerals

Patient handling Correct lifting technique - hoists - overhead hand grip (e.g. monkey pole) transfer devices

Patient comfort aids Real sheepskin - bed cradle

operating table theatre/A&E trolley 100 mm (4 ins) cover plus adequate protection

Skin care General hygiene, NO rubbing, cover with an appropriate dressing

WOUND GUIDELINES

Assessment Odor, exudate, measure/photograph position

WOUND CLASSIFICATION - EPUAP

Grade 1 Discoloration of intact skin not affected by light finger pressure (non-blanching erythema)
This may be difficult to identify in darkly pigmented skin

Grade 2 Partial thickness skin loss or damage involving epidermis and/or dermis
The pressure ulcer is superficial and presents clinically as an abrasion, blister or shallow crater

Grade 3 Full thickness skin loss involving damage of subcutaneous tissue but not extending to the underlying fascia
The pressure ulcer presents clinically as a deep crater with or without undermining of adjacent tissue

Grade 4 Full thickness skin loss with extensive destruction and necrosis extending to underlying tissue

Dressing guide Use local dressing formulary and/or www.worldwidewounds.com

IF TREATMENT IS REQUIRED, FIRST REMOVE PRESSURE

Figure A1.1.2 Waterlow Pressure Ulcer Prevention/Treatment Policy. Reproduced with permission from Judy Waterlow. © Judy Waterlow.

Braden scale for predicting pressure sore risk

Patient's Name _____ Evaluator's Name _____ Date of Assessment

	1	2	3	4			
SENSORY PERCEPTION Ability to respond meaningfully to pressure-related discomfort	**1. Completely Limited** Unresponsive (does not moan, flinch, or grasp) to painful stimuli, due to diminished level of con-sciousness or sedation. OR limited ability to feel pain over most of body	**2. Very Limited** Responds only to painful stimuli. Cannot communicate discomfort except by moaning or restlessness OR has a sensory impairment which limits the ability to feel pain or discomfort over ½ of body.	**3. Slightly Limited** Responds to verbal commands, but cannot always communicate discomfort or the need to be turned. OR has some sensory impairment which limits ability to feel pain or discomfort in 1 or 2 extremities.	**4. No Impairment** Responds to verbal commands. Has no sensory deficit which would limit ability to feel or voice pain or discomfort			
MOISTURE Degree to which skin is exposed to moisture	**1. Constantly Moist** Skin is kept moist almost constantly by perspiration, urine, etc. Dampness is detected every time patient is moved or turned.	**2. Very Moist** Skin is often, but not always moist. Linen must be changed at least once a shift.	**3. Occasionally Moist** Skin is occasionally moist, requiring an extra linen change approximately once a day.	**4. Rarely Moist** Skin is usually dry, linen only requires changing at routine intervals.			
ACTIVITY Degree of physical activity	**1. Bedfast** Confined to bed.	**2. Chairfast** Ability to walk severely limited or non-existent. Cannot bear own weight and/or must be assisted into chair or wheelchair.	**3. Walks Occasionally** Walks occasionally during day, but for very short distances, with or without assistance. Spends majority of each shift in bed or chair	**4. Walks Frequently** Walks outside room at least twice a day and inside room at least once every two hours during waking hours			
MOBILITY Ability to change and control body position	**1. Completely Immobile** Does not make even slight changes in body or extremity position without assistance	**2. Very Limited** Makes occasional slight changes in body or extremity position but unable to make frequent or significant changes independently.	**3. Slightly Limited** Makes frequent though slight changes in body or extremity position independently.	**4. No Limitation** Makes major and frequent changes in position without assistance.			
NUTRITION Usual food intake pattern	**1. Very Poor** Never eats a complete meal. Rarely eats more than ½ of any food offered. Eats 2 servings or less of protein (meat or dairy products) per day. Takes fluids poorly. Does not take a liquid dietary supplement OR is NPO and/or maintained on clear liquids or IV's for more than 5 days.	**2. Probably Inadequate** Rarely eats a complete meal and generally eats only about ½ of any food offered. Protein intake includes only 3 servings of meat or dairy products per day. Occasionally will take a dietary supplement. OR receives less than optimum amount of liquid diet or tube feeding	**3. Adequate** Eats over half of most meals. Eats a total of 4 servings of protein (meat, dairy products per day. Occasionally will refuse a meal, but will usually take a supplement when offered OR is on a tube feeding or TPN regimen which probably meets most of nutritional needs	**4. Excellent** Eats most of every meal. Never refuses a meal. Usually eats a total of 4 or more servings of meat and dairy products. Occasionally eats between meals. Does not require supplementation.			
FRICTION & SHEAR	**1. Problem** Requires moderate to maximum assistance in moving. Complete lifting without sliding against sheets is impossible. Frequently slides down in bed or chair, requiring frequent repositioning with maximum assistance. Spasticity, contractures or agitation leads to almost constant friction	**2. Potential Problem** Moves feebly or requires minimum assistance. During a move skin probably slides to some extent against sheets, chair, restraints or other devices. Maintains relatively good position in chair or bed most of the time but occasionally slides down.	**3. No Apparent Problem** Moves in bed and in chair independently and has sufficient muscle strength to lift up completely during move. Maintains good position in bed or chair.				
				Total Score			

Figure A1.1.3 Braden Scale for predicting pressure sore results. Reproduced with permission from B. Braden and N. Bergstrom. © Copyright Barbara Braden and Nancy Bergstrom, 1988. All rights reserved.

References

Bergstrom N, Braden BJ, Laguzza A, Holman V. 1987. The Braden scale for predicting pressure sore risk. *Nursing Research* 36: 205–210.

Ek AC, Bjurulf P. 1987. Interrater variability in a modified Norton scale. *Scandinavian Journal of Caring Science* 1: 99–102.

Norton D, McLaren R, Exton-Smith AN. 1962. *An Investigation of Geriatric Nursing Problems in Hospitals.* London, National Corporation for the Care of Old People.

Waterlow JA. 1985. A risk assessment card. *Nursing Times* 81: 49–55.

Further reading

NICE. 2005. NICE guidelines on pressure ulcer management including prevention. Available at: http://www.nice.org.uk/CG029 [Accessed October 2013]

Useful web sites

www.bradenscale.com/images/bradenscale.pdf [Accessed October 2013]

www.judy-waterlow.co.uk [Accessed October 2013]

Appendix 1.2 Conscious level

Sarah Stowe[1] and Amy Illsley[2]

[1] *Airedale NHS Foundation Trust, Keighley, UK*
[2] *Yorkshire and the Humber Deanery, Bradford, UK*

Key points

- The Glasgow Coma Scale is a 15-point score which was developed to allow an individual's conscious level to be reliably and objectively measured following trauma (Figure A1.2.1).
- This scale assesses motor and verbal responsiveness and eye opening and has become a universal tool in assessing coma severity and predicting mortality.
- The maximum score of 15 corresponds to a fully alert individual and the minimum score of 3 would be found in a deeply comatose person.
- Residents with cognitive impairment or speech difficulties may score less than 15 using the GCS – despite being fully alert.

Behaviour		Score (max 15)
Eye opening	Spontaneous	4
	To speech	3
	To pain	2
	None	1
Best verbal response	Orientated	5
	Confused	4
	Inappropriate	3
	Incomprehensible	2
	None	1
Best motor response	Obeying commands	6
	Localises to pain	5
	Flexion (withdrawal)	4
	Abnormal Flexion	3
	Extension	2
	None	1

Figure A1.2.1 The Glasgow Coma Scale. Reproduced from Teasdale and Jennett (1974) with permission from Elsevier.

Some aspects of the GCS can be difficult to assess for inexperienced healthcare professionals, such as the motor response to pain, and may lead to inappropriate scoring. Various studies have shown inexperienced personnel to miscalculate the GCS in 25–50% of cases.

A simpler tool to use is the 'AVPU' score, which was originally used in the assessment of victims of trauma, and is now in widespread use. This is a very quick and simple-to-perform assessment of alertness with four categories (Figure A1.2.2). This has been combined with standard observations to identify acutely ill adults in early warning scoring systems.

It is also important when assessing or monitoring a resident for reduced conscious level to examine and document the reactions of the pupils. Documenting pupil size, whether both are equal and whether they react to light, is an essential part of neurological observations.

The Care Home Handbook, First Edition. Edited by Graham Mulley, Clive Bowman, Michal Boyd and Sarah Stowe.
© 2015 John Wiley & Sons, Ltd. Published 2015 by John Wiley & Sons, Ltd.

Is the patient:-	Tick one
Alert & orientated	A
Responds to **v**oice	V
Responds to **p**ain	P
Unresponsive	U

Figure A1.2.2 The AVPU score. Reproduced from American College of Surgeons Committee on Trauma. *Advanced Trauma Life Support for Doctors*, 6th edn. Chicago: American College of Surgeons, 1997 with permission from the American College of Surgeons.

References

American College of Surgeons Committee on Trauma. 1997. *Advanced Trauma Life Support for Doctors*, 6th edn. Chicago, American College of Surgeons.

Teasdale G, Jennett B. 1974. Assessment of coma and impaired consciousness. *Lancet* 304: 81–84.

Namiki J, Yamazaki M, Funabiki T, Hori S. 2011. Inaccuracy and misjudged factors of Glasgow Coma Scale scores when assessed by inexperienced physicians. *Clinical Neurology Neurosurgery* 113(5): 393–398.

Further reading

Crossman J, Bankes M, Bhan A, Crockard, HA. 1998. The Glasgow Coma Score: reliable evidence? *Injury* 29(6): 435–437.

Appendix 1.3 Pain rating scales

Sarah Stowe[1] and Amy Illsley[2]

[1] *Airedale NHS Foundation Trust, Keighley, UK*
[2] *Yorkshire and the Humber Deanery, Bradford, UK*

Key points

* Pain is common among care home residents, yet it may be unrecognised and under-treated – especially in those with dementia (see Chapters 8.6 and 10.1).
* When a resident complains of pain, *it is essential to make an assessment of the nature and severity of their symptoms*. Response to treatment can be monitored by repeating assessments which objectively record their descriptions.
* It can be challenging to recognise, assess and treat pain in older people who have barriers to verbal communication such as language and cultural barriers, speech impairment or severe dementia. Many scales to assess pain are available and those with verbal descriptors or numerical scales are recommended for use in older people.

A comprehensive guide to assessing pain in older people was produced jointly by the British Pain Society, the British Geriatrics Society and the Royal College of Physicians in 2007. This resource is freely available online, and includes many assessment tools and a new algorithm (see Figure A1.3.1).

Huskisson (1974) first described the use of a *visual analogue scale*. This allows a resident to describe the severity of their pain using a vertical or horizontal scale, as demonstrated in Figure A1.3.2. Self-reporting scales, such as the visual analogue scale, have been shown to have high reliability and validity in older adults and they can be used those with mild to moderate cognitive impairment. The vertical tool may be preferable to the horizontal tool (Figure A1.3.3), as it avoids misinterpretation in patients with visuospatial neglect, for example hemianopia after a stroke.

The *Abbey pain scale* (Figure A1.3.4) is an observational pain assessment specifically developed to recognise and assess pain in care home residents with advanced dementia (Abbey et al., 2004). It can be used to ensure that residents who cannot verbalise receive good control of symptoms at the end of life. The Abbey tool is simple and only takes about a minute to administer. It is useful to assess residents with pain during movement, such as when turning for pressure area care or washing.

Other scales that can be used to assess pain in elderly care home residents with advanced dementia include the *Pain Assessment Checklist for Seniors with Limited Ability to Communicate (PACSLAC)* (Figure A1.3.5) and *DOLOPLUS-2 scales* (Figure A1.3.6) (Zwakhalen et al. 2006; see also Useful web sites). The DOLOPLUS-2 Scale was specifically designed to be a behavioural pain assessment in older adults with verbal communication problems. *These scales are the most appropriate scales currently available* when compared to other pain assessments, including the Abbey tool.

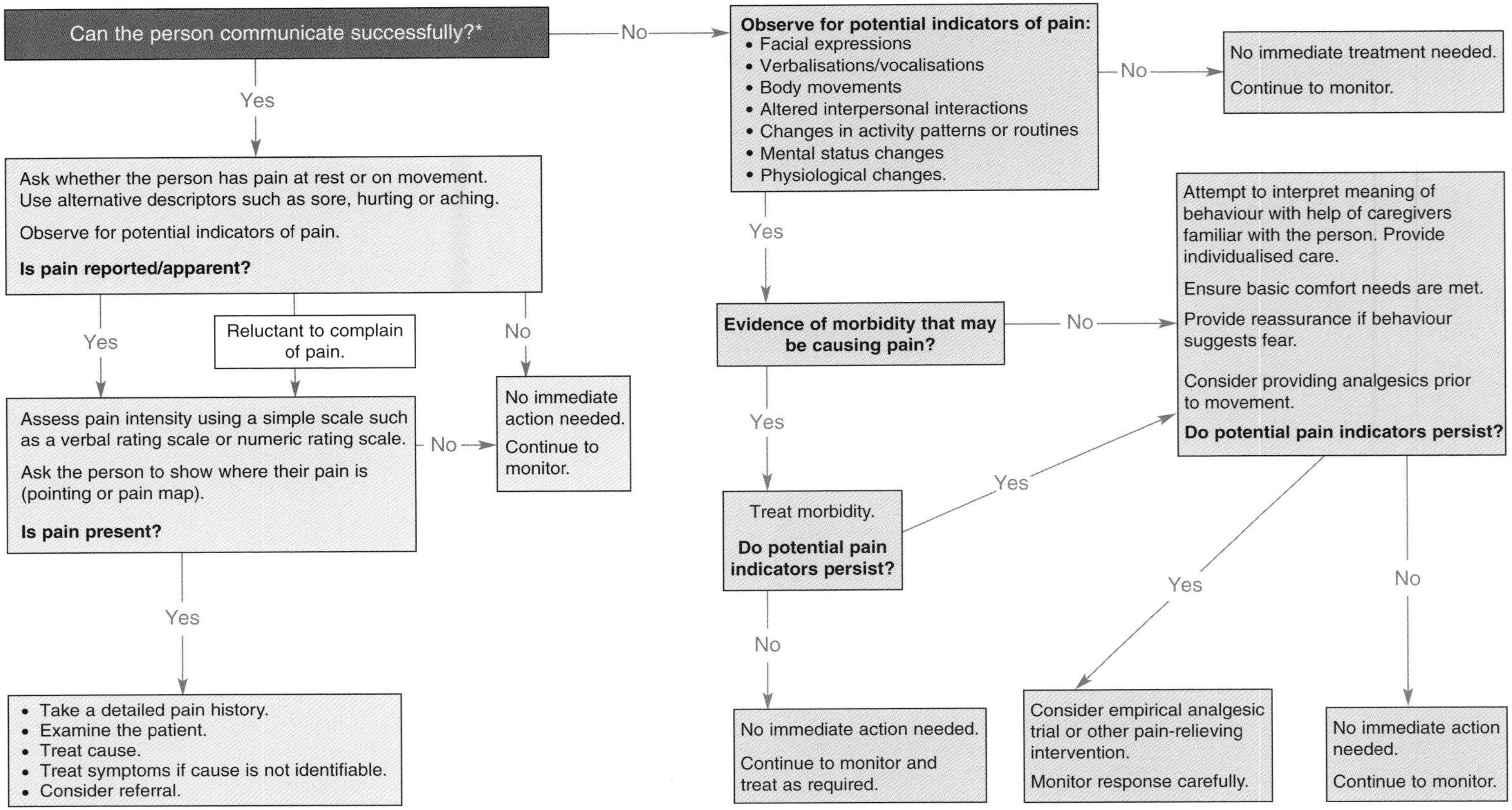

Can the person communicate successfully?*
No
Yes
Ask whether the person has pain at rest or on movement. Use alternative descriptors such as sore, hurting or aching.
Observe for potential indicators of pain.
Is pain reported/apparent?
Yes
Reluctant to complain of pain.
No
No immediate action needed.
Continue to monitor.
Assess pain intensity using a simple scale such as a verbal rating scale or numeric rating scale.
Ask the person to show where their pain is (pointing or pain map).
Is pain present?
No
Yes
• Take a detailed pain history.
• Examine the patient.
• Treat cause.
• Treat symptoms if cause is not identifiable.
• Consider referral.
Observe for potential indicators of pain:
• Facial expressions
• Verbalisations/vocalisations
• Body movements
• Altered interpersonal interactions
• Changes in activity patterns or routines
• Mental status changes
• Physiological changes.
No
No immediate treatment needed.
Continue to monitor.
Yes
Evidence of morbidity that may be causing pain?
No
Yes
Treat morbidity.
Do potential pain indicators persist?
Yes
No
No immediate action needed.
Continue to monitor and treat as required.
Attempt to interpret meaning of behaviour with help of caregivers familiar with the person. Provide individualised care.
Ensure basic comfort needs are met.
Provide reassurance if behaviour suggests fear.
Consider providing analgesics prior to movement.
Do potential pain indicators persist?
Yes
No
Consider empirical analgesic trial or other pain-relieving intervention.
Monitor response carefully.
No immediate action needed.
Continue to monitor.

*If there is doubt about ability to communicate, assess and facilitate as indicated in Recommendations 4 and 5 of the Guidelines.

Figure A1.3.1 Algorithm for the assessment of pain in older people. Reproduced from Royal College of Physicians, British Geriatrics Society and British Pain Society. The assessment of pain in older people: national guidelines. Concise guidance to good practice series, No 8. London: RCP, 2007 with permission from the Royal College of Physicians. Copyright © 2007 Royal College of Physicians.

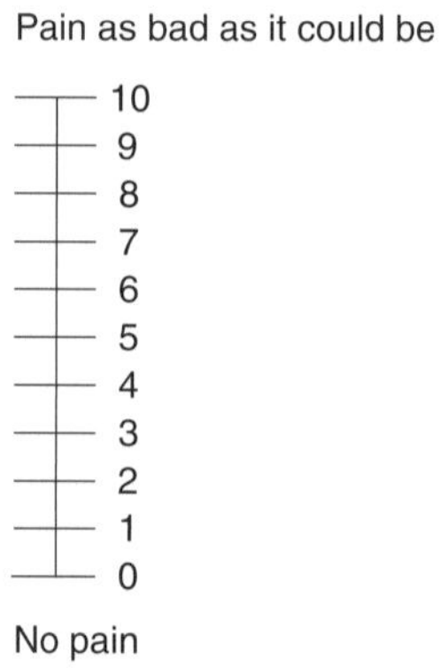

Pain as bad as it could be

— 10
— 9
— 8
— 7
— 6
— 5
— 4
— 3
— 2
— 1
— 0

No pain

Figure A1.3.2 Vertical visual analogue scale. Reproduced from Huskisson (1974) with permission from Elsevier.

Please mark the scale to show how intense your pain is

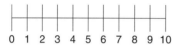

0 1 2 3 4 5 6 7 8 9 10

A zero (0) means no pain and ten (10) means extreme pain.
Ask the resident: "How *intense* is your pain now?"

Figure A1.3.3 Horizontal visual analogue scale. Reproduced from Huskisson (1974) with permission from Elsevier.

Abbey Pain Scale

For measurement of pain in people with dementia who cannot verbalize

How to use scale: While observing the resident, score questions 1 to 6.

Name of resident: ....

Name and designation of person completing the scale: ....

Date: .... Time: ....

Latest pain relief given was .... at ....hrs.

Q1.   Vocalisation

     e.g. whimpering, groaning, crying   Q1

     Absent 0   Mild 1   Moderate 2   Severe 3

Q2.   Facial expression

     e.g. looking tense, frowning, grimacing, looking frightened   Q2

     Absent 0   Mild 1   Moderate 2   Severe 3

Q3.   Change in body language

     e.g. fidgeting, rocking, guarding part of body, withdrawn   Q3

     Absent 0   Mild 1   Moderate 2   Severe 3

Q4.   Behavioural change

     e.g. increased confusion, refusing to eat, alteration in usual patterns   Q4

     Absent 0   Mild 1   Moderate 2   Severe 3

Q5.   Physiological change

     e.g. temperature, pulse or blood pressure outside normal limits, perspiring,
     flushing or pallor   Q5

     Absent 0   Mild 1   Moderate 2   Severe 3

Q6.   Physical changes

     e.g. skin tears, pressure areas, arthritis, contractures, previous injuries   Q6

     Absent 0   Mild 1   Moderate 2   Severe 3

Add scores for 1–6 and record here   ⟹   Total pain score

Now tick the box that matches
the total pain score   ⟹

0–2	3–7	8–13	14+
No pain	Mild	Moderate	Severe

Finally, tick the box which matches
the type of pain   ⟹

Chronic	Acute	Acute on chronic

Figure A1.3.4 The Abbey pain scale. Reproduced from Abbey et al. (2004) with permission from Mark Allen Healthcare Ltd.

How to complete the PACSLAC checklist

This is based on observations of the resident during activity or movement (such as transferring out of bed or walking) after a day-long shift of observation.

Determine the presence or absence of each behaviour on the checklist.

Determine the total score at each use.

Compare the total score after each use to the previous score documented.

An increased score suggests that an increase in pain is likely. On the other hand, a lower score suggests that the pain has decreased.

Facial expression	Present
Grimacing	
Sad look	
Tighter face	
Dirty look	
Change in eyes (Squinting, dull, bright, increased eye movements)	
Frowning	
Pain expression	
Grim face	
Clenching teeth	
Wincing	
Open mouth	
Creasing forehead	
Screwing up nose	

Social/personality/mood	Present
Physical aggression (e.g. pushing people and/or objects, scratching others, hitting others, striking, kicking).	
Verbal aggression	
Not wanting to be touched	
Not allowing people near	
Angry/mad	
Throwing things	
Increased confusion	
Anxious	
Upset	
Agitated	
Cranky/irritable	
Frustrated	

Activity/body movement	Present
Fidgeting	
Pulling away	
Flinching	
Restless	
Pacing	
Wandering	
Trying to leave	
Refusing to move	
Thrashing about	
Decreased activity	
Refusing medications	
Moving slow	
Impulsive behaviours (Repeat movements)	
Uncooperative/resistance to care	
Guarding sore area	
Touching/holding sore area	
Limping	
Clenching fist	
Going into fetal position	
Stiff/rigid	

Other (Physiological changes/eating sleeping changes/Vocal behaviours)	Present
Pale face	
Flushed, red face	
Teary eyed	
Sweating	
Shaking/trembling	
Cold clammy	
Changes in sleep routine (Please circle 1 or 2) 1) Decreased sleep ----------------------------------- 2) Increased sleep during the day	
Changes in appetite (Please circle 1 or 2) 1) Decreased appetite ----------------------------------- 2) Increased appetite	
Screaming/yelling	
Calling out (i.e. for help)	
Crying	
A specific sound of vocalisation For pain 'ow,' 'ouch'	
Moaning and groaning	
Mumbling	
Grunting	
Total Checklist Score	

Figure A1.3.5 The Pain Assessment Checklist for Seniors with Limited Ability to Communicate (PACSLAC). See: http://www.geriatricpain.org/Content/Assessment/Impaired/Pages/PACSLAC.aspx The PACSLAC is copyrighted by Shannon Fuchs-Lacelle and Thomas Hadjistavropoulos and is reprinted here with the permission of the copyright holders. The PACSLAC may not be reproduced without permission. For permission to reproduce the PACSLAC contact the worldwide copyright holders thomas.hadjistavropoulos@uregina.ca.

		DATES			
Somatic reactions					
1. Somatic complaints	No complaint	0	0	0	0
	Complaints expressed upon enquiry only	1	1	1	1
	Occasional involuntary complaints	2	2	2	2
	Continuous involuntary complaints	3	3	3	3
2. Protective body postures adopted at rest	No protective body posture	0	0	0	0
	The resident occasionally avoids certain postures	1	1	1	1
	Protective postures continuously and effectively sought	2	2	2	2
	Protective postures continuously sought, without success	3	3	3	3
3. Protection of sore areas	No protective action taken	0	0	0	0
	Protective actions attempted without interfering against any investigation or nursing	1	1	1	1
	Protective actions against any investigations and nursing	2	2	2	2
	Protective actions taken at rest, even when not approached	3	3	3	3
4. Expression	Usual expression	0	0	0	0
	Expression showing pain when approached	1	1	1	1
	Expression showing pain even without being approached	2	2	2	2
	Permanent and unusually blank look (voiceless, staring, looking blank)	3	3	3	3
5. Sleep pattern	Normal sleep	0	0	0	0
	Difficult to go to sleep	1	1	1	1
	Frequent waking (restlessness)	2	2	2	2
	Insomnia affecting waking times	3	3	3	3

Figure A1.3.6 The DOLOPLUS-2 Scale. Behavioural Pain Assessment in Elderly subjects (http://www.doloplus. com/index.php). Reproduced with permission from the DOLOPLUS group.

Psychomotor reactions					
6. Activities of daily living (washing &/or dressing)	Usual abilities unaffected	0	0	0	0
	Usual abilities slightly affected (careful but thorough)	1	1	1	1
	Usual abilities highly impaired, washing &/or dressing is laborious and incomplete	2	2	2	2
	Washing and/or dressing rendered impossible as the resident resists any attempt	3	3	3	3
7. Mobility	Usual abilities and activities remain unaffected	0	0	0	0
	Usual activities are reduced (the resident avoids certain movements and reduces his/her walking distance)	1	1	1	1
	Usual activities and abilities reduced (even with help, the resident cuts down on his/her movements)	2	2	2	2
	Any movement is impossible, the resident resists all persuasion	3	3	3	3
Psychosocial reactions					
8. Communication	Unchanged	0	0	0	0
	Heightened (the resident demands attention in an unusual manner)	1	1	1	1
	Lessened (the resident cuts him/herself off)	2	2	2	2
	Absence or refusal of any form of communication	3	3	3	3
9. Social life	Participates normally in every activity (meals, entertainment, therapy workshops)	0	0	0	0
	Participates in activities when asked to do so only	1	1	1	1
	Sometimes refuses to participate in any activity	2	2	2	2
	Refuses to participate in anything	3	3	3	3
10. Problems of behaviour	Normal behaviour	0	0	0	0
	Problems of repetitive reactive behaviour	1	1	1	1
	Problems of permanent reactive behaviour	2	2	2	2
	Permanent behaviour problems (without any external stimulus)	3	3	3	3
	SCORE				

Figure A1.3.6 (*Continued*)

References

Abbey J, Piller N, De Bellis A, et al. 2004. The Abbey Pain Scale: A one minute indicator for people with end stage dementia. *International Journal of Palliative Nursing* 10: 6–13.

Huskisson EC. 1974. Measurement of pain. *Lancet* 304: 1127–1131.

Royal College of Physicians, British Geriatrics Society and British Pain Society. 2007. The assessment of pain in older people: national guidelines. Concise guidance to good practice series, No 8. Appendix 2. Algorithm for the assessment of pain in older people. http://www.british-painsociety.org/book_pain_older_people.pdf [Accessed October 2013]

Zwakhalen SM, Hamers JP, Abu-Saad HH, Berger MP. 2006. Pain in elderly people with severe dementia: a systematic review of behavioural pain assessment tools. *BMC Geriatrics* 27(6): 3.

Useful web sites

http://www.doloplus.com/index.php [Accessed October 2013]

http://www.geriatricpain.org/Content/Assessment/Impaired/Pages/PACSLAC.aspx [Accessed October 2013]

Appendix 1.4 Wandering

Sarah Stowe

Airedale NHS Foundation Trust, Keighley, UK

Key points

- Residents with dementia may exhibit wandering and wandering-related activities which can result in injury and absconding from the care home and can cause concern to their caregivers (Chapter 10.1 and 18.3).
- Jan Dewing devised a screening tool (Table A1.4.1) to enable a person-centred risk assessment of wandering behaviour to be undertaken so that safe wandering can be facilitated. This identifies individuals who may wander so that appropriate interventions can be employed to maintain an appropriate balance between their safety and personal freedom.
- The tool (updated in 2008) is reproduced here with kind permission of the author and publisher.

Table A1.4.1 Screening for wandering.

Part A (pre-dementia)

- Does the person have a history of being a regular walker, whether as a hobby or as part of their daily life? Yes/No
- Has the person regularly used walking as a means of thinking things through, coping, dealing with stress or cooling off? Yes/No
- Does the person have a history of being extremely sociable or are they know to have an out-going personality? Yes/No

Part B (currently)

In the last year has the person:

- moved home (or been moved between or within a care setting)? Yes/No
- shadowed or closely followed a relative/carer around for prolonged periods? Yes/No
- moved around more frequently and had difficulty in sitting still for more than a few minutes? Yes/No
- entered into others' personal areas to investigate their belongings or to rummage? Yes/No
- made attempts to leave a safe place? (Note: the place must be well known to the person) Yes/No
- left a safe place and got lost? (Note: the place does not have to be known to the person) Yes/No

If the answer to any question in Part A is yes and there is a diagnosis of dementia (especially Alzheimer's), then the person is at risk of wandering or has the potential to wander if they become excessively under or over-simulated cognitively. Repeat the screening within a specified time period and implement a therapeutic plan to enable safe wandering.

If the answer to any question in Part B is yes, it is highly likely that the person is engaging in one type of wandering and may be at risk or have the potential to undertake a more risky type of wandering. Consider a full assessment, including detailed observation, and implement a therapeutic plan to enable safe wandering.

Reproduced from Dewing (2005) with permission from the RCN Publishing Company.

The Care Home Handbook, First Edition. Edited by Graham Mulley, Clive Bowman, Michal Boyd and Sarah Stowe.
© 2015 John Wiley & Sons, Ltd. Published 2015 by John Wiley & Sons, Ltd.

Another wandering scale is the Algase wandering scale, which has been validated on a care home population. (See Further reading for details.)

Reference

Dewing J. 2005. Screening for wandering among older persons with dementia. *Nursing Older People* 17(3): 20–24.

Further reading

Algase DL Beattie ER, Song JA, et al. 2004. Validation of the Algase wandering scale (version 2) in a cross-cultural sample. *Aging Mental Health* 8: 133–147.

Song JH, Algase D. 2008. Pre-morbid characteristics and wandering behaviour in persons with dementia. *Archives of Psychiatric Nursing* 22: 318–327.

Useful web site

www.wanderingnetwork.co.uk [Accessed October 2013]

Appendix 1.5 Mobility and falls risk assessments

Sarah Stowe

Airedale NHS Foundation Trust, Keighley, UK

Key points

- Many older people experience mobility impairments and it is important to perform a falls risk assessment in their usual environment.
- Multiple factors, such as muscle strength, continence, fear of falling, motivation, coordination, vision, and cognition contribute to an individual's mobility, gait and balance.
- Identifying areas for improvement with multi-disciplinary interventions can reduce falls and improve independence (see Chapter 6.6).

Tinetti (1986) described *a performance-orientated mobility assessment (POMA)* that can be used to identify abnormalities of strength and balance while performing daily functions, such as difficulty rising from a chair and bending down. See Table A1.5.1 for details of the assessment and potential causes of impairments.

Table A1.5.1 Performance-orientated evaluation of balance and gait.

Abnormal Manoeuvre	Possible Aetiologies*	Possible Therapeutic or Rehabilitative Measures†	Possible Preventive or Adaptive Measures†
Difficulty arising from chair	Proximal muscle weakness (many causes) Arthritides (especially involving hip, knees) Parkinson's syndrome Hemiparesis or paraparesis Deconditioning	Treatment of specific disease states (e.g., steroids, L-dopa) Hip and quadriceps exercises Transfer training	High, firm chair with arms Raised toilet seats Ejection chairs
Instability on first standing	Postural hypotension Cerebellar disease Multisensory deficits Lower extremity weakness or pain Foot pain leading to decreasing weight bearing	Treatment of specific diseases (e.g., adequate salt and fluid status, Fluorinef) Jobst stockings Hip and knee exercises Correct foot problems	Arise slowly Head of bed on blocks Supportive aid (e.g., walker, quadcane)

Abnormal Manoeuvre	Possible Aetiologies*	Possible Therapeutic or Rehabilitative Measures†	Possible Preventive or Adaptive Measures†
Instability with nudge on sternum	Parkinson's syndrome Back problems Normal pressure hydrocephalus ? Peripheral neuropathy Deconditioning	Treatment of specific diseases (e.g., L-dopa, shunt) Back exercises? Analgesia ? Balance exercises (e.g., Frankel's)	Obstacle free environment Appropriate walking aid (cane, walker) Night lights (more likely to fall if bump into object) Close observation with acute illness (high risk of falling) Avoid slippers
Instability with eyes closed (stable with eyes open)	Multisensory deficits Decreasing proprioception, position sense (e.g., B_{12} deficiency, DM, etc)	Treatment of specific diseases (e.g., B_{12}) Correct visual, hearing problem Remove cerumen ? Balance exercises	Bright lights Night lights Cane
Instability on neck turning or extension	Cervical arthritis Cervical spondylosis Vertebral-basilar insufficiency	? Anti-arthritic medication ?Cervical collar ? Neck exercises	Avoid quick turns Turn body, not just head Store objects in home low enough to avoid need to look up
Instability on turning	Cerebellar disease Hemiparesis Visual field cut Decreasing proprioception Mild ataxia	Gait training ? Proprioceptive exercises	Appropriate walking aid Obstacle-free environment
Unsafe on sitting down (misjudges distance or falls into chair)	Decreased vision Proximal myopathies Apraxia	Treatment of specific diseases ? Coordination training Leg strengthening exercises	High, firm chairs with arms, in good repair Transfer training
Decreased step height and length-bilateral (there will often be a flexed posture with all of these conditions)	Parkinson's syndrome Pseudobulbar palsy Myelopathy (usually spastic gait) Normal pressure hydrocephalus Advanced Alzheimer's disease (frontal lobe gait) Compensation for decreasing vision or proprioception Fear of falling Habit	Treatment of specific diseases (e.g., L-dopa) Correct vision Gait training (correct problems, suggest compensations, increase confidence)	Avoid throw rugs Good lighting Proper footwear (good fit, not too much friction or slip) Appropriate walking aid

Reproduced from Tinetti (1986) with permission of the author and Wiley.
*Not an exhaustive list.
†Most of these measures have not been subjected to clinical trials; evidence for effectiveness is usually anecdotal at best.

This can be useful as part of a multi-disciplinary assessment and may require some clinical expertise to interpret.

As a first line test, *the timed 'get up and go test'* is a quick and simple screening tool that needs no special equipment or training (Podsialdo and Richardson, 1991). This measures the time taken (in seconds) for individual to stand from an armchair, walk a distance of 3 metres, turn around, walk back and sit down. They walk with their usual footwear and walking aid where necessary. No physical assistance should be given unless there is a risk of injury.

Residents can have a 'practice run' to familiarise themselves with the test before being timed if they wish. The time taken to complete this test correlates well with overall functional abilities. Residents who can complete this test in ten to fourteen seconds or less are likely to be independently mobile. Time scores above 30 seconds are seen in individuals who will probably need assistance with activities such as transferring on and off the toilet.

This screening test can be used to identify residents who may benefit from referral to a specialist falls service for an individualised multi-factorial risk assessment linked to targeted interventions, such as strength and balance training.

A test of balance which is widely used by Physiotherapists is *the Berg Balance Test*. This does not require any special equipment and takes about 20 minutes to complete. (A shorter version is available.) The test is easy to do and has good inter-rater reliability. It is particularly useful in those with stroke (Thorbahn and Newton, 1996; Chou et al., 2006).

References

Chou CY Chien CW, Hsueh IP, et al. 2006. Developing a short from of the Berg Balance Test for people with stroke. *Physical Therapy* 86: 195–204.

Podsiadlo D, Richardson S. 1991. The timed "Up & Go": a test of basic functional mobility for frail elderly persons. *Journal of the American Geriatric Society* 39: 142–148.

Thorbahn LDB, Newton RA. 1996. Use of the Berg Balance Test to predict falls in elderly persons. *Physical Therapy* 76: 576–583.

Tinetti ME. 1986. Performance oriented assessment of mobility problems in elderly patients. *Journal of the American Geriatric Society* 34: 119–126.

Further reading

Harada N, Chiu V, Damron-Rodriguez J, et al. 1995. Screening for balance and mobility impairment in elderly individuals living in residential care facilities. *Physical Therapy* 75: 462–469.

NICE. 2004. The assessment and prevention of falls in older people NICE guideline. Available at: http://www.nice.org.uk/CG21 [Accessed October 2013]

Appendix 1.6 Single assessment process: MDS-RAI

Sarah Stowe

Airedale NHS Foundation Trust, Keighley, UK

Key points

- The minimum data set resident assessment instrument (MDS-RAI) is a standardised multi-disciplinary tool for assessing the strengths and needs of older people in care homes.
- It was originally developed in the USA to improve standards in care homes, where its use has been compulsory since 1997. A comprehensive assessment of a resident's needs over multiple domains provides a foundation for developing a detailed individualised care plan.

The MDS-RAI assesses each of the following:

- cognition
- communication
- activities of daily living
- continence
- social functioning
- disease diagnosis
- vision
- physical functioning
- health conditions and preventative health measures
- informal supportive services
- mood and behaviour
- nutrition/hydration status
- dental status
- skin condition
- environmental assessment
- service use in the last seven days.

Repeating the MDS assessment can provide information on changes in resident well-being which may have gone unnoticed. It can also be used as a tool to monitor quality indicators, such as pressure ulcer rates, and allow comparison between different care homes.

Although comprehensive, a significant disadvantage of the tool is its complexity, requiring extensive staff training and computer support to implement the tool. The validity and reliability of the tool are inconclusive and there is no section on residents' preferences or the views of care assistants. It also does not use commonly used assessment and screening tools and therefore the assessment results require training for interpretation.

Further reading

Hawes C, Morris JN, Phillips CD, et al. 1997. Development of the nursing home Resident Assessment Instrument in the USA. *Age and Ageing* 26-S2: 19–25.

Hutchinson HM. 2010. The RAI-MDS 2.0 quality indicators: a systematic review. *BMC Health Service Resources* 16: 166.

The Care Home Handbook, First Edition. Edited by Graham Mulley, Clive Bowman, Michal Boyd and Sarah Stowe.
© 2015 John Wiley & Sons, Ltd. Published 2015 by John Wiley & Sons, Ltd.

Appendix 1.7 Cognitive assessment

Amy Illsley

Yorkshire and the Humber Deanery, Bradford, UK

Key points

- Many care home residents will have some degree of cognitive impairment. It is therefore a good idea to know how to assess this by using some basic assessment tools.
- There are many cognitive assessment tools that have been developed for use among a variety of different patient groups.

One of the most commonly used in practice is the *Abbreviated Mental Test Score (AMTS)* which is discussed in more detail below.

Another commonly used test, both in primary and secondary care, is *the Mini Mental State Examination (MMSE)*. The MMSE is a 30-point test which includes similar questions to the AMTS but covers other cognitive functions not assessed by the AMTS, such as language, repetition and construction. The MMSE was first published in 1975 in the *Journal of Psychiatric Research* and copyright was held by the publisher. The scale was widely copied and distributed in organisations. It has since been bought by Psychological Assessment Resources Inc of Florida and users are required to pay for use of the MMSE, which has limited its availability (Powsner and Powsner, 2005). Because of cost we are, unfortunately, unable to reproduce the MMSE here.

As well as the AMTS, we have also reproduced the *Rowland Universal Assessment Scale (RUDAS)* below to give an example of a more in-depth cognitive assessment tool.

There are many other cognitive assessment tools available, such as the *Addenbrooke's Cognitive Examination Revised (ACER)*, but it is beyond the scope of this appendix to reproduce them all. We have tried to give an example of two brief, commonly used, cognitive assessments and a longer in-depth tool to show the scope of cognitive assessments.

Abbreviated Mental Test Score (AMTS)

One of the simplest and most commonly used tools is the Abbreviated Mental Test Score (AMTS) which was developed by Hodkinson et al. (1972) (Figure A1.7.1). This test consists of 10 validated questions on memory and orientation which can be easily remembered and quickly carried out to identify people who may have cognitive impairment. It is widely used across the U.K. A score of less than 8 prompts concern about cognitive function.

4-Point Abbreviated Mental Test (AMT)

A shorter, 4-point version of the AMTS, the 4-point Abbreviated Mental Test (4-point AMT) was developed by Swain and Nightingale (1997) (Figure A1.7.2). These four questions were found to have a similar efficacy to the 10-point AMTS in identifying cognitive impairment. There is a statistically significant correlation between score on the 4-point AMT and scores on the AMTS. Cognitive impairment is indicated by a score of less than 4.

The above tests ask question on memory and orientation. There are other areas of cognitive function that they do not cover.

Rowland Universal Dementia Assessment Scale (RUDAS)

For a more detailed cognitive assessment, a tool such as the Rowland Universal Dementia Assessment Scale (RUDAS) may be used (Figure A1.7.3). The RUDAS was developed by J. Rowland and his team in Australia in 2004 (Storey et al., 2004). The RUDAS looks at memory, visuo-spatial orientation, praxis, visuo-constructional drawing, situational judgement and language. It was developed to be a short

The Care Home Handbook, First Edition. Edited by Graham Mulley, Clive Bowman, Michal Boyd and Sarah Stowe.
© 2015 John Wiley & Sons, Ltd. Published 2015 by John Wiley & Sons, Ltd.

Question	Score one point for each correct answer
Age	
Time (to nearest hour)	
Address for recall at end of test – this should be repeated by the resident to ensure it has been heard correctly: 42 West Street	
Year	
Place (Name of hospital or care home)	
Recognition of two people (doctor, nurse, etc.)	
Date of birth	
Year of first world war	
Name of present Monarch	
Count backwards 20–1	

Figure A1.7.1 Abbreviated Mental Test Score. Reproduced from Hodkinson (1972) with permission from Oxford University Press.

Question	Score one point for each correct answer
Age	
Date of birth	
Place	
Year	

Figure A1.7.2 Four-point abbreviated mental test. Reproduced from Swain (1997) with permission from Sage Publications.

ITEM		Max score
Memory		
(Instructions) I want you to imagine that we are going shopping. Here is a list of grocery items. I would like you to remember the following items which we need to get from the shop. When we get to the shop in about 5 mins. Time I will ask you what it is that we have to buy. You must remember the list for me. **Tea, Cooking Oil, Eggs, Soap.** Please repeat this list for me (ask the person to repeat the list 3 times). (If person did not repeat all four words, repeat the list until the resident has learned them and can repeat them, or up to a maximum of five times.)		
Visuospatial Orientation		
I am going to ask you to identify/show me different parts of the body. *(Correct = 1).* Once the person correctly answers 5 parts of this question do not continue as the maximum score is 5.		
(1) Show me your right foot	...1	
(2) Show me your left hand	...1	
(3) With your right hand touch your left shoulder	...1	
(4) With your left hand touch your right ear	...1	
(5) Which is (indicate/point to) my left knee	...1	
(6) Which is (indicate/point to) my right elbow	...1	
(7) With your right hand indicate/point to my left eye	...1	
(8) With your left hand indicate/point to my left foot	...1	..../5
Praxis		
I am going to show you an action/exercise with my hands. I want you to watch me and copy what I do. Copy me when I do this... (One hand in fist, the other palm down on the table – alternate simultaneously.) Now do it with me: Now I would like you to keep doing this action at this pace until I tell you to stop – approximately 10 seconds. (Demonstrate at a moderate walking pace). Score as:		
Normal= 2 (Very few if any errors; self-corrected, progressively better; good maintenance; only very slight lack of synchrony between hands) *Partially adequate=1 (Noticeable errors with some attempt to self correct; some attempt at maintenance; poor synchrony)* *Failed=0 (cannot do the task; no maintenance; no attempt whatsoever)*		..../2
Visuoconstructional drawing		
Please draw this picture exactly as it looks to you (show cube). *(Yes=1)* Score as:		

Figure A1.7.3 Rowland Universal Dementia Assessment Scale. Reproduced from Storey et al. (2004) with permission from the authors.

...1
...1
...1
....../3

(1) Has the person drawn a picture based on a square?
(2) Do all internal lines appear in the person's drawing
(3) Do all external lines appear in the person's drawing?

Judgement

You are standing on the side of a busy street. There is a pedestrian crossing and no traffic lights. Tell me what you would do to get across to the other side of the road safely. (If the person gives an incomplete response that does not address both parts of the answer, use prompt: "Is there anything else you would do?") Record exactly what resident says and circle all parts of the response which were prompted.

....
....

Score as:
Did the person indicate that they would look for traffic? (*YES=2;YES PROMPTED=1;NO=0*)   ...2
Did the person make any additional safety proposals? (*YES=2;YES PROMPTED=1;NO=0*)   ...2

....../4

Memory Recall

(Recall) We have just arrived at the shop. Can you remember the list of groceries we need to buy? (Prompt: If person cannot recall any of the list, say "The first one was 'tea'." (*Score 2 points each for any item recalled which was not prompted – use only tea as a prompt.*)

Tea	...2
Cooking Oil	...2
Eggs	...2
Soap	...2

....../8

Language

I am going to time you for one minute. In that one minute, I would like you to tell me the names of as many different animals as you can. We'll see how many different animals you can name in one minute. (Repeat instructions if necessary). Maximum score for this item is 8. If person names 8 new animals in less than one minute there is no need to continue.

1...
2...
3...
4...
5...
6...
7...
8...

....../8

TOTAL SCORE   **/30**

Figure A1.7.3 (*Continued*)

screening instrument designed to minimise the effects of cultural learning and language diversity on the assessment of baseline cognitive performance.

The resident is encouraged to communicate in their first language and therefore relies on the use of an interpreter, where necessary. It is quick to administer and does not appear to be influenced by educational level or gender.

Six items are tested and a maximum score is 30. Any score of 22 or less should be considered as abnormal and prompt specialist referral.

References

Hodkinson EM. 1972. Evaluation of a mental test score for assessment of mental impairment in the elderly. *Age and Ageing* 1: 233–238.

Powsner S, Powsner D. 2005. Cognition, copyright, and the classroom. *American Journal of Psychiatry* 162: 627–628.

Storey JE, Rowland JT, Basic D, et al. 2004. The Rowland Universal Dementia Assessment Scale (RUDAS): A Multicultural Cognitive Assessment Scale. *International Psychogeriatrics* 16: 13–31.

Swain DG, Nightingale PG. 1997. Evaluation of a shortened version of the abbreviated mental test in a series of elderly patients. *Clinical Rehabilitation* 11: 243–248.

Further reading

Lam SC, Wong JJ, Woo J. 2010. Reliability and validity of the abbreviated mental test (Hong Kong version) in residential care homes. *Journal of the American Geriatric Society* 58: 2255–2257.

Appendix 1.8 Mood assessment

Amy Illsley

Yorkshire and the Humber Deanery, Bradford, UK

Key points

- Several assessment scales have been developed to assess mood in older people.
- One of the most commonly used scales is the Geriatric Depression Scale (GDS) which comes in a 30-point, 15-point, 10-point and 4-point format.
- As the 15-point scale is widely used, it is reproduced below.

Geriatric Depression Scale (GDS)

The Geriatric Depression Scale was developed by Yesavage (1982) in the USA as a screening questionnaire. The original scale consisted of 30 questions selected from a study looking at 100 potential questions, to be the most specific for depression.

The original scale is in the public domain due to it being partly the result of US Federal support and is freely available to download online.

The commonly used 15-point scale is shown in Figure A1.8.1. The resident is asked to state how they would answer when considering their feelings over the previous week. Answer in bold scores 1 point and a score of greater than 5 indicates the possibility of depression and merits a follow-up interview. If a resident scores greater than 10 on the GDS, their responses are indicative of depression and should therefore prompt a referral to a general practitioner.

The GDS has also been shown to be an effective screening tool for depression in dementia.

Question	Answers in bold score one point
Are you basically satisfied with your life?	YES / **NO**
Have you dropped many of your activities and interests?	**YES** / NO
Do you feel that your life is empty?	**YES** / NO
Do you often get bored?	**YES** / NO
Are you in good spirits most of the time?	YES / **NO**
Are you afraid that something bad is going to happen to you?	**YES** / NO
Do you feel happy most of the time?	YES / **NO**
Do you often feel helpless?	**YES** / NO
Do you prefer to stay at home, rather than going out and doing new things?	**YES** / NO
Do you feel you have more problems with memory than most?	**YES** / NO
Do you think it is wonderful to be alive now?	YES / **NO**
Do you feel pretty worthless the way you are now?	**YES** / NO
Do you feel full of energy?	YES / **NO**
Do you feel that your situation is hopeless?	**YES** / NO
Do you think that most people are better off than you are?	**YES** / NO

Figure A1.8.1 The Geriatric Depression Score. Reproduced from Brink (1982) with permission from Taylor and Francis.

The Care Home Handbook, First Edition. Edited by Graham Mulley, Clive Bowman, Michal Boyd and Sarah Stowe.
© 2015 John Wiley & Sons, Ltd. Published 2015 by John Wiley & Sons, Ltd.

References

Brink TL, Yesavage JA, Lum O, et al. 1982. Screening tests for geriatric depression. *Clinical Gerontologist* 1: 37–44.

Yesavage JA, Brink TL, Rose TL, et al. 1982. Development and validation of a geriatric depression screening scale: a preliminary report. *Journal of Psychiatric Research* 17: 37–49. Available at: http://www. stanford.edu/~yesavage/ GDS.english.short.score.html [Accessed October 2013]

Further reading

Burke WJ, Houston MJ, Boust SJ, Roccaforte WH. 1989. Use of the Geriatric Depression Scale in dementia of the Alzheimer type. *Journal of the American Geriatric Society* 37: 856–860.

Appendix 1.9 End of life pathway for the dying resident

Sangeeta Naraen

St James's Hospital, Leeds, UK

Key points

- Previously, there were concerns that the care of dying people was sometimes poor, with inadequate oral hygiene, thirst, poor symptom control and isolation as well as inappropriate medications and interventions and little attention to spiritual care.
- Locally developed pathways are currently being developed. These are to be used at the bedside to try and ensure that dying residents have high-quality care in the last hours and days of life.

Palliative care is the relief of symptoms in the final stages of life in order to prevent any unnecessary suffering or subjecting residents to inappropriate interventions. Good end of life care includes not only symptom control, but also dignified holistic care, tailored to each individual, with respect and kindness; good communication with the family and giving them emotional support; and co-ordination of care.

A pathway was developed in Liverpool which covered physical, social, spiritual and psychological aspects of dying. It aimed to ensure that death was dignified, pain-free and comfortable. It was to be used in those who were expected to live only a few hours or days. It allowed principles of hospice care to be applied in care homes and elsewhere and was meant to be initiated after discussions between the multidisciplinary team (who had been trained in its use), the resident (wherever possible) and the family.

Unfortunately, though the Liverpool Care Pathway was well intentioned, and often very useful, there were instances when the pathway was used without the patient or family being involved and without the staff being properly instructed in its use. There was widespread press coverage which blamed the pathway for accelerating death and causing distressing thirst and resulting in the excessive use of sedatives.

The pathway is now being phased out in the UK, New Zealand and other countries. Locally endorsed replacement pathways are being developed, with emphasis on an individualised approach to the end of life care.

The Care Home Handbook, First Edition. Edited by Graham Mulley, Clive Bowman, Michal Boyd and Sarah Stowe.
© 2015 John Wiley & Sons, Ltd. Published 2015 by John Wiley & Sons, Ltd.

Appendix 1.10 End of life: Gold Standards Framework (GSF)

Sangeeta Naraen

St James's Hospital, Leeds, UK

Key points

- About one in five people over 85 will spend some time in a care home and most residents will die there.
- People approaching end of life need the right care to be provided in the right place at right time. This can only be achieved if there is early identification, assessment of their need and good coordination between care homes, primary care and acute hospitals (see chapters in Section H).

The Gold Standards Framework (GSF) was originally developed to improve primary palliative care given by non-specialists in primary care.

It is a tool which records the individual's preferences and priorities in relation to end of life treatments and the basis of these decisions.

GSF is an evidence-based approach to provide best care – the 'Gold Standard' – for the resident nearing the end of life.
It improves:

- quality of care
- coordination of care and
- organisation of care.

GSF prognostic indicator guidance helps clinicians in:

- *Early identification* of individuals nearing the end of life who may need additional support. Once identified, people can be placed on a register (such as those held by GPs, hospital trigger systems or other local registers).
- They can then be *assessed* for current and future clinical and personal needs (including resuscitation decisions and advance care planning).

- *Plans* can then be made to provide appropriate care, with *improved coordination and communication* in their final days.

Use of the GSF can ensure that residents can die peacefully in their preferred place (so fewer will be admitted to hospital and die there) and can express the type of care they would like. They receive better symptom control.

Informal caregivers' needs (practical, supportive and financial) can also be considered.

Staff familiar with this system grow in confidence in terminal care and gain more job satisfaction.

Currently there is no standard form for recording residents' wishes on dying matters. Standardisation would be a major step forwards.

Further reading

www.goldstandardsframework.org.uk 2000 [Accessed October 2013]

Kinley J, Froggatt K, Bennett MI. 2012. The effect of policy on end-of-life practice within nursing care homes: a systematic review. *Palliative Medicine*: Jan 4epub.

Appendix 1.11 Constipation and diarrhoea stool scale

Sangeeta Naraen

St James's Hospital, Leeds, UK

Key points

- Constipation and diarrhoea are two of the most common conditions affecting elderly people.
- Bowels problems can cause distress to residents and their carers.
- The Bristol stool form scale (Figure A1.11.1) is a visual validated guide which classifies stools on the basis of shape, size and consistency in seven categories. It also provides information for detecting stool patterns or change in bowel habit.

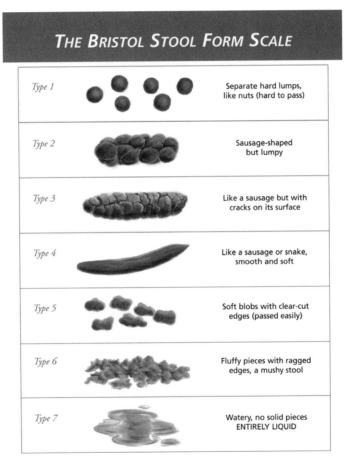

THE BRISTOL STOOL FORM SCALE

Type 1	Separate hard lumps, like nuts (hard to pass)
Type 2	Sausage-shaped but lumpy
Type 3	Like a sausage but with cracks on its surface
Type 4	Like a sausage or snake, smooth and soft
Type 5	Soft blobs with clear-cut edges (passed easily)
Type 6	Fluffy pieces with ragged edges, a mushy stool
Type 7	Watery, no solid pieces ENTIRELY LIQUID

Figure A1.11.1 Bristol stool chart. Types 1 and 2 are constipation. Types 3 and 4 are considered ideal stools. Types 5, 6 and 7 are tending towards diarrhoea. Reproduced by kind permission of Dr K.W. Heaton, Reader in Medicine at the University of Bristol. © 2000 Norgine Pharmaceuticals Ltd.

The Care Home Handbook, First Edition. Edited by Graham Mulley, Clive Bowman, Michal Boyd and Sarah Stowe.
© 2015 John Wiley & Sons, Ltd. Published 2015 by John Wiley & Sons, Ltd.

Reference

Lewis SJ, Heaton KW. 1997. Stool form scale as a useful guide to intestinal transit time. *Scandinavian Journal of Gastroenterology* 32 (9): 920–924.

Appendix 1.12 Nutrition

Sangeeta Naraen

St James's Hospital, Leeds, UK

Key points

Elderly people are at risk of malnutrition as a result of:

- Poor oral intake.
- Feeding or swallowing problems.
- Physical problems affecting eating, such as poor dentition, sore or dry mouth.
- Repeated investigations and treatments which require fasting.
- Side-effect of illness or medication.
- Psychological problems, such as isolation and depression.

Malnutrition in elderly residents is often under-diagnosed. Nutritional assessment is necessary for both a successful diagnosis and for the treatment plan for malnutrition.

The Malnutrition Universal Screening Tool (MUST) and the Mini Nutritional Assessment (MNA) are two well recognised tools for the assessment of malnutrition (see Figures A1.12.1 and A1.12.2).

MUST (as recommended by NICE) was initially developed to assess the risk of malnutrition in the community. However, it can also be used to assess risk in hospitals and may be useful in care homes.

It classifies malnutrition risk as low, medium, or high on the basis of BMI, history of unexplained weight loss and acute illness effect.

This tool has been reproduced with kind permission of BAPEN.

MNA was developed to evaluate the risk of malnutrition in elderly people at home, in nursing homes or in hospitals. The scoring is based on the following:

1. Reduced food intake in the preceding three months.
2. Weight loss during preceding three months.
3. Mobility.
4. Neuropsychological problems.
5. Suffering from psychological stress or acute disease in the past three months.
6. Body mass index.

Malnutrition is absent if patient score is 11 or more on the MNA.

The Care Home Handbook, First Edition. Edited by Graham Mulley, Clive Bowman, Michal Boyd and Sarah Stowe.
© 2015 John Wiley & Sons, Ltd. Published 2015 by John Wiley & Sons, Ltd.

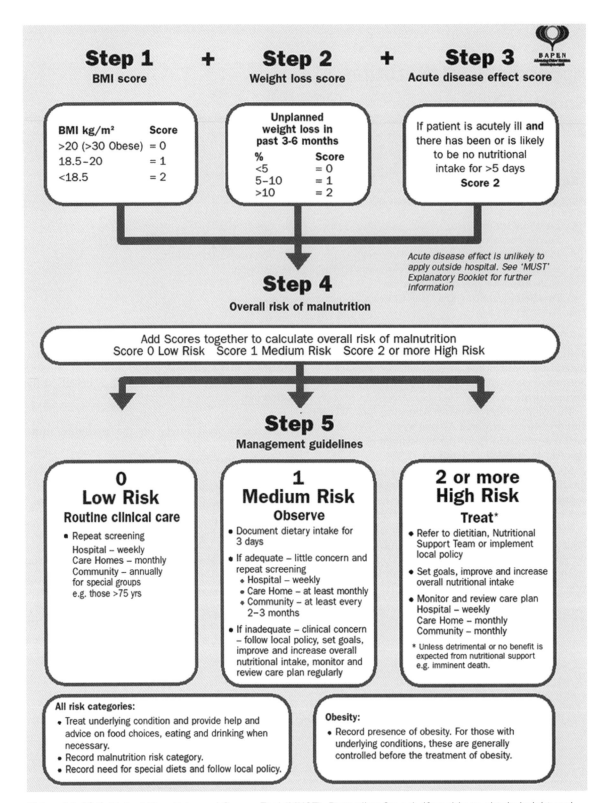

Figure A1.12.1 Malnutrition Universal Screen Tool (MUST). Regarding Step 1, if unable to obtain height and weight see 'MUST' Explanatory Booklet for alternative measurements and use of subjective criteria. The 'Malnutrition Universal Screening Tool' ('MUST') is reproduced here with the kind permission of BAPEN (British Association for Parenteral and Enteral Nutrition). For further information on 'MUST' see www.bapen.org.uk/

Screening

A Has food intake declined over the past 3 months due to loss of appetite, digestive problems, chewing or swallowing difficulties?
0 = severe decrease in food intake
1 = moderate decrease in food intake
2 = no decrease in food intake ☐

B Weight loss during the last 3 months
0 = weight loss greater than 3kg (6.6lbs)
1 = does not know
2 = weight loss between 1 and 3kg (2.2 and 6.6 lbs)
3 = no weight loss ☐

C Mobility
0 = bed or chair bound
1 = able to get out of bed / chair but does not go out
2 = goes out ☐

D Has suffered psychological stress or acute disease in the past 3 months?
0 = yes   2 = no ☐

E Neuropsychological problems
0 = severe dementia or depression
1 = mild dementia
2 = no psychological problems ☐

F Body Mass Index (BMI) (weight in kg) / (height in m^2)
0 = BMI less than 19
1 = BMI 19 to less than 21
2 = BMI 21 to less than 23
3 = BMI 23 or greater ☐

Screening score ☐☐
(subtotal max. 14 points)

12-14 points: Normal nutritional status
8-11 points: At risk of malnutrition
0-7 points: Malnourished

For a more in-depth assessment, continue with questions G-R

Assessment

G Lives independently (not in nursing home or hospital)
1 = yes   0 = no ☐

H Takes more than 3 prescription drugs per day
0 = yes   1 = no ☐

I Pressure sores or skin ulcers
0 = yes   1 = no ☐

Ref. Vellas B, Villars H, Abellan G, et al. *Overview of MNA® - Its History and Challenges.* J Nut Health Aging 2006; 10: 456-465.
Rubenstein LZ, Harker JO, Salva A, Guigoz Y, Vellas B. Screening for Undernutrition in Geriatric Practice: *Developing the Short-Form Mini Nutritional Assessment (MNA-SF).* J. Geront 2001; 56A: M366-377.
Guigoz Y. The Mini-Nutritional Assessment (MNA®) Review of the Literature – What does it tell us? J Nutr Health Aging 2006; 10: 466-487.
® Société des Produits Nestlé, S.A., Vevey, Switzerland, Trademark Owners
© Nestlé, 1994, Revision 2006. N67200 12/99 10M
For more information: www.mna-elderly.com

J How many full meals does the patient eat daily?
0 = 1 meal
1 = 2 meals
2 = 3 meals ☐

K Selected consumption markers for protein intake
• At least one serving of dairy products (milk, cheese, yoghurt) per day   yes ☐   no ☐
• Two or more servings of legumes or eggs per week   yes ☐   no ☐
• Meat, fish or poultry every day   yes ☐   no ☐
0.0 = if 0 or 1 yes
0.5 = if 2 yes
1.0 = if 3 yes ☐ . ☐

L Consumes two or more servings of fruit or vegetables per day?
0 = no   1 = yes ☐

M How much fluid (water, juice, coffee, tea, milk...) is consumed per day?
0.0 = less than 3 cups
0.5 = 3 to 5 cups
1.0 = more than 5 cups ☐ . ☐

N Mode of feeding
0 = unable to eat without assistance
1 = self-fed with some difficulty
2 = self-fed without any problem ☐

O Self view of nutritional status
0 = views self as being malnourished
1 = is uncertain of nutritional state
2 = views self as having no nutritional problem ☐

P In comparison with other people of the same age, how does the patient consider his / her health status?
0.0 = not as good
0.5 = does not know
1.0 = as good
2.0 = better ☐ . ☐

Q Mid-arm circumference (MAC) in cm
0.0 = MAC less than 21
0.5 = MAC 21 to 22
1.0 = MAC 22 or greater ☐ . ☐

R Calf circumference (CC) in cm
0 = CC less than 31
1 = CC 31 or greater ☐

Assessment (max. 16 points) ☐☐ . ☐

Screening score ☐☐ . ☐

Total Assessment (max. 30 points) ☐☐ . ☐

Malnutrition Indicator Score

24 to 30 points ☐   normal nutritional status

17 to 23.5 points ☐   at risk of malnutrition

Less than 17 points ☐   malnourished

Figure A1.12.2 Mini Nutritional Assessment (MNA). Please visit the MNA® website for further information: www.mna-elderly.com. With kind permission from Nestlé Health.

Useful web site

For further information on MUST, see: www.bapen.org.uk/ pdfs/must/must_full.pdf [Accessed October 2013]

Appendix 1.13 Functional assessment

Sangeeta Naraen

St James's Hospital, Leeds, UK

Key points

- Functional status is an ability to perform self-care, self-maintenance and physical activities.
- Many frail elderly residents have multiple health problems, accompanied by multiple medications which decrease the ability to carry out the activity of daily living
- A comprehensive review of an older person's daily activity is required to determine the current and future healthcare of the person.
- Functional capacity can be assessed by the Barthel Index or the Rivermead ADL Scale.

The *Barthel Index* (Figure A1.13.1) measures functional independence in the domains of personal care and mobility. It also includes continence. It monitors performance in chronic patients and long-term hospital patients with paralytic conditions before and after treatment. Two main versions exist: the original 10-item form and expanded 15-item versions.

The *Rivermead ADL Scale* was developed for assessing activities of daily living in stroke patients. A revalidation was done in 1990 to use the scale in those aged over 64 (Figure A1.13.2).

Rivermead ADL Index: guidelines

Self-care

- Drinking
A full cup of hot liquid, not spilling more than 1/8 of its contents.
- Clean teeth
Unscrewing toothpaste, putting toothpaste on brush, managing tap (faucet).
- Comb hair
To be presentable on completion.
- Wash face and hands
At basin (not with bowl), including putting in plug and managing taps and resident drying him/herself. (All materials to hand.)
- Make up or shave
Shaving to be done by resident's preferred method
- Eating
A slice of cheese on toast eaten with a knife and fork.

- Undress
Dressing gown, pyjamas, socks and shoes to be taken off.
- Indoor mobility
Moving from one room to another. Turns must be to the left. Distance of 10 m.
- Bed to chair
From lying covered, to chair with arm, within reach.
- Lavatory
- Mobility to WC (less than 10 m). To include managing pants and trousers, cleaning self and transferring.
- Outdoor mobility
To cover a distance of 50 m, and to include going up a ramp and through a door.
- Dressing
Does not involve fetching clothes. Clothes to be within reach in a pile, but not in any specific order. All essential fastenings to be done up by patient.
- Wash in bath
Showing movements, i.e. ability to wash all over. Ability to manage taps (faucets) and plugs.
- In and out of bath
A dry bath.
- Overall wash
Not in bath – at basin (not with bowl). Resident must be able to wash good arm, stand up and touch toes from sitting in order to be able to wash all over.
- Floor to chair
From lying to upholstered chair without arms, seat 45 cm (15 in) high.

The Care Home Handbook, First Edition. Edited by Graham Mulley, Clive Bowman, Michal Boyd and Sarah Stowe.
© 2015 John Wiley & Sons, Ltd. Published 2015 by John Wiley & Sons, Ltd.

Activity	Score
Bowels 0 = incontinent (or needs to be given enemata) 1 = occasional accident (once/week) 2 = continent	
Resident's score:	
Bladder 0 = incontinent, or catheterized and unable to manage 1 = occasional accident (max. once per 24 hours) 2 = continent (for over 7 days)	
Resident's score:	
Grooming 0 = needs help with personal care 1 = independent face/hair/teeth/shaving (implements provided)	
Resident's score:	
Toilet use 0 = dependent 1 = needs some help, but can do something alone 2 = independent (on and off, dressing, wiping)	
Resident's score:	
Feeding 0 = unable 1 = needs help cutting, spreading butter, etc. 2 = independent (food provided within reach)	
Resident's score:	
Transfer 0 = unable – no sitting balance 1 = major help (one or two people, physical), can sit 2 = minor help (verbal or physical) 3 = independent	
Resident's score:	
Mobility 0 = immobile 1 = wheelchair independent, including corners, etc. 2 = walks with help of one person (verbal or physical) 3 = independent (but may use any aid, e.g., stick)	
Resident's score:	
Dressing 0 = dependent 1 = needs help, but can do about half unaided 2 = independent (including buttons, zips, laces, etc.)	
Resident's score:	
Stairs 0 = unable 1 = needs help (verbal, physical, carrying aid) 2 = independent up and down	
Resident's score:	
Bathing 0 = dependent 1 = independent (or in shower) *Resident's* score	
Total score	

Scoring:
Sum the resident's scores for each item. Total possible scores range from 0–20, with lower scores indicating increased disability. If used to measure improvement after rehabilitation, changes of more than two points in the total score reflect a probable genuine change, and change on one item from fully dependent to independent is also likely to be reliable.

Figure A1.13.1 The Barthel Index. Reproduced from Shah et al. (1989) with permission from Elsevier.

Instructions
1. Decide where to start. If the resident can do that item, go back three to make sure that they can do these as well, and forward until three consecutive failures – then stop. This applies to each section.
2. All aids supplied or recommended to be stated on form are given below.

Scoring
3 = Independent with/without aid
2 = Verbal assistance only
1 = Dependent (i.e. if unfit, unassessable, unsafe or time is taken beyond practical bounds)

Item	Score	Equipment
Self-care		
Drinking		
Clean teeth		
Comb hair		
Wash face/hands		
Make up or shave		
Eating		
Undress		
Indoor mobility		
Bed to chair		
Lavatory		
Outdoor mobility		
Dressing		
Wash in bath		
In/out of bath		
Overall wash		
Floor to chair		
Household 1		
Preparation of hot drink		
Preparation of snack		
Cope with money		
Get in/out of car		
Prepare meal		
Carry shopping		
Crossing roads		
Transport self to shop		
Public transport		
Household 2		
Washing		
Ironing		
Light cleaning		
Hang out washing		
Bed-making		
Heavy cleaning		

Figure A1.13.2 The Rivermead ADL Scale. Reproduced from Lincoln and Edmans (1990) with permission from Oxford University Press.

Household 1

- Preparation of hot drink

Fill electric kettle, everything to be ready on working surface

- Preparation of snack

Cheese on toast – materials to be easily reached. Washing and cleaning work surface to be done easily.

- Cope with money

Match coins to packet of sugar, cornflakes and margarine. Ask for change (e.g. in the UK, of 34p from 50p; 72p from £1.00; £3.21 from £5.00)

- Get in and out of car

Front seat of any car except sports model.

- Preparation of meal

Peel one potato, fry sausage. Frozen vegetables from freezer. Open tin.

- Carry shopping

Half-pound of butter (250 g), 14 oz tin (500 g) and money.

- Crossing road

Cross at traffic lights with kerbs – no pedestrian crossing.

- Transport self to shop and back

Distance of 0.5 mile (1 km)

- Public transport

Travel on bus (not Park and Ride). Distance of at least 1 mile (2 km) with minimum three stops before destination.

Houshold 2

- Washing

Handwash underwear at sink.

- Ironing

Not with steam iron. Organise surface (board or table).

- Light cleaning

Cleaning and tidying surface – height 13–37 in (30–90 cm).

- Hang out washing

On rail indoors, away from sink, no pegs.

- Bed making

Putting on sheet and blanket, straightening and tucking in. Bed 21 in (50 cm) high.

- Heavy cleaning

Hoover (vacuum), sweep and dustpan/brush 11 ft (3 m) square room, moving dining room chairs only.

Further reading

Lincoln NB, Edmans JA. 1990. A revalidation of the Rivermead ADL scale for elderly patients with stroke. *Age and Ageing* 19, 19–24.

Shah S, Vanclay F, Cooper B . 1989. Improving the sensitivity of the Barthel Index for stroke rehabilitation. *Journal of Clinical Epidemiology* 42: 703–709.

Appendix 2: When to Request Urgent Medical Help

Graham Mulley

University of Leeds, Leeds, UK

Throughout this manual, we have identified signs, symptoms and situations when it is important to request urgent help – either from the GP or the emergency services.

Here, we briefly summarise the clinical presentations which warrant prompt referral and highlight the specific chapters in which you can find further details.

In general, it is helpful to report the resident's vital signs when you make an urgent referral: remember to give details on the pulse, blood pressure, temperature, respiratory rate as well as oxygen saturations, blood glucose and MEWS score if appropriate.

Abdominal pain
With absent bowel movements or faeculent vomiting: See Chapter 9.12 Nausea and vomiting
With peritonitis: See Chapter 13.8 Intra-abdominal infections
With abdominal infections: See Chapter 13.8 Intra-abdominal infections

Airway obstruction (stridor)
See Chapter 9.6 Dyspnoea

Angio-oedema
See Chapter 9.1 Anaphylaxis

Anaphylaxis
See Chapter 9.1 Anaphylaxis

Asthma
See Chapter 9.2 Asthma
With COPD exacerbation: See Chapter 13.6 Respiratory infections

Autonomic dysfunction
With fever, muscle stiffness and altered consciousness: Consider Neuroleptic malignant syndrome
See Chapter 10.4 Psychosis

Bleeding
With warfarin: See Chapter 9.3 Bleeding
With hypovolaemia: See Chapter 5.3 Hydration
After a fall: See Chapter 6.6

Blindness
Sudden loss of vision: See Chapter 7.1 Eye care; Chapter 8.1 Stroke

Bradycardia (> 50 bpm)
Consider shock: See Chapter 9.8
See Chapter 15.1 Pulse

Breathlessness
General: See Chapter 9.6 Dyspnoea, Chapter 13.6 Respiratory infections
Rapid respiratory rate: See Chapter 9.6 Dyspnoea; Chapter 13.6 Respiratory infection; Chapter 15.3 Respiratory rate and oximetry
With asthma (noisy, rapid, wheezing, cyanosis): See Chapter 9.2 Asthma
With COPD exacerbation: See Chapter 13.6 Respiratory infections
With stridor – anaphylaxis: See Chapter 9.1 Anaphylaxis
With heart failure – pulmonary oedema: See Chapter 8.6 Heart Failure, Chapter 9.8 Bradycardia and tachycardia
Oxygen: See Chapter 11.9

Calf that is hot, tender
Consider DVT

Cellulitis
Around IV access device
Around PEG tubes: See Chapter 14.1 Naso-gastric and PEG tubes
Around a cast: See Chapter 14.4 Fractures

Chest pain
Consider myocardial infarction (Chapter 8.6), pleurisy (Chapter 13.6), pulmonary embolus (Chapter 9.6), and anaphylaxis (Chapter 9.1)

Collapse
Generally: See Chapter 9.4 Collapse
Effect of medications: See Chapter 11.1 Reviewing medications
With anaphylaxis: See Chapter 9.1 Anaphylaxis
With chest pain: See Chapter 9.4 Collapse

The Care Home Handbook, First Edition. Edited by Graham Mulley, Clive Bowman, Michal Boyd and Sarah Stowe.
© 2015 John Wiley & Sons, Ltd. Published 2015 by John Wiley & Sons, Ltd.

With dyspnoea: See Chapter 9.4 Collapse

With heart failure: See Chapter 9.8 Bradycardia and tachycardia

With hypoglycaemia: See Chapter 8.5 Diabetes

With seizures: See Chapter 9.4 Collapse, Chapter 9.5 Seizures

Coma/altered consciousness

With features of stroke: See Chapter 8.1 Stroke

With seizures: See Chapter 9.5 Seizures

With delirium: See Chapter 10.2 Delirium

With pyrexia, rigid muscles, autonomic dysfunction: See Chapter 10.4 Psychosis

With cardiac arrest: See Chapter 9.7 Cardiac arrest

With raised intra-cranial pressure: See Chapter 9.8 Bradycardia and tachycardia

With blockage of tracheostomy: See Chapter 14.2 Tracheostomy

Confusion

See Chapter 10.2 Delirium

Cyanosis

Consider asthma (Chapter 9.2), respiratory infection (Chapter 13.6), COPD exacerbation (Chapter 13.6)

Deafness

Sudden deafness

Consider ear infection: See Chapter 7.2 Hearing impairment

Deep vein thrombosis (DVT)

Consider in casts for fracture: See Chapter 14.4 Fractures

Delirium (acute confusion)

See Chapter 10.2 Delirium

Depression (severe or persistent)

See Chapter 10.3 Anxiety and Depression

Diarrhoea

Watery: See Chapter 13.4 *C. difficile*

With blood or mucus: See Chapter 13.7 Diarrhoea

With vomiting: See Chapter 13.2 Norovirus

Prolonged (>48 hours)

With pyrexia: See Chapter 13.2 *C. difficile*, Chapter 13.7 Diarrhoea

With jaundice: See Chapter 13.7 Diarrhoea, Chapter 13.8 Intra-abdominal infections

With abdominal pain or tenderness: See Chapter 13.4 *C. difficile*, Chapter 13.7 Diarrhoea

With dehydration: See Chapter 5.3 Hydration

Consider *C. difficile*: See Chapter 13.7 Diarrhoea

With diverticular abscess: See Chapter 13.8 Intra-abdominal infections

Drowsiness

Consider hypoglycaemia (Chapter 8.5), asthma (Chapter 9.2), delirium (Chapter 10.2) and raised intra-cranial pressure (Chapter 9.8)

Drug error

See Chapter 11.13 Mistakes with medication: what to do

Dysphagia

See Chapter 5.1 Swallowing difficulties and associated problems

Dyspnoea – see Breathlessness

Ear discharge

See Chapter 7.2 Hearing impairment

Eye redness and pain

Consider eye infection: See Chapter 7.1 Eye care

Eye – loss of vision

Consider stroke, glaucoma: See Chapter 7.1 Eye care, Chapter 8.1 Stroke

Facial weakness

See Chapter 7.1 Eye care; Chapter 8.1 Stroke

Fever

See Chapter 15.4 Temperature

With chest infection: See Chapter 13.6 Respiratory infections

With rigid muscles, autonomic dysfunction and fluctuating consciousness (neuroleptic malignant syndrome): See Chapter 10.4 Psychosis

With influenza: See Chapter 13.1

With abdominal infections: See Chapter 13.8

With Norovirus: See Chapter 13.2

Fits

Prolonged or multiple seizures (status epilepticus) or serious injury: See Chapter 9.5 Seizures

Flu: see Influenza

Fracture

Consider if limb is swollen, deformed, red, warm, numb, has crepitus, if pain on weight-bearing: See Chapter 14.5 Fractures

Haematemesis (vomiting blood)

Consider bleeding peptic ulcer: See Chapter 9.3

Haemoptysis

Consider lung cancer, chest infection, pulmonary embolus: See Chapter 9.3 Bleeding, Chapter 9.6 Dyspnoea, Chapter 13.6 Respiratory infection

Head injury with altered consciousness
See Chapter 15.6 Head injury observations

Hearing impairment
Sudden loss of hearing
Consider ear infection: See Chapter 7.2 Hearing
  impairment

Hypertension
If BP very high (>200 mm systololic and >110 mm
  diastolic) consider stroke (Chapter 8.1), A-V block
  (Chapter 9.8) and raised intra-cranial pressure
  (Chapter 9.8)

Hypotension
If BP is very low (< 80 mm systolic) consider bleed-
  ing (Chapter 9.3), asthma (Chapter 9.2), shock
  (Chapter 9.8), myocardial infarction (Chapter
  9.8), anaphylaxis (Chapter 9.1), I.V. access
  (Chapter 11.6)

Hypothermia
With loss of consciousness: See Chapter 9.9
  Hypothermia
Consider underlying infection: See Chapter 9.8
  Bradycardia and tachycardia, Chapter 13.6 respira-
  tory infections

Hypoxia
See Chapter 15.4 Temperature
See Chapter 15.3 Respiratory rate and oximetry
With respiratory infection: See Chapter 13.6 Respira-
  tory infections
With tracheostomy tube: See Chapter 14.2
  Tracheostomy

Influenza
See Chapter 13.1 Influenza

Jaundice
Consider intra-abdominal infection: See Chapter 13.7
  Diarrhoea

Joints that are hot, swollen or tender
Consider infection and gout: See Chapter 9.10 Hot
  painful joints

Leg ischaemia (acute)
Consider occlusion of leg artery: See Chapter 9.11
  Acute limb ischaemia

Light intolerance: see Photophobia

Medication error
If potential harm known or you are uncertain: See
  Chapter 11.13 Mistakes with medication: what to
  do

MEWS score > 5
See Chapter 15.9 Modified early warning score

Mobility – sudden change
Consider stroke: See Chapter 8.1 Stroke
Consider fracture: See Chapter 14.4 Fractures, casts
  and splints
See Chapter 6.1 Exercise and mobility

Modified early warning score
See Chapter 15.9 MEWS

Muscle stiffness
Consider neuroleptic malignant syndrome: See
  Chapter 10.4 Psychosis

Nausea
Consider Norovirus: See Chapter 13.2 Norovirus

Pain
On weight-bearing
Consider fracture: See Chapter 14.4 Fractures, casts
  and splints
Chest pain on breathing
Consider pneumonia: See Chapter 13.6 Respiratory
  infection
Central chest pain
Consider myocardial infarction: See Chapter 8.6
  Heart failure, Chapter 9.8 Bradycardia and
  Tachycardia
Leg pain (acute)
Consider acute ischaemia: See Chapter 9.11 Acute
  limb ischaemia
Due to a cast
See Chapter 14.4 Fractures, casts and splints

PEG site infections
See Chapter 14.1 Naso-gastric and PEG tubes

Photophobia (intolerance of light)
Consider meningitis: See Chapter 9.12 Nausea and
  vomiting

Physical decline
Consider influenza (Chapter 13.1); chest infection
  (Chapter 13.6); urinary infection (Chapter 13.9);
  neuroleptic malignant syndrome (Chapter 10.4
  Psychoses); stroke (Chapter 8.1)

Pleurisy
See Chapter 13.6 Respiratory infections

Pneumonia
See Chapter 13.6 Respiratory infections
With aspiration: See Chapter 5.2 Swallowing difficul-
  ties and associated problems

Pulse
Fast or slow (< 50 bpm) or irregular
See Chapter 9.8 Bradycardia and tachycardia
See Chapter 15.1 Pulse

Pyrexia: see Fever

Rectal bleeding
Consider colitis, bowel cancer, and piles: See Chapter 9.3 Bleeding

Respiratory rate
See Chapter 13.6 Respiratory infections
See Chapter 14.2 **Tracheostomy**

Rigidity
See Chapter 10.4 Psychoses

Seizures
If status epilepticus (fits lasting >30 minutes), frequent seizures, associated severe injury, breathing difficulties after the seizure has stopped: See Chapter 9.5 Seizures

Sputum production
Consider pneumonia, lower respiratory tract infection: See Chapter 9.6 Dyspnoea, Chapter 13.6 Respiratory infections
If bloody, consider infection, pulmonary embolus: See Chapter 9.3 Bleeding

Skin infection – cellulitis
Infection around a PEG
Consider necrotizing fasciitis: See Chapter 14.1 Nasogastric (NG) and percutaneous endoscopic gastrostomy (PEG) tubes
Around IV access device

Status epilepticus
See Chapter 9.5 Seizures

Stridor
See Chapter 9.6 Dyspnoea
Consider asthma (Chapter 9.2), anaphylaxis (Chapter 9.1), airways obstruction (Chapter 9.6)

Stroke
If acute and treatment is appropriate: See Chapter 8.1 Stroke

Swelling of limb
Consider DVT (see above)
With a cast: See Chapter 14.4 Fractures, casts and splints

Swelling of lips and tongue (angio-oedema)
Consider anaphylaxis: See Chapter 9.1 Anaphylaxis

Tachycardia
Consider shock: See Chapter 9.8 Bradycardia and tachycardia
See Chapter 15.1 Pulse

Temperature
Raised: Chest symptoms
See Chapter 9.6 Dyspnoea
Lowered: Hypothermia
See Chapter 9.9 Hypothermia

Tender calf: consider DVT (see above)
Tracheostomy
Tube falls out or becomes blocked: See Chapter 14.2 Tracheostomy

Unrousable resident
See Chapter 15.6 Head injury observations, Appendix 1.2 Conscious level

Upper respiratory tract infection (severe)
See Chapter 9.6 Dyspnoea, Chapter 13.6 Respiratory infections

Visual disturbance
Sudden loss of vision: See Chapter 7.1 Eye care

Vomiting
With bowels not open
Vomiting blood: See Chapter 9.3 Bleeding
With diarrhoea: See Chapter 9.12 Nausea and vomiting
With fever: See Chapter 9.12 Nausea and vomiting
With pain and tenderness: See Chapter 9.12 Nausea and vomiting
With headache: Consider meningitis or raised intracranial pressure: See Chapter 9.12 Nausea and vomiting

Weight bearing difficulty or pain
Consider fracture

Wheezing
Consider asthma (Chapter 9.2), pulmonary oedema (Chapters 8.6, 9.6), anaphylaxis (Chapter 9.1)

Index

The Care Home Handbook, First Edition. Edited by Graham Mulley, Clive Bowman, Michal Boyd and Sarah Stowe.
© 2015 John Wiley & Sons, Ltd. Published 2015 by John Wiley & Sons, Ltd.